THE WASHINGTON MANUAL™

Nephrology   Subspecialty Consult

Second Edition

Editor

David Windus, MD
Professor of Medicine
Assistant Medical Director of the
Chromalloy American Kidney Center
Washington University School of Medicine
St. Louis, Missouri

Series Editors

Katherine E. Henderson, MD
Instructor in Medicine
Department of Internal Medicine
Division of Medical Education
Washington University School of Medicine
Barnes-Jewish Hospital
St. Louis, Missouri

Thomas M. De Fer, MD
Associate Professor of Internal Medicine
Washington University School of Medicine
St. Louis, Missouri

Wolters Kluwer | Lippincott Williams & Wilkins
Health
Philadelphia · Baltimore · New York · London
Buenos Aires · Hong Kong · Sydney · Tokyo

Acquisitions Editor: Ave McCracken
Managing Editor: Michelle LaPlante
Project Manager: Bridgett Dougherty
Marketing Manager: Kimberly Schonberger
Senior Manufacturing Manager: Benjamin Rivera
Design Coordinator: Risa Clow
Cover Designer: Joseph DePinho
Production Service: Aptara, Inc.

Second Edition

Library of Congress Cataloging-in-Publication Data

The Washington manual nephrology subspecialty consult / editor, David Windus. — 2nd ed.
    p. ; cm.
    Includes bibliographical references and index.
    ISBN 978-0-7817-9149-6 (pbk. : alk. paper)
    1. Kidneys—Diseases—Diagnosis—Handbooks, manuals, etc. 2. Nephrology—Handbooks, manuals, etc. I. Windus, David. II. Title: Nephrology subspecialty consult.
    [DNLM: 1. Kidney Diseases—diagnosis—Handbooks. 2. Kidney Diseases—therapy—Handbooks. 3. Nephrology—methods—Handbooks. WJ 39 W319 2008]
    RC904.W27 2008
    616.6'1—dc22   2008001322

The Washington Manual™ is an intent-to-use mark belonging to Washington University in St. Louis to which international legal protection applies. The mark is used in this publication by LWW under license from Washington University.

Care has been taken to confirm the accuracy of the information present and to describe generally accepted practices. However, the authors, editors, and publisher are not responsible for errors or omissions or for any consequences from application of the information in this book and make no warranty, expressed or implied, with respect to the currency, completeness, or accuracy of the contents of the publication. Application of this information in a particular situation remains the professional responsibility of the practitioner; the clinical treatments described and recommended may not be considered absolute and universal recommendations.

The authors, editors, and publisher have exerted every effort to ensure that drug selection and dosage set forth in this text are in accordance with current recommendations and practice at the time of publication. However, in view of ongoing research, changes in government regulations, and the constant flow of information relating to drug therapy and drug reactions, the reader is urged to check the package insert for each drug for any change in indications and dosage and for added warnings and precautions. This is particularly important when the recommended agent is a new or infrequently employed drug.

Some drugs and medical devices presented in this publication have Food and Drug Administration (FDA) clearance for limited use in restricted research settings. It is the responsibility of health care providers to ascertain the FDA status of each drug or device planned for use in their clinical practice.

To purchase additional copies of this book, call our customer service department at **(800) 638-3030** or fax orders to **(301) 223-2320**. International customers should call **(301) 223-2300**.

Visit Lippincott Williams & Wilkins on the Internet: http://www.lww.com. Lippincott Williams & Wilkins customer service representatives are available from 8:30 am to 6:00 pm, EST.

RRS1006

Table of Contents

Contributing Authors   **vi**
Chairman's Note   **viii**
Preface   **ix**

PART I. GENERAL APPROACH TO KIDNEY DISEASE

1. Art and Science of Urinalysis   **1**
   Anton A. M. Cabellon

2. Assessment of Kidney Function   **8**
   Sijie Zheng

3. Renal Biopsy   **15**
   Imran A. Memon

4. Approach to Proteinuria   **21**
   Kabeya Mwintshi

5. Approach to Hematuria   **27**
   Rouba Ghoussoub

PART II. ELECTROLYTES AND ACID-BASE DISORDERS

6. Disorders of Water Balance: Hyponatremia and Hypernatremia   **35**
   Andrew Siedlecki and Matthew J. Koch

7. Disorders of Potassium Balance   **48**
   Matthew J. Koch

8. Disorders of Calcium Metabolism   **62**
   Jawad Munir

9. Disorders of Phosphorus Metabolism   **71**
   Jawad Munir

10. Acid-Base Disorders   **78**
    Bala P. Sankarapandian

PART III. ACUTE KIDNEY INJURY AND CONTINUOUS RENAL REPLACEMENT

11. Overview and Management of Acute Kidney Injury and Acute Tubular Necrosis **94**
    Anitha Vijayan

12. Prerenal and Postrenal Acute Kidney Injury **107**
    Alexis Argoudelis and Anitha Vijayan

13. Intrinsic Causes of Acute Kidney Injury **121**
    Kamalanathan Sambandam

14. Contrast-Induced Nephropathy **144**
    Ethan Hoerschgen and Anitha Vijayan

15. Renal Replacement Therapy in Acute Kidney Injury **151**
    Anitha Vijayan

PART IV. CAUSES OF KIDNEY DISEASE

16. Overview and Approach to the Patient with Glomerular Disease **159**
    Rasa Kedainis

17. Primary Glomerulopathies **171**
    David Windus

18. Glomerulonephritis in Multisystem Disorders **183**
    Nadine D. Tanenbaum

19. Diabetic Nephropathy **193**
    Steven Cheng

20. Renal Artery Stenosis and Renovascular Hypertension **202**
    Matthew C. Lambert

21. Cystic Diseases of the Kidney **212**
    Michele Cabellon

PART V. PREGNANCY AND NEPHROLITHIASIS

22. Renal Diseases in Pregnancy **223**
    Drew C. Heiple

23. Nephrolithiasis: Physicochemical Principles and
    General Management 235
    Sreedhara B. Alla

PART VI. CHRONIC KIDNEY DISEASE

24. Management of Chronic Kidney Disease 250
    Daniel O. Young

25. Hemodialysis 260
    Steven Cheng

26. Peritoneal Dialysis 273
    Seth Goldberg

27. Principles of Drug Dosing in Renal Impairment 286
    Christine Spaeth-Kelso

28. Care of the Renal Transplant Patient 293
    Andrew Siedlecki and Matthew J. Koch

   Appendixes
   A. Red Flag Drugs That May Cause Renal Impairment 301
   B. Mechanisms of Nephrotoxicity and Alternatives to Some
      Common Drugs 302
   C. Common Medications with Active Metabolites 304
   D. Dosing Adjustments for Antimicrobials 305
   E. Dosing Adjustments for Antiretrovirals 309

Index 311

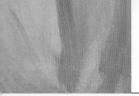

Contributing Authors

Sreedhara B. Alla, MD
Clinical Fellow
Department of Internal Medicine
Renal Division
Washington University School of Medicine
Barnes-Jewish Hospital
St. Louis, Missouri

Alexis Argoudelis, MD
Clinical Fellow
Department of Internal Medicine
Renal Division
Washington University School of Medicine
Barnes-Jewish Hospital
St. Louis, Missouri

Anton A. M. Cabellon, DO
Clinical Fellow
Department of Internal Medicine
Renal Division
Washington University School of Medicine
Barnes-Jewish Hospital
St. Louis, Missouri

Michele Cabellon, MD
Assistant Professor of Medicine
Department of Internal Medicine
Renal Division
Washington University School of Medicine
Barnes-Jewish Hospital
St. Louis, Missouri

Steven Cheng, MD
Assistant Professor of Medicine
Department of Internal Medicine
Renal Division
Washington University School of Medicine
Barnes-Jewish Hospital
St. Louis, Missouri

Rouba Ghoussoub, MD
Clinical Fellow
Department of Internal Medicine
Renal Division
Washington University School of Medicine
Barnes-Jewish Hospital
St. Louis, Missouri

Seth Goldberg, MD
Clinical Fellow
Department of Internal Medicine
Renal Division
Washington University School of Medicine
Barnes-Jewish Hospital
St. Louis, Missouri

Drew C. Heiple, MD
Clinical Fellow
Department of Internal Medicine
Renal Division
Washington University School of Medicine
Barnes-Jewish Hospital
St. Louis, Missouri

Ethan Hoerschgen, MD
Attending Physician
Barnes-Jewish Hospital
St. Louis, Missouri

Rasa Kedainis, MD
Clinical Fellow
Department of Internal Medicine
Renal Division
Washington University School of Medicine
Barnes-Jewish Hospital
St. Louis, Missouri

Mathew J. Koch, MD
Assistant Professor of Medicine
Department of Internal Medicine
Renal Division
Washington University School of Medicine
Barnes-Jewish Hospital
St. Louis, Missouri

Matthew C. Lambert, MD
Clinical Fellow
Department of Internal Medicine
Renal Division
Washington University School of Medicine
Barnes-Jewish Hospital
St. Louis, Missouri

Imran A. Memon, MD
Clinical Fellow
Department of Internal Medicine & Pediatrics
Renal Division
Washington University School of Medicine
Barnes-Jewish Hospital and St. Louis
Children's Hospital
St. Louis, Missouri

Jawad Munir, MD
Attending Physician
Western Kentucky Kidney Specialists
Paducah, Kentucky

Kabeya Mwintshi, MD
Clinical Fellow
Department of Internal Medicine
Renal Division
Washington University School of Medicine
Barnes-Jewish Hospital
St. Louis, Missouri

Kamalanathan Sambandam, MD
Clinical Fellow
Department of Internal Medicine
Renal Division
Washington University School of Medicine
Barnes-Jewish Hospital
St. Louis, Missouri

Bala P. Sankarandian, MD
Clinical Fellow
Department of Internal Medicine
Renal Division
Washington University School of Medicine
Barnes-Jewish Hospital
St. Louis, Missouri

Andrew Siedlecki, MD
Clinical Fellow
Department of Internal Medicine
Renal Division
Washington University School of Medicine
Barnes-Jewish Hospital
St. Louis, Missouri

Christine Spaeth-Kelso, PharmD, BCPS, AE-C
Ambulatory Care Clinical Pharmacist
Department of Pharmacy
Barnes-Jewish Hospital
St. Louis, Missouri

Nadine D. Tanenbaum, MD
Assistant Professor of Medicine
Department of Internal Medicine
Renal Division
Washington University School of Medicine
Barnes-Jewish Hospital
St. Louis, Missouri

Anitha Vijayan, MD
Associate Professor of Medicine
Department of Internal Medicine
Renal Division
Washington University School of Medicine
Barnes-Jewish Hospital
St. Louis, Missouri

David Windus, MD
Professor of Medicine
Department of Internal Medicine
Renal Division
Washington University School of Medicine
Barnes-Jewish Hospital
St. Louis, Missouri

Daniel O. Young, MD
Clinical Fellow
Department of Internal Medicine
Renal Division
Washington University School of Medicine
Barnes-Jewish Hospital
St. Louis, Missouri

Sijie Zheng, MD, PhD
Clinical Fellow
Department of Internal Medicine
Renal Division
Washington University School of Medicine
Barnes-Jewish Hospital
St. Louis, Missouri

Chairman's Note

Medical knowledge is increasing at an exponential rate, and physicians are being bombarded with new facts at a pace that many find overwhelming. The Washington Manual™ Subspecialty Consult Series was developed in this context for interns, residents, medical students, and other practitioners in need of readily accessible practical clinical information. They, therefore, meet an important unmet need in an era of information overload.

I would like to acknowledge the authors who have contributed to these books. In particular, the series editors, Katherine E. Henderson, MD and Thomas M. De Fer, MD, for their oversight of the project. I'd also like to recognize Melvin Blanchard, MD, Chief of the Division of Medical Education in the Department of Medicine at Washington University for his guidance and advice. The efforts and outstanding skill of the lead authors are evident in the quality of the final product. I am confident that this series will meet its desired goal of providing practical knowledge that can be directly applied to improving patient care.

Kenneth S. Polonsky, MD
Adolphus Busch Professor
Chairman, Department of Medicine
Washington University School of Medicine
St. Louis, Missouri

Preface

T he first edition of *The Washington University Nephrology Subspecialty Consult* achieved the goal of the "subspecialty" series because it was well-written, well-organized, and served as an efficient bedside resource for residents and students. The hope of this and future editions is to build on that success by updating content with new developments while maintaining the original high standards.

The challenge and excitement of nephrology results from the need of the learner to master three intersecting domains. The first of these is electrolyte and acid-base disorders. Physicians, regardless of career path, must have a solid working knowledge of underlying physiology, assessment, and management of these disorders. The second domain is the diagnosis and management of acute and chronic kidney diseases. These diseases can result from genetic defects, immune dysfunction, toxic injury, and other systemic processes. The differential diagnosis for persons with abnormal urinary findings or loss of kidney function can be broad. The efficient assessment and proper management of these cases requires a good understanding of the diseases causing kidney injury. Lastly, the appropriate management of progressive chronic kidney disease, dialysis and kidney transplant looms ever more important with the growth of this population worldwide.

Several changes in content were made with the second edition. New chapters, covering renal replacement therapy for acute kidney injury, cystic kidney diseases, and the management of chronic kidney diseases, were added. In addition, photographs of key urinalysis findings were included. Drug dosing information was also reviewed and updated in the appendices.

I would like to acknowledge and thank the authors and the editors of the first and current editions for the great amount of interest and effort they put into this project. In addition, I would like to thank the current series editor, Katherine Henderson, MD, for the extraordinary amount of care she gave in her review of the material.

—DWW

Art and Science of Urinalysis

Anton A. M. Cabellon

1

INTRODUCTION

The urinalysis is a key aspect in the evaluation of renal and urinary tract disease, and therefore should be performed by the renal consultant as part of the initial exam of the patient. It is rarely used as a screening tool, except in pregnancy, and its greatest value is assessment and follow-up of renal and urinary tract disease. Proper examination of the urine consists of two parts: (a) the urine dipstick and (b) the sediment evaluation by light microscopy. The urine dipstick gives insight into the physical and chemical parameters of the urine, while microscopic analysis allows for sediment evaluation. The presence or absence of certain features on urinalysis can be useful in narrowing diagnostic possibilities.

SPECIMEN COLLECTION

Regardless of the source, urine should ideally be examined immediately or no longer than 2 hours after collection. Specimens that are allowed to stand longer are notoriously inaccurate for changes in the sediment. This happens because the urine becomes progressively more alkaline (urea is broken down, generating ammonia). The higher pH dissolves casts and promotes cell lysis. If delay is inevitable, urine can be preserved for up to 6 hours if refrigerated at $+2$ to $+8°C$. Refrigeration may result in precipitation of phosphates or crystals. Preservatives such as formaldehyde, glutaraldehyde, "cellFIX," and tubes containing lypophilized borate-formate sorbitol powder have been used to maintain the urine sample's formed elements. The method for preparing a urine sample is given in Table 1-1.

PHYSICAL PROPERTIES

Visual inspection and notation of other general physical characteristics of a urine sample can yield important diagnostic information. The main physical properties to be determined include color, clarity, odor, and specific gravity.

Color

Normal urine is pale to yellow in color, and the hue varies with urine concentration. Dilute urine appears lighter, and concentrated urine attains a darker yellow to amber shade. *Red* urine may be noted with hematuria. A positive dipstick for blood without evidence of RBCs on microscopy is a clue to the presence of free hemoglobin or myoglobin in the urine. This could be suggestive of conditions such as sickle cell anemia, ABO incompatible blood transfusion, or rhabdomyolysis. Red urine is also noted in patients ingesting large amounts of foodstuffs with red pigments (e.g., beets, rhubarb, blackberries), the presence of excess urates, certain drugs (e.g., phenytoin, rifampin), and occasionally with

TABLE 1-1	PROCEDURE FOR URINE SPECIMEN COLLECTION, DIPSTICK TESTING, AND MICROSCOPIC ANALYSIS

Collect midstream urine catch of first or second morning urine specimen in clean container.
- Bladder catheterization may be used (risk of hematuria).
- Suprapubic catheterization is also acceptable though rarely used.
- Avoid collecting urine from the Foley bag (may collect fresh specimen from Foley catheter itself).

Perform dipstick testing and record results.
Centrifuge 10 mL aliquot at 1500–3000 rpm (400–450 g) for 5–10 minutes.
Remove 9.5 mL of supernatant urine.
Gently resuspend sediment using pipette in remaining 0.5 ml of supernatant.
Using pipette, apply one drop of resuspended urine onto clean slide and cover with coverslip.
Examine urine under phase-contrast light microscopy at 160× and 400×.
- Polarized light may help with lipids and crystal examination.

porphyria. *Green or blue* urine can be seen with *Pseudomonas* UTI, biliverdinuria, as well as exposure amitriptyline, IV cimetidine, IV promethazine, methylene blue, and triamterene. *Orange* urine is typically seen with rifampin, phenothiazines and phenazopyridine. Urine which turns black upon standing is classically described in homogentisic acid oxidase deficiency (alkaptonuria). *Brown or black* urine is also seen in conditions such as copper or phenol poisoning, excessive L-dopa excretion, and with excess melanin excretion in melanoma.

Clarity

Normal urine is typically clear. It may appear turbid if cellular elements, casts, or organisms are present. Although decreased urine clarity is most commonly noted with urinary tract infections (pyuria), the urine may appear hazy with other renal diseases as well. Two other frequent causes of increased turbidity include heavy hematuria and contamination from genital secretions. Other considerations include the presence of phosphate crystals in an alkaline urine, chyluria, lipiduria, hyperoxaluria, and hyperuricosuria.

Odor

Normal urine typically does not have a strong odor. Bacterial urinary tract infections may be associated with a pungent odor. Diabetic ketoacidosis can cause urine to have a fruity or sweet odor. Other conditions with characteristic odors include maple-syrup urine disease (maple-syrup odor), phenylketonuria (musty odor), isovaleric acidemia (sweaty feet odor), hypermethioninemia (rancid butter/fishy odor), gastrointestinal-bladder fistulas (fecal odor), and cystine decomposition (sulfuric odor). Finally, different medications (e.g., penicillin) and diet (e.g., asparagus, coffee) can also contribute to different urine odors.

Specific Gravity

Specific gravity is the most common method used to assess the relative density of urine. It is typically measured using an ionic reagent strip because of its simplicity. Though commonly used, ion exchange strips typically provide falsely low results with urine pH values >6.5 and falsely high results with protein levels of >7 g/L. In general, values ≤1.010 indicate a state of relative hydration, and values ≥1.020 point toward dehydration. A very low specific gravity (≤1.005) may be indicative of diabetes insipidus or water intoxication.

A very high specific gravity (≥ 1.032) may be suggestive of glucosuria, and even higher values may indicate the presence of an extrinsic osmotic agent such as contrast. Generally speaking, the relative density of urine is best determined by measuring osmolality or by refractometry.

CHEMICAL PROPERTIES

Urine pH

Urine pH can be measured very accurately and is quite reproducible. Normally, urine pH is in the range of 4.5 to 7.8. A low urine pH can be observed in patients with large protein consumption, metabolic acidosis, and volume depletion. A high urine pH may be seen in renal tubular acidosis (especially distal) and in persons consuming vegetarian diets. In addition to prolonged storage of urine (allowing generation of ammonia from urea), infection with urea-splitting organisms (e.g., *Proteus*) is an important cause of high urinary pH.

Hemoglobin

The presence of hemoglobin by dipstick may be indicative of hematuria or point to other pathology such as intravascular hemolysis or rhabdomyolysis. A discussion of hematuria and hemoglobinuria can be found in Chapter 5.

Glucose

Urine glucose measurement is sensitive but not specific enough for quantification by usual methods. Most labs give out a semiquantitative readout (e.g., + for present to + + + + for present in large amounts), but correlation with blood glucose levels is approximate and varies with the concentration of the urine. Glucose in the urine may be seen in diabetes, pancreatic and liver disease, Cushing syndrome, and Fanconi syndrome. False negative results may be seen with the presence of ascorbic acid, uric acid, and bacteria. False positive results can be observed in the presence of levodopa, oxidizing detergents, and hydrochloric acid.

Protein

Proteinuria is an important marker of kidney disease. Traditionally, a urine specimen is checked for protein using a dipstick. Details of the methodology and more quantitative methods are found in Chapter 4.

Leukocyte Esterase and Urine Nitrite

- The *leukocyte esterase* test depends on esterases released from lysed granulocytes in urine reacting with the reagent strip. Esterase produced from granulocyte lysis in longstanding urine or contaminating vaginal cells may cause false positives. False negatives occur when the esterase reaction with granulocytes is inhibited, such as with hyperglycemia, albuminuria, tetracycline, cephalosporins, and oxaluria.
- The presence of *nitrites* in the urine depends on the ability of bacteria to convert nitrate into nitrite which then reacts with the reagent test strip. This reaction is inhibited by ascorbic acid and high specific gravity. Low levels of urinary nitrate secondary to diet, degradation of nitrites secondary to prolonged storage, and inadequate conversion of nitrates to nitrites due to rapid transit in the bladder may contribute to false negatives despite the presence of urinary infection. Certain bacteria (e.g., *Streptococcus faecalis*, *Neisseria gonorrhoeae*, and *Mycobacterium tuberculosis*) do not convert nitrate to nitrite.

- Specificity for infection is best when both leukocyte esterase and nitrites are positive. However, even if both tests are negative, infection cannot be completely ruled out, and the clinical context must be considered.

Ketones

Ketones are detected using a nitroprusside reaction. The routine dipstick test detects only acetoacetic acid and not beta-hydroxybutyrate. Ketones are mainly seen in diabetic and alcoholic ketoacidosis, but can also be observed in pregnancy, carbohydrate-free diets, starvation, vomiting, and strenuous exercise. The presence of free sulfhydryl groups, levodopa metabolites, or highly pigmented urine can give false-positive results.

MICROSCOPIC EXAM

Urine microscopic examination of the sediment is a very important and an underutilized tool to evaluate renal pathology. The urine sediment can contain cells, casts, crystals, bacteria, fungi, and contaminants.

Cells

RBCs

More than two RBCs per high-power field is abnormal and suggests bleeding from some point in the genitourinary system. RBCs are typically 4 to 7 µm in diameter and have a characteristic red pigment with central opacity and smooth borders. Dysmorphic RBCs are associated with glomerular disease and are best seen on phase-contrast microscopy. These should be distinguished from swollen (ghost) cells or shrunken (crenated) cells, which are normal RBCs that have been altered by osmolality of the urine. Crenated cells have spiked borders and can be mistaken for small, granulated cells. Ghost cells often require phase-contrast microscopy for viewing.

WBCs

WBCs are characterized by their cytoplasmic granulation. WBCs can be distinguished from crenated RBCs by their lack of pigment and their large size (10–12 µm in diameter) compared to crenated cells, which are much smaller than normal RBCs (5 µm in diameter). Phase-contrast microscopy also affords the opportunity to view the brownian motion of the granules in WBCs and distinguish them from other cells. WBCs in the urine are associated with infection and inflammation. The presence of eosinophils in urine used to be thought of as a marker for allergic interstitial nephritis; however, it is now considered a nonsensitive and a nonspecific marker. It can be seen in cholesterol embolism, glomerulonephritis, prostatitis, chronic pyelonephritis, and urinary schistosomiasis. Urine eosinophils are not easily identified unless special staining (Hansel or Wright) is used.

Epithelial Cells

Four major epithelial cell groups must be distinguished: squamous cells, transitional cells, renal tubular cells, and fat bodies. *Squamous epithelial cells* have large, flat, irregular cytoplasm of 30 to 50 µm in diameter and a nucleus-to-cytoplasmic ratio of 1:6. They are present in the urine due to shedding from the distal genital tract and essentially are contaminants. *Transitional epithelial cells* are 20 to 30 µm in diameter, are pear or tadpole shaped, and have a nucleus-to-cytoplasmic ratio of 1:3. They are usually seen intermittently with bladder catheterization or irrigation. Occasionally, they may be associated with malignancy, especially if irregular nuclei are noted. *Renal tubular epithelial cells* are only slightly larger than leukocytes and have a large, eccentrically placed round nucleus that takes up half the area of the cytoplasm. Their presence in significant numbers (>15 cells in ten high-power fields) may be seen with tubular injury. Tubular epithelial cells from the proximal tubule tend to be very granulated. *Oval fat bodies* are renal epithelial cells that are filled with lipids. They also appear granulated but are distinguished by characteristic "Maltese crosses" seen under polarized light, reflecting their cholesterol content. Oval fat bodies are typically seen in nephrotic syndrome and indicate lipiduria.

Casts

Casts are formed when proteins secreted in the lumen of renal tubules (typically the Tamm-Horsfall protein) trap cells, fat, bacteria, or other inclusions at the time of amalgamation and then are excreted in the urine. Thus, a cast provides a snapshot of the milieu of the tubule at the time of this amalgamation.

Hyaline Casts

Renal tubules secrete a protein called Tamm-Horsfall protein (uromodulin). Under certain circumstances, the protein amalgamates on its own without any other tubular inclusions, forming hyaline casts. It is easy to miss them with plain microscopy and they are better seen with phase-contrast microscopy. Hyaline casts are seen in concentrated, acidic urine. They are not associated with proteinuria and can be seen with various physiologic states, such as strenuous exercise or dehydration.

Granular Casts

Granular casts are made of Tamm-Horsfall protein filled with breakdown debris of cells and plasma proteins that appear as granules. Granular casts are nonspecific and appear with many glomerular or tubular diseases. Large numbers of "muddy brown" granular casts are typically seen in acute tubular necrosis. They have also been reported after vigorous exercise.

Waxy Casts

Waxy casts represent the last stage in degeneration of hyaline, granular, and cellular casts. They have smooth, blunt ends, are easily detected by light microscopy (unlike hyaline casts), and are usually seen with chronic kidney disease rather than acute processes. Polarized light should be used to distinguish waxy casts from artifacts. Artifacts tend to polarize, whereas true casts do not.

Fatty Casts

Fatty casts contain lipid droplets that are very refractile. They may be confused with cellular casts, but polarized light demonstrates the characteristic Maltese cross appearance. They are associated with nephrotic syndrome, mercury poisoning, and ethylene glycol poisoning.

Red Cell Casts

Red cell casts are identified by their orange-red color on bright-field microscopy and well-defined cellular elements. They are best seen in fresh urine. At times, they may appear fractured. Red cell casts signify glomerular hematuria and are an important finding suggesting potentially serious glomerular disease. Detection of red cell casts should trigger further rigorous evaluation of the patient.

White Cell Casts

White cell casts contain WBCs trapped in tubular proteins. Sometimes, WBCs appear in the urine in clumps, and it is important not to confuse them with casts. Phase-contrast microscopy is useful to demonstrate protein matrix of the cast, which is not seen in white cell clumps or pseudocasts. White cell casts are associated with interstitial inflammatory processes, such as pyelonephritis.

Epithelial Cell Casts

Epithelial cell casts are characterized by epithelial cells of various shapes, haphazardly arranged in a protein matrix representing desquamation from different portions of the renal tubules.

Crystals

- Crystals are a striking finding on urinalysis. However, cooling of urine allows many normally dissolved substances to precipitate at room temperature. Thus, most crystals are present as artifacts. The following crystals may be present in the urine without an underlying disease:
- *Crystals in acidic urine:* uric acid, monosodium urate, amorphous urates, and calcium oxalate
- *Crystals in alkaline urine:* triple phosphate, ammonium biurate, calcium phosphate, calcium oxalate, and calcium carbonate
- Crystals produced from pathologic excess of metabolic products (e.g., cystine, tyrosine, leucine, bilirubin, and cholesterol) are all seen more frequently in acidic urine. Similarly, drug-associated crystals (e.g., acyclovir, indinavir, sulfonamides, and ampicillin) are seen in more acidic concentrated urine. Uric acid crystals come in various forms, including rhomboid, rosettes, lemon shaped, and four-sided "whetstones." Other urate forms are very tiny crystals, spheres, or needles that are hard to distinguish.
- *Calcium oxalate* crystals appear in characteristic octahedral "envelope" shapes. They may also take rectangular, dumbbell, and ovoid shapes—the last of which may cause them to be confused with RBCs. *Triple phosphate* crystals are usually three- to six-sided prisms in "coffin-lid" form but may present as flat, fern leaf–like sheets. *Calcium phosphate* crystals are usually small rosettes. *Calcium carbonate* usually presents as tiny spheres in pairs or crosses. *Ammonium biurate,* which is usually seen in aged urine, is usually a dark, yellow sphere with a "thorn apple" shape. *Cystine* crystals are hexagons that can polarize and are confused with uric acid crystals. *Tyrosine* and *leucine* crystals usually occur together. The former forms fine needles arranged in rosettes, whereas the latter forms spheres with concentric striations like the core of a tree. *Bilirubin* crystals occur in many shapes but are usually distinguished by the bilirubin color. *Cholesterol* crystals are usually flat with a corner notch and are sometimes confused with crystals of contrast medium, which also have a corner notch. *Sulfonamide* crystals appear as spheres or needles. *Ampicillin* crystals usually take a long, slender needle shape. *Acyclovir* crystals have a similar needle-like shape but display negative birefringence under polarized light.

Organisms

Bacteria

Bacteria are frequently seen in urine specimens given the fact that urine is typically collected under nonsterile conditions. To delineate the different bacteria that may cause an infectious process is beyond the scope of this manual, however gram negative organisms such as *E. coli* tend to predominate in uncomplicated UTI, followed by *S. saprophyticus,* and occasionally by *Proteus, Klebsiella,* enterococci, Group B streptococci, *Pseudomonas aeruginosa,* and *Citrobacter* species. Complicated UTI may be caused by a myriad of organisms. Identification and susceptibilities of these organisms typically requires high-powered magnification, staining, culture, and in vitro testing against antibiotics.

Fungal

The presence of *Candida* in urine is typically thought to be a contaminant from genital secretions or, in the presence of a long, indwelling bladder catheter, colonization. *Candida* urinary tract infections can cause similar symptoms to that seen with a bacterial infection. *Candida* species are the most frequent cause of fungal urinary tract infections with *C. albicans* as the most common, followed by *C. glabrata* and *C. tropicalis. Candida* may have the appearance of yeast (spherical cells), budding yeast, and pseudohyphae depending on reproductive cycle. Other infectious fungal agents, including *Aspergillus, Cryptococcus,* and *Histoplasmosis,* can be seen in the chronically ill or immunocompromised.

Parasites

The presence of *Trichomonas vaginalis* and *Enterobius vermicularis* in urine are typically thought of as contaminants stemming from genital secretions. Trichomonads are single-celled, flagellated protozoans characterized by their "corkscrew" motility which can cause a sexually transmitted disease with white vaginal discharge and itching as part of its symptoms. *Enterobius vermicularis* (human pinworm) do not typically reside in the urinary tract, but may occasionally be found in the vagina leading to urine contamination. Another parasitic disease characterized by painful hematuria with exposure to fresh river waters in endemic areas is *Schistosoma haematobium*. The large, abundant ova can be detected in a fresh urine sample with the urine tending to be dark in color.

KEY POINTS TO REMEMBER

- Patients should be meticulously briefed about specimen collection technique to avoid contamination of the sample.
- Abnormalities detected on routine screening should be confirmed with repeat testing.
- Exam of the urine sediment is an important part of urinalysis. For this purpose, it is best to study a fresh sample of the first morning void.
- Use of phase-contrast microscopy greatly enhances appreciation of abnormalities during sediment exam.

REFERENCES AND SUGGESTED READINGS

Feehally J, Floege J, Johnson RJ. Urinalysis. In: *Comprehensive Clinical Nephrology*. 3rd ed. Philadelphia: Mosby Elsevier; 2007:35–50.

Lorincz AE, Kelly DR, Dobbins GC, et al. Urinalysis: current status and prospects for the future. *Ann Clin Lab Sci.* 1999;29:169.

Massry SG, Glassock RJ, eds. *Massry & Glassock's Textbook of Nephrology*. Philadelphia: Lippincott Williams & Wilkins; 2001:1765.

McClatchey KD, ed. *Clinical Laboratory Medicine*. 2nd ed. Philadelphia: Lippincott Williams & Wilkins; 2002:519.

Misdraji J, Nguyen PL. Urinalysis. When—and when not—to order. *Postgrad Med.* 1996;100:173.

Phillips CM, et al. Urinalysis tutor CD-ROM. Department of Laboratory Medicine, Center for Bioengineering. Seattle: University of Washington; 1995.

Rasoulpour M, Banco L, Laut JM, Burke GS. Inability of community-based laboratories to identify pathologic casts in urine samples. *Arch Pediatr Adolesc Med.* 1996; 150:1201.

Ringsrud KM, Linne JJ. *Urinalysis and Body Fluids: A Color Text and Atlas*. St. Louis: Mosby; 1995.

Rose BD. Clinical assessment of renal function. In: *Pathophysiology of Renal Disease*. 2nd ed. New York: McGraw-Hill; 1987:1–40.

Simerville JA, Maxted WC, Pahira JJ. Urinalysis: a comprehensive review. *Am Fam Physician.* 2005;71:1153–1162.

Van Nostrand JD, Junkins AD, Bartholdi RK. Poor predictive ability of urinalysis and microscopic examination to detect urinary tract infection. *Am J Clin Pathol.* 2000;113:709.

Assessment of Kidney Function

2

Sijie Zheng

INTRODUCTION

Assessing kidney function is a critical step in recognition and monitoring of acute and chronic kidney diseases. Creatinine measurement has become the preferred method for routine clinical monitoring of renal function. Creatinine determinations are most valuable when the underlying assumptions and pitfalls regarding this marker are well understood.

PHYSIOLOGIC PRINCIPLES OF CREATININE PRODUCTION AND ELIMINATION

Creatinine is a metabolic product of creatine and the major sources are skeletal muscle cells and dietary meat. Thus, persons with larger muscle mass have a higher creatinine production and level than do those with a smaller muscle mass. Typical daily production rates are 20 to 25 mg/kg/day in males and 15 to 20 mg/kg/day in females. To a lesser extent, meat consumption can affect appearance of creatinine in the urine and plasma. Aging and weight loss lead to reduced creatinine production rates. The kidney eliminates creatinine by glomerular filtration and proximal tubular secretion. In persons with normal renal function, glomerular filtration accounts for >90% of creatinine elimination and tubular secretion accounts for the rest. As renal function declines, the proportion entering the urine via tubular secretion of creatinine can increase up to 50%. Therefore, all creatinine-based glomerular filtration rate (GFR) equations tend to overestimate renal function due to tubular secretion of creatinine. Furthermore, the measurement of creatinine has not been standardized in different laboratories, leading to intralaboratory variation in plasma creatinine level for a given GFR.

CREATININE AS A MARKER FOR KIDNEY FUNCTION

Persons with a stable weight and dietary intake will have a constant creatinine production rate. With constant production, plasma creatinine concentration will be inversely related to kidney function. However, when using creatinine to assess kidney function, four factors need to be kept in mind:

1. Creatinine concentration must be interpreted in the context of the patient's characteristics. For example, creatinine of 1.1 mg/dL in a 100-kg muscular bodybuilder will be consistent with normal GFR whereas that same creatinine concentration in a 40-kg octogenarian represents significant renal impairment.
2. Change in plasma creatinine does not correlate with decline in renal function in a linear fashion (Fig. 2-1). A small increase in creatinine at a lower creatinine level

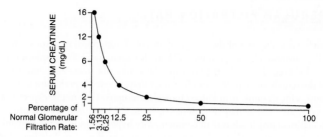

FIGURE 2-1. The nonlinear relationship between rise in plasma creatinine and fall in the glomerular filtration rate. (From Lazarus JM, Brenner BM, eds. *Acute renal failure.* 3rd ed. New York: Churchill Livingstone; 1993:133.)

signals a greater decline in renal function as compared with the same increase in creatinine when the baseline creatinine level is high. For example, a change of 1.0 to 1.4 represents a greater decline in renal function than does a change of 3.0 to 3.4.

3. One should account for changes in creatinine for an individual over time. In most laboratories, normal creatinine range is reported between 0.4 to 1.5 mg/dL. If a person's baseline creatinine has been around 0.7 mg/dL for some time and suddenly increases to 1.4 mg/dL, this change represents a significant decrease in kidney function despite the value remaining in the normal range.

4. In acute kidney injury, creatinine levels are a poor reflection of renal function. With sudden changes of GFR, re-equilibration must take place. Therefore, an anuric patient can have a very low creatinine level even though his or her renal function has completely shut down. Rapid increases in volume status can also mask deteriorating renal function because of dilution of the creatinine concentration.

CONDITIONS THAT INCREASES PLASMA CREATININE LEVEL WITHOUT GFR CHANGES

Trimethoprim and *cimetidine* block proximal tubular secretion of creatinine. They can increase plasma creatinine level as much as 0.5 mg/dL. This effect is more pronounced in chronic kidney disease when baseline creatinine is already elevated. *Cefoxitin* and *flucytosine* interfere with the creatinine assay, giving a false elevation of plasma creatinine levels. *Acetoacetate* in diabetic ketoacidosis can be falsely recognized by the colorimetric assay as creatinine and may elevate creatinine by as much as 0.5 to 2 mg/dL. *Hypothyroidism* increases plasma creatinine levels and *hyperthyroidism* decreases plasma creatinine level.

UREA AND UREA CLEARANCE

The elimination of urea by the kidney is more complex than creatinine, which renders the blood urea nitrogen (BUN) a less useful marker of kidney function when evaluated in isolation. Plasma urea level is influenced by many factors other than GFR. The three most common nonrenal etiologies of an increased BUN are gastrointestinal bleeding, steroid usage, and total parenteral nutrition. For practical purposes, the BUN is most useful when the BUN-to-creatinine ratio (BUN/Cr) is higher than normal (normal = 10–20) or increasing. This finding is suggestive of a prerenal state. However, one must exclude gastrointestinal bleeding and steroid usage. Malnutrition and liver disease can lower BUN level due to reduced urea generation rates.

GLOMERULAR FILTRATION RATE

GFR is defined as the sum of the filtration rates of all functional nephrons. The usual average GFR is around 125 mL/minute/1.73 m^2 for men and 100 mL/minute/1.73 m^2 for women. However, decline in nephron numbers may not necessarily result in decline in GFR, as the remaining nephrons can increase filtration rate (hyperfiltration) to compensate for the loss. One example is in kidney transplant donors. One might expect a 50% reduction of GFR after the kidney donation. However, the measured GFR is often at 80% of their prenephrectomy levels due to compensatory hyperfiltration in the remaining kidney. GFR is measured from urinary clearance of a marker by Equation 2 (below). **Clearance** is generally considered to be the number of mL per minute cleared of a marker substance. An ideal marker should be biologically inert, freely and completely filtered by the glomerulus, neither secreted nor absorbed by tubules, and not degraded by the kidney.

Equation 1 describes the relationship between GFR, marker concentration, and urinary appearance of the marker in a 24-hour sample.

Equation 1:
plasma concentration of a marker (P_{marker}) × GFR = urine concentration of a marker (U_{marker}) × urine flow rate (24-hour volume)/1440 minutes

where U = urine and P = plasma

This formula can be rearranged to yield the standard clearance or GFR formula:

Equation 2:
GFR = (U_{marker}/ P_{marker}) × urine flow rate (24-hour urine volume)/1440 minutes

Inulin was the classic gold standard marker for such measurements as it is freely filtered, neither secreted nor absorbed by tubules, and not metabolized by the kidney. This marker has been superseded by other radioactive and nonradioactive substances such as iothalamate, DTPA, EDTA, and iohexal when very accurate GFR measurements are needed. Occasionally, clinical questions require their use, but creatinine is still used routinely.

ESTIMATES OF CREATININE CLEARANCE AND GFR BY CREATININE-BASED EQUATIONS

- Two widely used creatinine-based equations are currently used for estimates of kidney function in adults. Other estimates are available for children. The **Cockcroft-Gault** formula is an estimate of creatinine clearance and the abbreviated **Modification of Diet in Renal Disease study (MDRD)** equation is an estimate of GFR. Online calculators are readily available using standard search software.
- *Cockcroft-Gault equation:*

  est. creatinine clearance = (140 − age) × weight × 0.85 (if female)/72 × plasma creatinine

- *MDRD equation:*

  est. GFR = 170 × $[Pcr]^{-0.999}$ × $[Age]^{-0.175}$ × [0.762 if female] × [1.180 if African American] × $[BUN]^{-0.170}$ × $[Alb]^{+0.318}$

- *Abbreviated MDRD equation:*

  est. GFR (mL/minute/1.73 m^2) = 186 × $(S_{cr})^{-1.154}$ × (age in yrs)$^{-0.203}$ × (0.742 if female) × (1.21 if African American)

- The Cockcroft-Gault equation was originally developed in a male inpatient population but has been found to be reasonably accurate in other populations. The main pitfalls of this estimate are determining the patient's actual lean body weight and overestimation of true GFR by creatinine clearance with lower levels of kidney function.
- The MDRD equation was developed in established outpatient CKD patients using ^{125}I-iothalamate renal clearance as a reference. The estimated GFR best correlates with the true GFR in the population under original study. In CKD patients with **measured** GFR less than 60 mL/minute/1.73 m^2, the MDRD equation correlates well. It has not been well validated in other patient populations. For instance, it is not useful in persons with normal renal function and was not validated in persons over the age of 70 years or in hospitalized or malnourished patients. In renal transplant donors, both the MDRD and the Cockcroft-Gault equation significantly underestimates measured GFR by as much as 9% to 29%. The MDRD equation has an adjustment factor for African American populations but not for Hispanic or Asian populations. The K/DOQI guidelines define chronic kidney disease as an **estimated** GFR <60 mL/minute/1.73 m^2, and separate chronic kidney disease (CKD) into five stages (Table 2-1). However, one should keep in mind that this is an imperfect system. CKD is a progressive disease with a variable rate of decline. A GFR of 30 mL/minute/1.73 m^2 has half of the renal function as a GFR of 60 mL/minute/1.73 m^2, even though they are both classified as stage III CKD. A GFR of 29 mL/minute/1.73 m^2 has virtually the same renal function as a GFR of 30 mL/minute/1.73 m^2, even though one is classified as stage IV and the other is classified as stage III. A decline from a previous GFR of 120 mL/minute/1.73 m^2 to 80

TABLE 2-1	CKD STAGES	
	GFR (mL/Min/1.73 m^2)	**Description**
CKD Stage 1	≥90	Normal kidney function but urine findings or structural abnormalities or genetic trait point to kidney disease
CKD Stage 2	60–89	Mildly reduced kidney function, and other findings (as for stage 1) point to kidney disease
CKD Stage 3	30–59	Moderately reduced kidney function
CKD Stage 4	15–29	Severely reduced kidney function
CKD Stage 5	<15 (or dialysis)	Very severe, or end-stage kidney failure (sometimes called *established renal failure*)

TABLE 2-2	SITUATIONS IN WHICH A 24-HOUR URINE COLLECTION IS MORE ACCURATE THAN MDRD EQUATION

1. GFR >60 mL/minute/1.73 m^2
2. Age <18 or >70
3. Extreme body size
4. Severe malnutrition
5. Pregnancy
6. Skeletal muscle disease
7. Paraplegia or quadriplegia
8. Vegetarian
9. Rapid changing renal function

mL/minute/1.73 m^2 is a significant decline in renal function, even though it in not considered CKD.

TWENTY-FOUR HOUR CREATININE CLEARANCE

- The 24-hour urine collection has been used as a semi-gold standard to evaluate kidney function in the clinical setting (Table 2-2). It can be measured by collecting a 24-hour urine sample and using the following formula:

$$Ccr \text{ mL/minute} = (U_{Creatinine} / P_{Creatinine}) \times 24\text{-hour urine volume in mL}/1440 \text{ minutes}$$

where Ccr is the creatinine clearance.
- Meticulous volume collection is important to prevent overcollection (thus overestimating Ccr) or undercollection (thus underestimating Ccr). Table 2-3 lists the steps needed for collecting a 24-hour urine sample. One can estimate the adequacy of the collection by calculating the amount of creatinine collected in 24 hours. In the ICU setting, shorter timed collection (e.g., 8 or 12 hours) can also be done to decrease collection errors.

NEWER MARKERS OF KIDNEY FUNCTION

There is an active ongoing search for newer markers which will accurately predict GFR and detect early loss of renal function. *Cystatin C* holds promise as it has a constant daily production and is excreted by the kidney.

TABLE 2-3	PROPER STEPS IN 24-HOUR URINE COLLECTION

1. After waking up in the morning, empty the bladder completely and discard urine.
2. Save all subsequent urine samples during the rest of the day and through the night.
3. The next morning, save the first urine sample.

KEY POINTS TO REMEMBER

- Plasma creatinine can be misleading as a surrogate for renal function if used in isolation. An estimated clearance using the Cockcroft-Gault or MDRD equation should be calculated.
- Creatinine is a useful marker of GFR in the *steady state only*. In cases of acute renal failure, it does not accurately reflect the true GFR.
- When measuring a 24-hour creatinine clearance, patients should be thoroughly briefed in the routine for collection of the specimen. In addition, the amount of creatinine excreted per kilogram body weight should be estimated on the sample to ensure an adequate collection.
- Cockcroft-Gault and abbreviated MDRD equations are imperfect as they can underestimate GFR with normal renal function and overestimate GFR with severe renal dysfunction.
- Always keep in mind conditions that can elevate or depress BUN or creatinine values.

REFERENCES AND SUGGESTED READINGS

Baumann TJ, Staddon JE, Horst HM, et al. Minimum urine collection periods for accurate determination of creatinine clearance in critically ill patients. *Clin Pharm.* 1987;6:393–398.

Berg KJ, Gjellestad A, Nordby G, et al. Renal effects of trimethoprim in ciclosporin- and azathioprine-treated kidney-allografted patients. *Nephron.* 1989;53:218–222.

K/DOQI clinical practice guidelines for chronic kidney disease: evaluation, classification, and stratification, part 5. Evaluation of laboratory measurements for clinical assessment of kidney disease. *Am J Kidney Dis.* 2002;39[Suppl 1]:S76–S110.

Kainer G, Rosenberg AR. Effect of co-trimoxazole on the glomerular filtration rate of healthy adults. *Chemotherapy.* 1981;27:229–232.

Knight EL, Verhave JC, Spiegelman D, et al. Factors influencing serum cystatin C levels other than renal function and the impact on renal function measurement. *Kidney Int.* 2004;65:1416–1421.

Kos J, Stabuc B, Cimerman N, et al. Serum cystatin C, a new marker of glomerular filtration rate, is increased during malignant progression. *Clin Chem.* 1998;44:2556–2557.

Kreisman SH, Hennessey JV. Consistent reversible elevations of serum creatinine levels in severe hypothyroidism. *Arch Intern Med.* 1999;159:79–82.

Levey AS, Bosch JP, Lewis JB, et al. A more accurate method to estimate glomerular filtration rate from serum creatinine: a new prediction equation. Modification of Diet in Renal Disease Study Group. *Ann Intern Med.* 1999;130:461–470.

Markantonis SL, Agathokleous-Kioupaki E. Can two-, four- or eight-hour urine collections after voluntary voiding be used instead of twenty-four-hour collections for the estimation of creatinine clearance in healthy subjects? *Pharm World Sci.* 1998;20:258–263.

Mitchell EK. Flucytosine and false elevation of serum creatinine level. *Ann Intern Med.* 1984;101:278.

Molitch ME, Rodman E, Hirsch CA, et al. Spurious serum creatinine elevations in ketoacidosis. *Ann Intern Med.* 1980;93:280–281.

Palvesky P, Murray P. Acute kidney injury and critical care nephrology. In: NephSAP, March 2006;5(2).

Poggio ED, Wang X, Greene T, et al. Performance of the modification of diet in renal disease and Cockcroft-Gault equations in the estimation of GFR in health and in chronic kidney disease. *J Am Soc Nephrol.* 2005;16:459–466.

Rahn KH, Heidenreich S, Bruckner D. How to assess glomerular function and damage in humans. *J Hypertens.* 1999;17:309–317.

Rocci ML, Jr., Vlasses PH, Ferguson RK. Creatinine serum concentrations and H2-receptor antagonists. *Clin Nephrol.* 1984;22:214–215.

Rose BD. Clinical assessment of renal function. In: *Pathophysiology of Renal Disease.* 2nd ed. New York: McGraw-Hill; 1987:1–40.

Rule AD, Larson TS, Bergstralh EJ, et al. Using serum creatinine to estimate glomerular filtration rate: accuracy in good health and in chronic kidney disease. *Ann Intern Med.* 2004;141:929–937.

Saah AJ, Koch TR, Drusano GL. Cefoxitin falsely elevates creatinine levels. *JAMA.* 1982;247:205–206.

Verhelst J, Berwaerts J, Marescau B, et al. Serum creatine, creatinine, and other guanidino compounds in patients with thyroid dysfunction. *Metabolism.* 1997;46:1063–1067.

Renal Biopsy

Imran A. Memon

3

INTRODUCTION

Diagnosis of many kidney diseases depends on histologic evaluation of tissue. Early biopsy methods were done with manual needle systems and without the benefit of imaging resulting in higher complication rates and poor tissue yield. Modern techniques now use accurate ultrasound imaging and semiautomatic needle biopsy devices to obtain samples of renal cortex for histopathologic exam to aid in the specific diagnosis of renal diseases.

INDICATIONS

Generally, patients who benefit most from renal biopsy and subsequent pathologic diagnosis have nephrotic syndrome, a nephritic presentation, acute renal failure, proteinuria and hematuria, or renal allograft dysfunction (Table 3-1). Several studies have shown that about half of patients subjected to renal biopsy will have a change of diagnosis or management based on the results of the biopsy. Adult patients with **nephrotic syndrome** generally require a kidney biopsy because treatment algorithms vary for the disorders depending on the pathology. Patients with **acute renal failure** without clear etiology need to be evaluated for interstitial nephritis and acute nephritic syndromes or systemic disorders, such as SLE or small-vessel vasculitis. The management of **proteinuria or hematuria** of unclear etiology can be affected by biopsy results, although the decision process is more complex depending on other clinical features. In the **evaluation of renal allograft dysfunction**, renal transplant biopsy is invaluable in diagnosing acute rejection or acute tubular necrosis in the immediate posttransplant period. Deterioration in previously stable renal function can also be evaluated when distinguishing acute or chronic rejection from cyclosporine nephrotoxicity or infection.

PREPROCEDURE EVALUATION FOR RENAL BIOPSY

Planning a biopsy requires assessing risks with a good history and physical, laboratory assessment, and imaging (Table 3-2). **Renal imaging** should be performed to ensure that the patient has two kidneys of normal size and shape. Native kidney biopsy is relatively contraindicated for atrophic kidneys <9 cm in size, as the risk of capsular hemorrhage increases in fibrotic kidneys (as does the risk of a low-yield biopsy result). Renal biopsy of a **solitary native kidney** should be undertaken only when absolutely necessary to preserve renal function as there is a risk of marked bleeding leading to nephrectomy. It has been suggested that surgically performed open renal biopsy should be the procedure of choice in this setting, but the risk of percutaneous biopsy is so low that it may be lower than the risk of general anesthesia and surgery. **Blood pressure** should be optimally controlled, with diastolic BP <95 mm Hg to minimize bleeding complications. **Urine culture** should be

TABLE 3-1	COMMON CURRENT INDICATIONS FOR RENAL BIOPSY

Major

Acute renal failure—diagnosis not apparent by clinical data
Nephrotic syndrome
Nephritic syndrome of unclear etiology
RPGN (Rapidly progressive glomerulonephritis)
Acute or chronic renal allograft dysfunction

Relative indications depending on other clinical features

Asymptomatic hematuria
Asymptomatic proteinuria

sterile before a biopsy attempt. **Blood coagulation parameters** should be normalized as much as possible before renal biopsy. Systemic anticoagulants, including antiplatelet therapy, aspirin, and NSAIDs, should be discontinued ≥5 days before renal biopsy. PT should be <1.2 times control; activated PTT should be <1.2 times control. The role for bleeding time or other functional platelet testing remains unclear but is usually done to screen for unsuspected aspirin use or other platelet disorders. In a patient with renal insufficiency and an elevated BUN with a prolonged bleeding time, DDAVP, 0.4 mcg/kg IV, 2 to 3 hours, is usually given before biopsy.

The diagnostic and therapeutic utility of a renal biopsy in patients needing **chronic anticoagulation** should be carefully considered and balanced with the risk of reversal of anticoagulation and of postbiopsy bleeding. Consultation with cardiology and hematology colleagues may be needed. One approach is to allow the INR to decline to 1.5 over several days or to reverse the anticoagulation with vitamin K depending on the urgency of the biopsy. Intravenous or subcutaneous unfractionated heparin should be stopped at least 6 hours prior to the procedure and should not be resumed until at least 18 to 24 hours after the procedure.

Informed consent should be obtained from the patient by the physician(s) performing the biopsy. Risks, benefits, possible complications, and alternatives to the procedure should always be discussed in detail with the patient. **Difficult or high-risk biopsies** (e.g., single kidney, morbid obesity, requirement for ongoing systemic anticoagulation) should be given careful consideration as to whether risks outweigh benefits. The main contraindications for renal biopsy are given in Table 3-3. Consideration may be given to CT-guided biopsy, transjugular biopsy, or open biopsy, depending on local center expertise.

TABLE 3-2	PREBIOPSY CHECKLIST

History and physical

Laboratory data
    Complete blood count with platelets
    Basic chemistry panel
    Coagulation assessment (INR, aPTT, platelet function)
    Urinalysis and/or urine culture

Baseline kidney ultrasound

Hold antiplatelet and antithrombotic agents at least 1–2 weeks prior to biopsy

TABLE 3-3	CONTRAINDICATIONS FOR RENAL BIOPSY

Absolute Contraindications

Uncooperative patient
Bleeding diathesis or anticoagulation
Uncontrolled hypertension

Relative Contraindications

Small kidneys (<9 cm)
Multiple, bilateral cysts or a renal tumor
Hydronephrosis
Active renal infection
Medium to large vessel vasculitis with multiple intrarenal aneurysms
Anatomical abnormalities of the kidneys (e.g., horseshoe kidney)
Pregnancy

PROCEDURE FOR PERCUTANEOUS NATIVE BIOPSY OF KIDNEY

Patient Positioning

The patient should lie prone on the exam table, with or without a support under the upper abdomen. If the patient is **pregnant** or **very obese**, biopsy can be performed in the seated or lateral decubitus position. The decision to biopsy the left or right kidney depends on imaging quality, presence of cysts, and operator preference. **Ultrasound guidance** should be used to localize the lower pole of the kidney and mark the overlying skin site; with particular attention paid to the depth and angle of the renal cortex in relation to the skin entry site of the biopsy needle (this will minimize the risk of puncturing a major vessel). The amount and direction of movement of the kidney in relation to inspiration and expiration should be carefully noted, especially if real-time ultrasound is not used during the actual biopsy.

Sterile technique should be followed to prepare the skin entry site with Betadine and to drape the field with sterile towels. **Local anesthetic** (e.g., 1% lidocaine + bicarbonate) should be injected with a small-gauge needle to raise a skin wheal and then infiltrated down to the capsule of the kidney along the anticipated biopsy tract with a larger needle. A scalpel should be used to make a small stab incision at the skin site. A variety of biopsy needles are commercially available. Most commonly, 16- or 18-gauge needles are used as sample size is poor with smaller needle gauges. The incidence of major bleeding complications is lower with a spring-loaded needle under ultrasound guidance compared with manual needles. The biopsy needle should be advanced (either with or without real-time ultrasound guidance with a sterile probe) just short of the depth of the renal capsule. The patient may breathe normally during this phase.

The kidney normally moves up and down with the respiratory cycle. When **obtaining the renal biopsy,** the patient should be asked to hold his or her breath as the biopsy needle is slowly advanced through the capsule. Once the biopsy needle is appropriately positioned in the renal cortex, clear movement of the needle should be obvious with the patient's normal breathing. The patient should again be asked to hold his or her breath while the biopsy gun is fired to obtain the core sample. The biopsy needle can then be withdrawn and the core recovered for pathologic exam. A pathology technician is invaluable for examining the core of tissue under an operating microscope to determine if sufficient glomeruli are present. Usually, two to three cores suffice for an adequate biopsy, with one core fixed in formalin for light microscopy and the remainder divided for electron microscopy, immunofluorescence, and special studies. An adequate sample is usually obtained when a total of 10 to 15 glomeruli are present.

ROUTINE POSTBIOPSY CARE

The major complication rate (bleeding severe enough to require transfusion or invasive procedure, septicemia, acute renal obstruction or failure, or death) is 6.4%; while the rate of minor complications is 6.6% (the rate of complications would likely be higher among clinicians with less experience). Clinical recognition of a major complication occurs within 8 to 24 hours among 67% and 91% of patients, respectively. Observation of patients for about 24 hours is usually done to avoid missing most complications. Typically, the patient should remain supine for 6 hours and then remain at bed rest overnight. To help detect bleeding and other complications, vital signs are closely monitored and complete blood counts are obtained at various time points postbiopsy. To minimize the risk of bleeding, blood pressure should ideally be well controlled (goal <140/90 mm Hg). In low-risk patients (e.g., serum creatinine concentration <2 mg/dL [177 micromol/L], blood pressure <140/90 mm Hg, and no evidence of coagulopathy), a shorter observation period may be reasonable.

COMPLICATIONS

The main complications after biopsy are due to bleeding and to pain (Table 3-4). **Hematuria** and the formation of a perinephric hematoma occur to some degree in all patients after renal biopsy, although only approximately 3% to 10% of patients experience gross hematuria. Serial exam of urine specimens for clearing of visible blood is useful in these cases. CBC should be monitored every 6 hours in all patients after renal biopsy. A fall in hemoglobin of approximately 1 g/dL is average after an uncomplicated renal biopsy. **Blood loss requiring transfusion** occurs in 1 to 3 out of 1000 cases. This will depend in part on prebiopsy hemoglobin and risk. The most common site of significant blood loss is

TABLE 3-4	POSTBIOPSY COMPLICATIONS

Bleeding
   Into collecting system—microscopic to gross hematuria
   Subcapsular—pressure tamponade and pain
   Perinephric space—hematoma formation and fall in hematocrit

Colicky pain due to ureteral obstruction from a blood clot from bleeding

Arteriovenous fistula

"Page Kidney"—chronic hypertension due to pressure-induced ischemia from a large subcapsular hematoma

Perinephric soft tissue infection

Puncture of other organs (i.e., liver, pancreas, or spleen)

TABLE 3-5	COMMON INDICATIONS FOR RENAL ALLOGRAFT BIOPSY

Failure of graft function 1 week postengraftment
Rapid deterioration after initial good function, before antirejection Rx
Slow allograft function deterioration
New onset of nephrotic range proteinuria

into the perinephric space, leading to a large perinephric hematoma. Subcapsular bleeds usually tamponade themselves. Significant bleeding into the urinary collecting system may also occur, which manifests as gross hematuria and may lead to ureteral obstruction. **Intervention to control bleeding** is required in 0.1% to 0.4% of cases and **nephrectomy** may be necessary in 0.06% of cases.

Hypotension after renal biopsy can occur in 1% to 2% of patients and is usually fluid responsive. **Arteriovenous fistulas** can be detected radiologically in up to 15% of cases but are rarely of clinical significance and usually resolve spontaneously. The diagnosis is suggested by development of hypotension, high-output heart failure, or persistent hematuria and can be confirmed by color-flow Doppler ultrasound. **Persistent pain** at the biopsy site may result from a subcapsular or perinephric hematoma or from renal colic as blood clots pass through the collecting system. **Biopsy of nonrenal tissues** (most commonly liver or spleen) can occur inadvertently during an intended renal biopsy. Serious complications are rare in these instances. Mortality rate was reported to be 0.2% in one large series but is substantially lower using modern techniques.

RENAL ALLOGRAFT BIOPSY

Biopsy of a transplanted kidney is simplified by the superficial abdominal location of the allograft. Standard indications are summarized in Table 3-5. Biopsy can be done as an outpatient, as risk of significant bleeding is much less than with native biopsy. Transplant biopsies are usually done with real-time ultrasound guidance, as the kidney does not move with the respiratory cycle. After the core tissues are obtained, direct pressure should be applied to the biopsy site for ≥15 minutes to control local bleeding, with a sandbag placed at the site afterward. Patients are usually observed for 6 hours and may then go home in the absence of complications or other factors.

KEY POINTS TO REMEMBER

- Renal biopsy is generally a safe procedure and should be used with confidence when indicated.
- Serious complications are unusual and can be minimized by meticulous prebiopsy preparation (review of coagulation profile, cessation of antiplatelet therapy a few days before the biopsy, and so forth). However, bleeding after a biopsy is unpredictable, and vital signs and hemoglobin should be monitored closely.

REFERENCES AND SELECTED READINGS

Appel GB. Renal biopsy: how effective, what technique, and how safe. *J Nephrol.* 1993;6:4.

Ball RP. Needle aspiration biopsy. *J Tenn Med Assoc.* 1934;27:203.

Iverson P, Brun C. Aspiration biopsy of the kidney. *Am J Med.* 1951;11:324.

Parrish AE. Complications of percutaneous renal biopsy: a review of 37 years' experience. *Clin Nephrol.* 1992;38:135.

Renal Physicians Association. RPA position on optimal length of observation after percutaneous renal biopsy. *Clin Nephrol.* 2001;56:179.

Approach to Proteinuria

Kabeya Mwintshi

4

DEFINITION

Increased protein in the urine is a common sign of kidney disease. Typically, urinary protein is described in terms of total protein or as albumin. Normal individuals excrete <150 mg of total protein and <30 mg of albumin in urine every 24 hours. Other proteins found in the urine are either secreted by tubules (Tamm-Horsfall protein) or are small filtered proteins that have escaped reabsorption or degradation by renal tubule cells. Any level of protein excretion in the urine above 150 mg per 24 hours is abnormal and merits further evaluation. The urine dipstick is the most common initial screening test for proteinuria, but is only sensitive for protein concentrations >20 mg/dL (roughly equivalent to 300 mg per 24 hours). **Nephrotic syndrome** is defined as a urine protein excretion of >3 g per 24 hours associated with hypoalbuminemia, hyperlipidemia, and edema. The same level of proteinuria without the other features is referred to as a **nephrotic range proteinuria.** The approach to the patient with proteinuria is determined by the amount of protein, other renal manifestations, and the overall clinical picture.

WHY TEST FOR PROTEINURIA?

Measuring protein in the urine has become more than just a diagnostic test. Even relatively small increases in protein or albumin in the urine can be early signs of kidney disease and often precede a detectable change in GFR. Protein in the urine is more than a simple marker of disease, as persistently high levels may cause further kidney damage and result in faster progression of the kidney disease. In addition, proteinuria is a strong and independent risk factor for cardiovascular disease and death, mostly in people with diabetes, hypertension, and chronic kidney disease. Interventions that reduce the amount of proteinuria also tend to retard the progression of kidney disease and improve the prognosis of cardiovascular disease.

DETECTION AND QUANTIFICATION OF PROTEINURIA

Urine Dipstick

The simplest and least expensive method of detecting proteinuria is by **routine dipstick.** This dye-impregnated paper uses tetrabromophenol blue as a pH indicator. Urine albumin binds to the reagent and changes its pH, which then results in a spectrum of color changes depending on the degree of pH change. This test is less sensitive to other proteins, such as light chains. False-positive results may occur when highly alkaline urine overwhelms the dye's buffer. A typical scale for a positive test is shown in Table 4-1. The lower threshold concentration for detection of protein by the routine dipstick is around 15 to 20 mg/dL. This is roughly equivalent to a 24-hour urine protein of 300 to 500 mg. **False positive and**

TABLE 4-1	SCALE FOR DETECTING PROTEINURIA ON ROUTINE URINE DIPSTICK
Negative	
Trace: 15–30 mg/dL	
1+: 30–100 mg/dL	
2+: 100–300 mg/dL	
3+: 300–1000 mg/dL	
4+: >1000 mg/dL	

negative tests occur because these semiquantitative estimates of proteinuria are concentration values, and their significance is greatly influenced by urinary concentration. Highly concentrated urine may show an abnormal result even when the absolute daily protein excretion is normal. Similarly, highly dilute urine may show normal or only modestly elevated results for protein concentration when abnormal amounts of protein are excreted. Even with 30 mg/dL of protein, the dipstick can be negative up to 50% of the time. The dipstick will not detect nonalbumin proteins, such as immunoglobulins, as the reaction is relatively specific for albumin. False positives can occur if the patient received radiocontrast up to 24 hours before the test or if the urine is very concentrated.

Test strips that are more sensitive to **albumin** are also available (Albustix). Dye-impregnated strips and special immunoassays are available that can detect albumin concentrations to as low as 30 mg/day, which is far below the 300 mg per 24 hours threshold of the standard dipstick. These strips can be used to screen for microalbuminuria, and their sensitivity and specificity range from 80% to 97% and 33% to 80%, respectively.

Quantitative Methods

Spot Urine Protein-to-Creatinine Ratio

The amount of dilution of the urine will directly affect protein concentration. The concentration of creatinine in the urine serves as an internal control for urine dilution. The ratio of protein to creatinine is independent of urine concentration, as concentration affects both parameters equally. There is evidence that untimed or spot urine specimen is adequate for quantification of proteinuria. Since the rate of creatinine excretion remains fairly constant, the ratio of protein to creatinine on a random specimen is a good estimate of amount of protein excreted. It is important to note the units in which the laboratory reports protein and creatinine, as equivalent units should be used to generate a valid ratio. The protein-to-creatinine ratio in a normal person is <0.2 and is roughly equivalent to an excretion of <0.2 g/24 hours/1.73 m^2. For instance, a ratio of 2 roughly translates to a 24-hour urinary protein excretion of 2 g. The accuracy of the total protein-to-creatinine ratio is related to the assumption that daily creatinine excretion is only slightly >1000 mg (8.8 mmol)/24 hours/1.73 m^2. The accuracy of the ratio is diminished when creatinine excretion is either markedly increased in a muscular man (the ratio will underestimate proteinuria) or markedly reduced in a cachectic patient (the ratio will overestimate proteinuria).

Urinary Albumin Evaluation

The presence of increased amounts of urinary albumin is an important marker for early kidney disease. Validation of this concept is strongest in early diabetic kidney disease but may also apply to other forms of kidney disease. In addition, urinary albumin is a marker for cardiovascular risk. The term *microalbuminuria* resulted from early studies that used more sensitive assays for albumin and detected the presence despite negative results for usual dipstick tests for protein. Methods for assessing urinary albumin excretion include untimed and timed collection methods. The urinary albumin is most often assessed using the albumin (microalbumin)-to-creatinine ratio on an untimed or "spot" specimen.

Microalbumin-to-Creatinine Ratio

The microalbumin-to-creatinine ratio can be used in same way as the urine protein-to-creatinine ratio, although a sensitive assay for albumin is used instead of the usual protein assay. A value <30 mcg/g of creatinine is considered normal, whereas values from 30 to 300 mcg/g creatinine indicate microalbuminuria. Values above 300 mcg/g are detected by the routine dipstick and fall in the category of overt proteinuria (macroalbuminuria) in persons with diabetes. Microalbumin-to-creatinine ratio is the preferred routine screening tool for all diabetics for detection of early nephropathy. A single first-morning voided specimen has a sensitivity and specificity of >90% when compared with a 24-hour collection, but this varies when the urine samples are taken at other times of the day. In addition, falsely elevated values may be obtained with hyperglycemia, vigorous exercise, infections, and ketoacidosis.

24-Hour Urine Protein Collection

The 24-hour urine collection has been the definitive method of collection but is used less often because of problems with collection errors, patient inconvenience, and the increased use of the protein-to-creatinine ratio. However, this test is still useful as a baseline in persons with proteinuria even though ratio methods are used for ongoing follow-up. This test is also probably preferred in patients where urine creatinine excretion is less reliable (changing renal function, high and low muscle mass). To verify proper collection, 24-hour urine creatinine should always be measured in the same urine specimen. Excretion of creatinine in male patients during a 24-hour period should be roughly 20 to 25 mg/kg; for female patients, it should be approximately 15 to 20 mg/kg. If the amount of creatinine in the urine sample is quite different from the expected range, an error in collection of the sample should be suspected.

GENERAL MECHANISMS OF PROTEINURIA

Proteinuria can occur due to glomerular or tubular dysfunction. **Glomerular proteinuria** results from a disruption of the glomerular barrier leading to increased filtration of plasma proteins in amounts that exceed tubular reabsorptive capacity. If the amount of protein in 24 hours exceeds 2 g, a glomerular disease is usually present. **Tubular proteinuria** is a consequence of inadequate reabsorption of filtered low-molecular-weight proteins (e.g., $beta_2$-microglobulin or lysozyme), which then appear in the urine. It can coexist with glomerular proteinuria or in isolation in the setting of a defective proximal tubule function. Typically, tubular proteinuria is <2 g per 24 hours. **Overflow proteinuria** occurs when there is excessive systemic production of abnormal proteins (of small molecular weight) that exceeds the capacity of the tubule for reabsorption. A prime example is the increased urinary excretion of light chains in myeloma. Occasionally, lysozymuria appears in acute monocytic leukemia. **Tissue proteinuria** is associated with an inflammatory or neoplastic process within the urinary tract.

Classification of Proteinuria

Proteinuria can be divided into three categories: transient, orthostatic, and persistent.

Transient Proteinuria

Transient proteinuria is primarily seen in children and adolescents who are healthy and asymptomatic with normal urinary sediment. It is believed to result from alteration in renal hemodynamics. It disappears on repeat testing and requires no further evaluation. Some individuals have recurrent episodes of transient proteinuria, which often goes into permanent remission within a few years. Some studies of this group have reported a histological association and progression toward renal insufficiency and hypertension. It is therefore recommended to monitor this subgroup yearly. Finally, transient proteinuria can occur reversibly in hyperadrenergic states like fever, exercise, congestive heart failure, seizures, use of vasopressors, pregnancy, and obstructive sleep apnea. A 10% incidence of functional proteinuria has been reported among ER admissions, with the most common causes being congestive heart failure, seizures, and fever. The proteinuria resolves within hours to days after the precipitating event is removed, usually without consequence. Pathogenesis is believed to be secondary to increased glomerular permeability and decreased tubular reabsorption of proteins, possibly due to angiotensin II or norepinephrine.

Orthostatic Proteinuria

This syndrome is characterized by the excretion of abnormal quantities of protein in the upright position, with normal levels of protein excretion while supine. It is present in up to 3% to 5 % of adolescents and young men, mostly <30 years old. Most patients have rates of protein excretion <2 g per 24 hours in the upright position, although higher rates have been reported. The diagnosis can be made with 24-hour split urine collections in the supine and upright positions. The 24-hour collection is divided into a 16-hour daytime portion and an 8-hour overnight portion. Long-term follow-up of these patients shows no deterioration in renal function, with spontaneous resolution in 50% of patients 10 years after diagnosis.

Persistent Proteinuria

Persistent proteinuria is present regardless of position, activity level, or functional status. It is established by confirming proteinuria on subsequent testing a week or two after the first positive test. It may result from an isolated kidney disease or may be part of a multisystem process with renal involvement. Patients with persistent proteinuria are typically classified as having nephrotic or non-nephrotic range proteinuria and by the presence or absence of features of the nephrotic syndrome. Higher amounts of proteinuria are predictive of an underlying kidney disease.

CLINICAL APPROACH TO PROTEINURIA

Once proteinuria has been detected on a dipstick, the next step is to confirm the abnormal result by repeat measurement after several weeks with a freshly voided specimen. However, no confirmatory test is needed if the proteinuria is heavy on dipstick. Once confirmation is done, the next step is to quantify protein excretion by a protein- or albumin-to-creatinine ratio or timed collection.

The **history and physical** examination should include a search for symptoms and signs attributable to kidney disease, as well as complications and risk factors of kidney disease. Key issues to be addressed are:

- The presence and duration of common causes of kidney disease such as **diabetes** and **hypertension.**
- Features suggestive of a **connective tissue disorder** such as arthralgias, arthritis, skin rashes, and constitutional symptoms.
- Clinical features of **malignancy** should be sought. For example, solid organ malignancies have been associated with membranous nephropathy, whereas lymphomas have been associated with minimal change disease.
- Features suggestive of **infections** such as hepatitis, endocarditis, syphilis, or HIV should be explored. These disorders can lead to many different forms of glomerular disease.
- A complete history of **drugs**, both prescription and over the counter should be taken. For example, NSAIDs can cause nephrotic syndrome.

• **Family history** of kidney disease including hereditary nephritis, nail-patella syndrome, or polycystic kidney disease.

Additional testing is determined by the context. In all cases, a urine sediment, GFR estimation, CBC, basic metabolic profile, and serum albumin are appropriate. Urine protein electrophoresis (UPEP) and serum protein electrophoresis (SPEP) should be ordered if there is suspicion of an overflow proteinuria from myeloma, amyloidosis, or other immunoglobulin diseases. Dysmorphic red cells in the sediment, or a nephrotic range proteinuria would favor a kidney biopsy. An evaluation of the anatomy of the urinary tract is usually not needed unless there is significant hematuria, or history of recurrent urinary tract infection (Fig. 4-1).

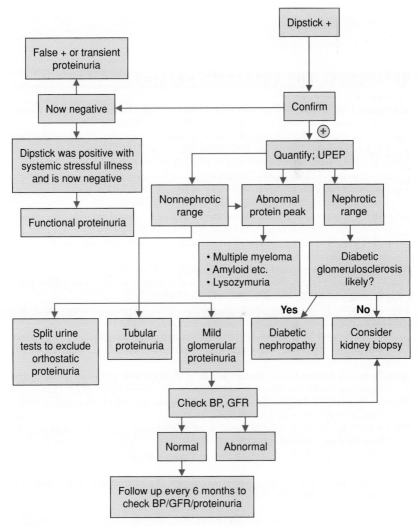

FIGURE 4-1. Evaluation of proteinuria. ⊕, positive; GFR, glomerular filtration rate; UPEP, urine protein electrophoresis.

KEY POINTS TO REMEMBER

- The dipstick detects albumin only from a level of 300 mg per 24 hours. Special dipsticks are required to detect microalbuminuria.
- In a patient with a negative standard dipstick but with kidney or cardiovascular disease risk factors, a spot urine albumin-to-creatinine ratio must be done looking for microalbuminuria.
- Spot urine protein-to-creatinine ratio is as good as a 24-hour protein sample.
- It is important to detect and quantify proteinuria, as it is linked to kidney disease progression as well as cardiovascular disease prognosis.
- Nephrotic range proteinuria is often of glomerular origin and in most cases warrants a kidney biopsy.

REFERENCES AND SUGGESTED READINGS

Damsgaard EM, Froland A, Jorgensen OD, Mogensen CE. Microalbuminuria as predictor of increased mortality in elderly people. *BMJ.* 1990;300:297–300.

Grimm RH, Svendsen KH, Kasiske B, et al. Proteinuria is a risk factor for mortality over 10 years follow up. *Kidney Int.* 1997;52:10–14.

Gross, JL, de Azevedo, MJ, Silveiro, SP, et al. Diabetic nephropathy: diagnosis, prevention, and treatment. *Diabetes Care.* 2005;28:164.

Larrsson SO, Thysell H. Four years' follow up of asymptomatic isolated proteinuria diagnosed in general health survey. *Acta Med Scand.* 1969;186:375.

Lemann J Jr, Doumas BT. Proteinuria in health and disease assessed by measuring the urinary protein/creatinine ratio. *Clin Chemistry.* 1987;33:297–299.

Levitt JI. The prognostic significance of proteinuria on young college students. *Ann Intern Med.* 1967;66:685.

Muth RG. Asymptomatic mild proteinuria. *Arch Intern Med.* 1965;115:569.

Park YH, Choi JY, Chung HS, et al. Hematuria and proteinuria in a mass school urine screening. *Pediatr Nephrol.* 2005;20(8):1126–1130.

Robinson, RR. Isolated proteinuria in asymptomatic patients. *Kidney Int.* 1980; 18:395.

Rytand DA, Spreiter S. Prognosis in postural (orthostatic) proteinuria: forty to fifty-year follow up of six patients after diagnosis by Thomas Addis. *N Engl J Med.* 1981;305: 618.

Springberg PD, Garrett LE Jr, Thompson AL, et al. Fixed and reproducible orthostatic proteinuria: results of a 20-year follow up study. *Ann Intern Med.* 1982;97:516.

Wagner DK, Harris T, Madans JH. Proteinuria as a biomarker risk of subsequent morbidity and mortality. *Environ Res.* 1994;66:160–172.

Wagner MD, Smith FG, Tinglof BO, et al. Epidemiology of proteinuria: a study of 4807 school children. *J Pediatr.* 1968;73:825.

Wingo CS, Clapp WL. Proteinuria: potential causes and approach to evaluation. *Am J Med Sci.* 2000;320:188.

Wolman IJ. The incidence, causes and intermittency of proteinuria in young men. *Am J Med Sci.* 1945;210:765.

Approach to Hematuria

5

Rouba Ghoussoub

INTRODUCTION AND DEFINITION

Hematuria, or blood in the urine, can be a sign of serious underlying pathology of the kidney or urinary tract. Therefore, it is important to identify and, if necessary, to treat the disease lurking behind it at an early stage. Hematuria can be either gross or microscopic. **Gross hematuria** is, as the name implies, blood in the urine that is grossly visible to the eye. The American Urological Association (AUA) has defined **microscopic hematuria** as 3 or more RBCs per high-power field (HPF) on microscopic examination of urinary sediment from 2 out of 3 properly collected urine specimens in average or low-risk patients, and from 1 out of 3 specimens in high-risk patients (delineated below).

Epidemiology

Gross hematuria is estimated to have a community prevalence of 2.5%. The prevalence of microscopic hematuria, according to population-based studies, varies widely depending on age and sex distribution of the populations at hand, and on the method of detection that was utilized. The prevalence in the general population ranges from 0.18% to 16.1%. It is unclear whether there is a higher prevalence with increasing age.

SCREENING

Screening for asymptomatic microscopic hematuria is generally not recommended and is usually an incidental finding on urinalysis dipstick testing. The presence of a positive dipstick dictates microscopic analysis of the urine sediment for RBCs as this test cannot differentiate between RBCs, myoglobin, and hemoglobin. Further investigation may be warranted depending on the clinical scenario and risk for serious underlying disease.

DETECTION OF HEMATURIA

In gross hematuria, urine may appear red, cola-colored, or brown. In microscopic hematuria, it will appear clear and diagnosis is usually made by dipstick (incidentally). The following points should be considered in order to do an accurate assessment of microscopic hematuria.

Urine Collection

Should be a freshly voided, clean-catch, midstream urine specimen.

Dipstick Testing

- Highly sensitive (91%–100%) but less specific (65%–99%)
- False negatives can be due to ingestion of large amounts of ascorbic acid or other reducing agents, low pH, or the presence of formaldehyde.

- When positive, the urine sample should be centrifuged and the sediment examined microscopically to count the number of RBCs per HPF (see Chapter 1 about urine centrifugation)

Microscopic Analysis

- Allows for examination of RBC morphology and the detection of RBC casts.
- Dysmorphic RBCs and RBC casts are indicative of a glomerular pathology and a renal cause for hematuria.
- Dysmorphic urinary RBCs are best seen by phase-contrast microscopy and are variable in size and shape, having irregular borders compared with the normal, doughnut-shaped RBCs. If >80% of urinary RBCs are dysmorphic, hematuria is more likely due to a glomerular cause. If >80% of urinary RBCs are normal, this indicates a lower urinary tract source of bleeding. Note that dysmorphic RBCs are seen in hematuria of nonglomerular origin and isomorphic (normal morphology) RBCs in hematuria of glomerular origin, but it is the relative abundance of each that is key.
- Acanthocytes, or doughnut-shaped RBCs with membrane blebs, have also been used as a marker for glomerular bleeding, whereas crenated RBCs (with spicules) are not usually relevant and indicate concentrated urine.

CAUSES OF HEMATURIA

Hematuria can be glomerular or nonglomerular in origin. Nonglomerular hematuria can be further divided into upper and lower urinary tract. The various etiologies of hematuria are listed in Table 5-1. In persons <50 years of age, the most common glomerular causes are IgA nephropathy and thin basement membrane disease (recent data suggests similar frequency), whereas nephrolithiasis, pyelonephritis, cystitis, prostatitis, and urethritis are the most common nonglomerular causes in that age group. In persons >50 years of age, renal, prostate, and transitional cell cancers (bladder/ureteral) are more common nonglomerular sources of bleeding while IgA nephropathy continues to be the leading cause of glomerular hematuria.

EVALUATION OF HEMATURIA

History

Obtaining a thorough history is crucial in the evaluation of hematuria. Medications should be carefully reviewed as certain commonly prescribed drugs can be the culprits (NSAIDs, busulfan, aspirin, oral contraceptives, and warfarin). Over-anticoagulation with warfarin may cause hematuria if excessive, but still warrants further investigation as it may be unmasking underlying pathology. Risk factors for significant disease should also be investigated, as increasing age (>40 years), cigarette smoking, occupational exposure to chemicals, and high doses of cyclophosphamide increase the risk of transitional cell cancers of the bladder and the urinary tract. Gross hematuria is four times more likely than microscopic hematuria to be associated with urothelial cancers, and is by itself considered a risk factor for serious pathology. Table 5-2 lists the various risk factors for significant urologic disease. Patients should also be checked for signs of glomerular pathology or systemic disease, for instance edema, purpura, and skin rashes. Fever, dysuria, and flank pain are suggestive of pyelonephritis/complicated urinary tract infection. Travel history may uncover a risk for schistosomiasis. A family history of hematuria can be significant in Alport syndrome and thin basement membrane disease.

Physical Examination

This should include measurement of BP, pulse, and volume status. Hypertension (HTN) could be a manifestation of glomerulonephritis. Edema may be a sign of proteinuria. Fever, castrovertebral angle (CVA) tenderness, and suprapubic tenderness are suggestive of an

TABLE 5-1	CAUSES OF MICROSCOPIC HEMATURIA

Origin			Causes
Glomerular			IgA nephropathy
			Thin basement membrane disease (benign familial hematuria)
			Hereditary nephritis (Alport syndrome)
			Mild focal glomerulonephritis of other causes (primary glomerulonephritis [e.g., MCD, membranous, MPGN, FSGS, etc.] versus secondary glomerulonephritis [e.g., SLE, HIVAN, amyloid/LCDD, SBE, etc.])
Nonglomerular	*Upper urinary tract (renal, vascular, and ureteral)*		Nephrolithiasis
			Pyelonephritis
			Renal cell cancer
			Polycystic kidney disease
			Medullary sponge kidney
			Hypercalciuria, hyperuricosuria, or both, without documented stones
			Renal pelvis or ureteral transitional cell cancer
			Renal trauma
			Interstitial nephritis
			Papillary necrosis
			Renal infarction/arteriovenous malformation/renal vein thrombosis
			Ureteral stricture and hydronephrosis
			Sickle cell trait or disease
			Renal tuberculosis
	Lower urinary tract (bladder, prostate, and urethra)		Cystitis, prostatitis, urethritis
			Bladder cancer
			Prostate cancer/benign prostatic hypertrophy
			Benign bladder and ureteral polyps and tumors
			Urethral and meatal strictures
			Schistosoma haematobium in North Africans
			Trauma (catheterization/blunt urethral or bladder trauma)
Uncertain			Exercise hematuria
			Menstrual contamination
			Over-anticoagulation (usually with warfarin)
			Sexual intercourse
			"Benign hematuria" (unexplained microscopic hematuria)

TABLE 5-2	RISK FACTORS FOR SIGNIFICANT UROLOGIC PATHOLOGY IN PATIENTS WITH MICROSCOPIC HEMATURIA

Age >40 years
History of smoking
History of gross hematuria
Occupational exposure to chemicals or dyes (benzenes or aromatic amines)
Recurrent urinary tract infections
Irritative voiding symptoms
History of high-dose cyclophosphamide
Pelvic irradiation
Analgesic abuse

infectious etiology. A nonblanching purpuric rash may be evidence of vasculitis. Cardiovascular exam may reveal atrial fibrillation or murmurs due to endocarditis—both sources for renal emboli. Abdominal exam may reveal a mass, enlarged bladder, or polycystic kidneys. A detailed genitourinary exam should be performed to look for local sources of bleeding and to exclude rectal or vaginal bleeding.

Laboratory Evaluation

This should begin with urine dipstick and microscopic examination of the urine sediment. If **pyuria** or **bacteruria** is present, urine culture should be obtained to look for infection. If urine culture is positive, appropriate treatment with antibiotics should be given and urine dipstick and microscopy repeated 6 weeks later to ensure resolution of hematuria. If the hematuria has resolved, no further evaluation is needed. If dipstick is positive for *protein*, quantification of the proteinuria is necessary. A ratio of urinary protein to urinary creatinine in a spot urine specimen of more than 0.3 or a 24-hour urinary protein excretion of more than 300 mg suggests a renal source of bleeding and warrants evaluation by a nephrologist. **Serum creatinine** should be checked and an abnormal value should prompt a work-up for renal disease. CBC, electrolytes, and BUN should also be obtained. **Dysmorphic RBCs, RBC casts,** or **acanthocytes** in the urine suggest glomerular bleeding and should be followed by a glomerulonephritis workup including measurement of ANA, ANCA, anti-GBM antibodies, complement levels, cryoglobulins, serology for hepatitis B and C viruses, and HIV antibody test. A renal biopsy would often be indicated at this point. **Urine cytology** is indicated in those at risk for bladder cancer (Table 5-2). This test has only about 66% to 79% sensitivity but very high specificity (95%–100%). Sensitivity is improved if the urine is collected on 3 consecutive days from the first voiding in the morning. Its sensitivity is higher for carcinoma in situ and high-grade bladder cancer than for cancers of low histologic grade, and is insensitive for renal cell cancer.

If a careful history and examination were suggestive of a benign source of hematuria, urinalysis should be repeated 48 hours after cessation of the precipitating cause (e.g., menstruation, vigorous exercise, sexual activity, or trauma). If the hematuria has resolved no further workup is necessary.

Stepwise Approach to Evaluation

There is no consensus as to a standard protocol to be followed when encountering a hematuria workup. The AUA published recommendations in 2001, which are incorporated

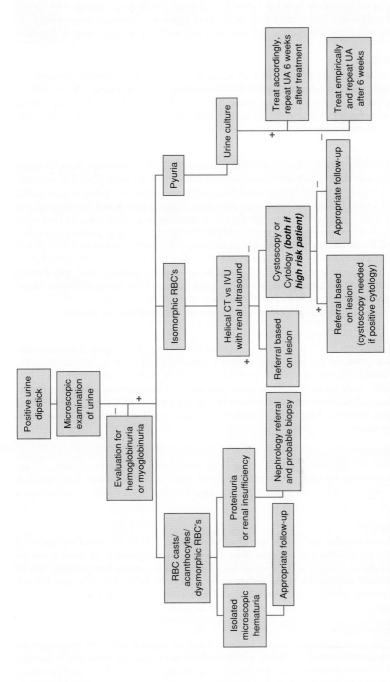

FIGURE 5-1. Algorithm for microscopic hematuria evaluation. IVU, intravenous urography.

partly in the algorithm shown in Figure 5-1. Although the optimal imaging study for the initial evaluation of the urinary tract has not been agreed on, computed tomography (CT) is being used increasingly due to high sensitivity and specificity in a wide range of diagnoses.

Imaging

If infection and a glomerular source of bleeding are ruled out, imaging of the upper urinary tract should be obtained to look for renal cell cancer or transitional cell cancer of the ureter and the renal pelvis, stones, cystic disease, or obstructive lesions. CT scan is being used more frequently now as the initial study although traditionally intravenous urography (IVU) had been recommended as the initial modality of choice.

CT Scan

This is the best modality for the detection of stones (94%–98% sensitivity) and solid masses of the urinary tract, as well as renal and perirenal infections or abscesses. If possible, the unenhanced helical CT should be done first to evaluate for stones; then if negative or if the patient has risk factors for renal or transitional cell cancer, it should be followed by enhanced contrast CT (CT urography). Although the CT is more expensive than either IVU or ultrasound, these tests are often followed by additional imaging resulting in greater expense than if the CT scan had been done initially. In addition, CT scan detects masses <3 cm in size, which can be missed by IVU or ultrasound. High detection rates for transitional cell carcinoma have also been reported for CT scans, including in the bladder, which may decrease the need for cystoscopy, but there is no statistical analysis of the data available yet. Disadvantages are expense, the risk of contrast nephropathy (which can also occur with IVU), and availability. Note that in pregnancy, ultrasound is the preferred imaging modality.

IVU

Traditionally the IVU has been the initial modality of choice for imaging of the upper urinary tract; however it is being replaced by CT scans if available. IVU is more sensitive than ultrasound for detection of transitional cell cancer in the kidney or the ureter, but it cannot differentiate between solid and cystic components. Thus it is often followed by further imaging such as ultrasound or CT scan. IVU is less costly than CT and is more widely available, but it also has the risk of contrast nephropathy and may miss upper tract lesions <3 cm in size.

Ultrasound

Excellent for characterizing solid versus cystic components but can miss lesions <3 cm (82% sensitivity for masses between 2 and 3 cm). It is the preferred test used in pregnancy as it is the safest. However, its use is becoming more limited in the evaluation of hematuria since the advent of CT scans.

Cystoscopy

It is recommended that cystoscopy should be done as part of the initial evaluation of microscopic hematuria in all adults older than 40 years of age and in all those at risk for bladder cancer (Table 5-2). Cystoscopy has a lower yield in patients younger than 40 years and in those with no risk factors for malignancy. It can be deferred in these cases but urinary cytology should be performed instead. Disadvantages are that it is an invasive procedure and can result in infection and patient discomfort.

Ureterorenoscopy

Once the above radiologic tests are performed and are negative, fiberoptic imaging of the upper urinary tract and the kidney is now available and performed frequently in urologic clinics. Ureterorenoscopy is mostly done in patients who have benign essential hematuria or unilateral hematuria, where they have recurrent macroscopic hematuria with negative radiologic/laboratory workup, with the hematuria localizing to one side of the bladder on cystoscopy. Discrete vascular lesions like arteriovenous malformations or hemangiomas that can be fulgurated are found in 0.50% of cases. Renal calculi or upper tract transitional cell carcinomas are found in 5% to 10%. No diagnosis is made in 10% of patients. Biopsies of lesions suspicious for neoplasms can be taken in the ureters or the kidneys with partial nephrectomy performed for those with high suspicions of renal cell cancer. Vascular lesions can be treated with the Holmium:YAG laser successfully. Calculi can be extracted. Thus ureterorenoscopy provides a novel technique that is useful for diagnosis and treatment of what was otherwise claimed to be "benign hematuria."

FOLLOW-UP

Some patients who initially have a negative workup for microscopic hematuria eventually develop significant disease (although most do not). For this reason, patient follow-up is recommended. Microscopic hematuria can precede bladder cancer and certain glomerulonephritides by years, initially demonstrating a negative evaluation. Repeating BP measurements, urinalysis, and voided-urine cytology at 6, 12, 24, and 36 months are recommended. Of course, in patients who develop worrisome signs such as irritative voiding symptoms or gross hematuria, further evaluation with imaging and cystoscopy is warranted. Positive cytology should naturally be followed by cystoscopy and possibly imaging. After 3 years, if follow-up is negative, no further monitoring is recommended. Another important point to remember is that immediate referral to a nephrologist should be done if proteinuria, hypertension, or renal insufficiency were to develop during follow-up as they may be indicative of glomerular disease. In cases of isolated microscopic hematuria that is persistent, renal biopsy is controversial as available data does not suggest that identification of the disease may alter management or outcome (e.g., IgA or thin basement membrane disease).

KEY POINTS TO REMEMBER

- Hematuria can be glomerular or nonglomerular in origin, so microscopic examination of urinary sediment is crucial in the evaluation.
- Nonglomerular hematuria can be of upper or lower urinary tract in origin, and has numerous causes, most commonly urinary stones, cysts, or malignancy.
- History is important in excluding "benign" causes of hematuria and drug/toxin-induced etiologies.
- Dysmorphic RBCs, RBC casts, and acanthocytes, as well as proteinuria and renal insufficiency point to a renal etiology of hematuria and should indicate prompt referral to a nephrologist and consideration for renal biopsy.
- CT scan is becoming the preferred imaging modality for upper urinary tract abnormalities.
- Follow-up over 3 years is indicated for patients with a negative workup as they may eventually develop significant disease.

REFERENCES AND SELECTED READINGS

Cohen RA, Brown RS, et al. Microscopic hematuria. *New Eng J Med.* 2003;348:2330.
Dooley RE, Pietrow PK. Ureteroscopy for benign hematuria. *Urol Clin North Am.* 2004;31(1):137–143.

Grossfield G, Wolf JS, Litwin M, et al. Asymptomatic microscopic hematuria in adults: summary of the AUA best practice policy recommendations. *Am Fam Physician.* 2001;63:1145.

Jaffe JS, Ginsberg PC, Harkaway RC, et al. A new diagnostic algorithm for the evaluation of microscopic hematuria. *Adult Urology.* 2001;57:889.

Khadra MH, Pickard RS, Charlton M, et al. A prospective analysis of 1,930 patients with hematuria to evaluate current diagnostic practice. *J Urol.* 2000;163:524.

McDonald MM, Swagerty D, Wetzel L, et al. Assessment of microscopic hematuria. *Am Fam Physician.* 2006;73:1748.

Van Savage JG, Fried FA. Anticoagulant-associated hematuria: a prospective study. *J Urol.* 1995;153:1594–1596.

Disorders of Water Balance: Hyponatremia and Hypernatremia

6

Andrew Siedlecki and Matthew J. Koch

INTRODUCTION

Disorders of sodium (hypo- or hypernatremia) reflect abnormalities in water homeostasis. They can cause acute morbidity if the change in the plasma sodium occurs rapidly or reaches an extreme level over a prolonged period. The rapid correction of either a hypo- or hypernatremic state can cause significant morbidity as well. Measured plasma osmolality reflects the combined effects of all soluble particles in the plasma component of the extracellular fluid (ECF). Much of the osmolality of the ECF (95%) is derived from the sodium and chloride content of the plasma. Further, as body compartments are in osmotic equilibrium, the osmolality of the intracellular fluid (ICF) compartment is equal to the ECF. The membranes that separate these components are described as *semipermeable*. Our developing knowledge of the water channels (*aquaporins*) has modified our characterization of these barriers to now include a ubiquitous number of membrane-crossing channels that regulate water diffusion.

Antidiuretic hormone (ADH), also known as *arginine vasopressin* (AVP) is a polypeptide released from the supraoptic and paraventricular nuclei of the hypothalamus and is the main determinant of renal water regulation and free water balance. It is normally released in response to minor increases in effective osmoles as detected by osmoreceptors in the hypothalamus. In addition, decrease in mean arterial pressure is a potent stimulus for ADH release and is sensed by baroreceptors in the vasculature and the heart. Other stimuli for ADH release include nausea and pain. The primary site of action for ADH is the collecting duct of the kidney. ADH stimulates insertion of aquaporin-2 water channels into the apical membrane of principal cells in this location resulting in more water reabsorption. Under normal circumstances, an acute water load can be excreted within 1 to 2 hours.

HYPONATREMIA

Hyponatremia is defined as a serum or plasma sodium concentration [Na^+] <135 mmol/L. The prevalence is reported to be around 30% of hospitalized patients and 7% in ambulatory care clinics. The approach to a patient with hyponatremia includes an assessment of the acuity (acute vs. chronic) of the decreased [Na^+] and the severity of symptoms. This aids in decision making regarding the appropriate rate of correction. **Acute hyponatremia** is defined as a fall in [Na^+] over a period of <48 hours. Remember that the sodium level as measured in mmol/L does not provide any information about the actual sodium content, as it is only the ratio of sodium to the amount of ECF in which it is contained. Total body sodium can be low, normal, or elevated in the presence of hyponatremia. Hyponatremia is the result of either solute loss with free water replacement or free water gain due to impaired water excretion. Within several hours of a change of plasma osmolality, intracellular osmolality again achieves equilibrium with the extracellular space in an attempt to maintain cell volume.

Neurologic Complications of Hyponatremia

As plasma sodium and tonicity drops, cells in the brain must readjust intracellular osmolality by lowering the osmotic content. If changes occur rapidly or in the face of severe hyponatremia, this adaptation fails leading to cerebral edema, altered mental status, and seizures. Hyponatremia can be fatal should brainstem herniation result. Patients with underlying metabolic disorders or preexisting neurologic disease, as well as children and young women, may be at particular risk of severe complications without rapid reversal of acute hyponatremia. As the brain swells, the restricted volume of the calvarium reduces blood supply and modifies the excitatory potential of neurons. *Central pontine myelinolysis* (osmotic demyelination) is thought to be due to rapid a correction of chronic hyponatremia. The adaptation to the hyponatremic condition by the cells results in cellular dehydration when the $[Na^+]$ is increased too rapidly. Cognitive, behavioral, and movement disorders due to the occurrence of osmotic demyelination may not be apparent for days after the correction of hyponatremia, and visible changes on MRI may take weeks to appear. Alcoholic patients and those with severe malnutrition appear to be at particular risk for osmotic demyelination due to rapid sodium correction. Osmotic demyelination does not appear to be a major concern in the correction of acute hyponatremia; however, there is no apparent benefit in a rapid return to normal sodium level in this situation once symptoms have been controlled.

Clinical Evaluation of Hyponatremia

A thorough **history** should include the estimated duration of inciting factors and an assessment of signs or symptoms suggesting that immediate intervention may be necessary (mental status change, lethargy, coma, seizure). Management of a patient with hyponatremia depends on whether the process is considered to be *acute* or *chronic* and the severity of symptoms. It usually is asymptomatic until $[Na^+]$ <125 mmol/L, but fatalities have been reported with an extremely rapid decrease from a normal $[Na^+]$ to the 120- to 128-mmol/L range. Symptoms include CNS effects, such as confusion, weakness, obtundation, or seizures. Chronic hyponatremia (developing over >48 hours) is generally fairly well tolerated. Symptoms include cognitive defects as well as nausea, vomiting, weakness, and headache. The **physical exam** should be geared toward assessing the volume status of the patient. Elevated blood pressure, an S3 heart sound, or increased jugular venous pressure indicate volume excess often in the setting of early congestive heart failure. Edema in the lower extremities or presacral region or evidence of pulmonary edema indicates increased ECF volume in heart failure and kidney disease. Conversely, orthostatic hypotension, decreased skin turgor, dry mucosal membranes, and decreased jugular venous pressure suggest intravascular volume depletion.

Laboratory Evaluation

The overall clinical context will guide the significance of laboratory testing. The following approach first briefly identifies nonhypotonic hyponatremia, leaving more extensive evaluation for the category of hypotonic hyponatremia. This latter type of hyponatremia describes the majority of presentations and will be discussed in the most detail.

Plasma Osmolality: Calculated, Measured, and Effective
Calculated plasma osmolality (P_{osm}) is obtained using plasma sodium $[Na^+]$ (mmol/L), blood urea nitrogen (BUN, mg/dL), and serum glucose (mg/dL):

$$\text{Calculated } P_{osm} = 2 \times [Na] + (BUN/2.8) + (glucose/18)$$

TABLE 6-1   COMMON CAUSES OF SIADH

CNS disorders	Hemorrhage, psychosis, infection, alcohol withdrawal
Malignancy (ectopic ADH)	Small-cell lung carcinoma (most commonly implicated), CNS disease, leukemia, Hodgkin disease, duodenal cancer, pancreatic cancer
Pulmonary	Infection, acute respiratory failure, mechanical ventilation
Miscellaneous	Pain, nausea (powerful stimulator of ADH), HIV (multifactorial), general post-op state
Pharmacologic agents (either mimic or enhance ADH)	Cyclophosphamide, vincristine, vinblastine, NSAIDs, tricyclics and related agents, selective serotonin reuptake inhibitors, chlorpropamide, nicotine, bromocriptine, oxytocin, DDAVP

ADH, antidiuretic hormone.

(Dividing BUN by 2.8, glucose by 18, and ethanol [when present] by 4.6 converts the measurements from mg/dL to mmol/L).

Measured P_{osm} should be obtained to evaluate for the presence of an osmolar gap (measured P_{osm} − calculated P_{osm}) and to calculate effective osmolality (E_{osm}).

The normal *effective* serum osmolality (sodium plus anions and glucose) is approximately 285 mOsm/kg (275–290). Urea and ethanol are not confined to the ECF, thus are not effective osmoles and do not affect the tonicity of the ECF. The concentration of these substances (expressed in mmol/L) should be subtracted from the measured P_{osm} to obtain the E_{osm}:

$$E_{osm} = \text{measured } P_{osm} - (BUN/2.8 + ethanol/4.6)$$

From these calculations, it is apparent that uremia or alcohol intoxication provide ineffective osmoles and can present with a normal or elevated P_{osm} but a low E_{osm} (see Table 6-1). On the other hand, glucose and several other sources of carbohydrate are retained in the ECF inducing a hypertonic hyponatremia.

Urine Osmolality
Urine osmolality (U_{osm}) <100 mOsm/kg in the setting of hyponatremia is rare, but suggests primary polydipsia or reset osmostat. In the presence of ADH (appropriate or inappropriate), the U_{osm} is usually significantly >100 mOsm/kg.

Urine Sodium
In the presence of intact renal function, urine sodium (U_{Na}) will be low (<20 mmol/L) in the face of volume depletion due to extrarenal loss of sodium (vomiting, diarrhea, sweating). Avid renal sodium reabsorption is triggered by the expected neurohumoral response to this state. An elevated U_{Na} (>20 mmol/L) can be seen with tubular dysfunction, diuretics, the presence of osmotically active particles in the urine, or sodium-losing nephropathies.

Causes of Hyponatremia
Pseudohyponatremia
Apparent hyponatremia with normal osmolality has classically been caused by severe elevations of plasma lipids or proteins. Standard laboratory analyzers assume that the water

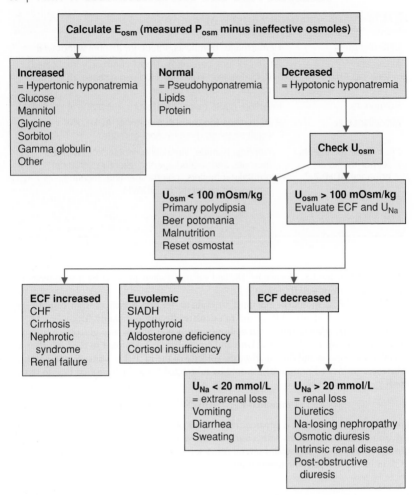

FIGURE 6-1. Evaluation of hyponatremia. CHF, congestive heart failure; ECF, extracellular fluid; E_{osm}, effective osmolality; P_{osm}, plasma osmolality; U_{Na}, urine sodium; U_{osm}, urine osmolality.

phase of plasma is 93% of total volume. The presence of large quantities of plasma protein or lipid makes this assumption false and may cause the apparent sodium concentration to be lowered. Alternative measurement with ion-specific electrode methods can provide a more accurate assay. This form of hyponatremia has no clinical significance and its importance lies only in recognizing the underlying condition and avoiding unnecessary treatment.

Hypertonic Hyponatremia
When hyponatremia is present but the E_{osm} is elevated, hypertonic hyponatremia is present. In this case, ICF moves to the ECF due to an increased E_{osm}, decreasing the $[Na^+]$. These patients are at risk for cellular dehydration, just as a patient with hypernatremia is. **Hyperglycemia** lowers the $[Na^+]$ by 2.4 mmol/L for every 100 mg/dL increase in the

plasma glucose. Osmotic diuresis can cause water loss, which may ultimately result in converting hyponatremia to hypernatremia. **Hypertonic mannitol** solutions (mmol/L = mg/dL divided by 18.2) are important because mannitol is usually excreted without incident in the presence of normal renal function. However, extreme amounts can cause acute renal failure and require dialysis unrelated to the hyponatremia. As with hyperglycemia, osmotic diuresis can be severe with mannitol and may lead to hypernatremia. Bladder or uterine irrigants, such as sorbitol or glycine, used during urologic or gynecologic procedures have the potential to be absorbed in large volumes and can cause acute hypertonic hyponatremia. Glycine initially is an effective osmole but, with time, accumulates equally in the ECF and the ICF. Its toxicity most likely is due to its metabolism to ammonia, and symptoms are probably best treated with hemodialysis. Sorbitol is metabolized leaving a state of hypotonic hyponatremia after the initial increased E_{osm} effect. Some gamma globulin infusions contain sucrose and can also cause hypertonic hyponatremia in patients with renal insufficiency that prevents timely elimination of the molecule.

Hypotonic Hyponatremia

The most common form of hyponatremia is due to reduced plasma tonicity or osmolality. The first steps in evaluating the cause of hyponatremia once a low plasma osmolality is established are assessment of urine osmolality and volume status. The critical underlying principle is assessing whether an effect of ADH can be found. Normally, a hypotonic state will completely suppress ADH production. In this case, the urine osmolality should be maximally dilute (<100 mOsm/kg). The finding of a urine osmolality >100 mOs/Kg is strong evidence for continued production of ADH, even if urine osmolality is less than plasma osmolality.

Hypotonic Hyponatremia with a Low Urine Osmoality (Urine Osmolality <100 mOsm/kg)

A urine osmolality <100 mOsm/kg is characteristic of **primary polydipsia**, **severe malnutrition**, and **beer potomania**. Many patients with primary polydipsia actually lack full ADH suppression due to the effects of psychiatric medications or an innate defect in free water elimination; therefore, they cannot produce maximally dilute urine. Depending on the severity to which the countercurrent multiplier is affected by beer potomania or severe malnutrition, the final U_{osm} likewise varies. Acute hyponatremia has recently been seen in association with excess hypotonic fluid intake during **marathon running** and with the use of ecstasy. **Ecstasy** can cause severe hyponatremia due both to inappropriate ADH effect and by the extreme thirst that it induces. In addition, the use of **large volume irrigation solutions** during transurethral resection or laparoscopic procedures has been a reported cause of hyponatremia.

Reset osmostat technically is a form of syndrome of inappropriate ADH (SIADH), but the $[Na^+]$ remains stable at a level of 125 to 135 mmol/L. Free water excretion occurs at the newly set "normal" $[Na^+]$, and progressive hyponatremia does not occur without an additional insult. As such, it does not require attempts at treatment, as the only result is increased thirst and an eventual return to the new "normal" $[Na^+]$ once treatment is stopped. The possible causes should be evaluated as with SIADH (see below).

Hypotonic Hyponatremia with an Increased Urine Osmolality (Urine Osmolality >100 mOsm/kg)

Increased urine osmolality is evidence that ADH activity is present despite hyponatremia. The next step is to determine if this is an appropriate or inappropriate ADH production by assessing ECF volume and considering other clinical factors associated with increased ADH production. This is not always obvious, as free water replacement in the face of prior significant solute loss can often mask the initial condition and make the patient appear euvolemic. Conversely, severe hyponatremia can affect baroreceptor response and cause a euvolemic patient to appear volume depleted.

Hypotonic Hyponatremia in the Presence of Volume Excess

In congestive heart failure, cirrhosis, and sometimes nephrotic syndrome, the ADH secretion is physiologically appropriate due to a decrease in the effective circulating volume (ECV) and the U_{Na} is low as well. Hyponatremia in these conditions tends to remain stable at levels >125 mmol/L and usually does not require treatment directed at resolving a low [Na^+]. In chronic kidney disease, the kidney has limited ability to increase the excretion of excess sodium, and an excessive intake of water compared with sodium results in hyponatremia.

Congestive Heart Failure. In congestive heart failure, loop diuretics (to increase free water clearance) combined with appropriate fluid restriction are the treatment of choice for increasingly severe hyponatremia.

Cirrhosis. Excess vasodilation as a result of liver disease creates a state of decreased ECV. Extremely low levels of plasma albumin can contribute as well. The treatment depends on the U_{Na} and the presence or absence of refractory ascites.

Renal Failure and Nephrotic Syndrome. In renal failure, the intake of excess water relative to sodium causes the dilutional hyponatremia with increased ECV. The U_{Na} is often fixed, and free water restriction combined with diuretics can be used. In nephrotic syndrome, the ECV can be decreased despite marked edema, and diuretics must be used with caution. Nephrotic syndrome often coexists with renal insufficiency, in which case hypervolemia may be present.

Hypotonic Hyponatremia in the Face of Volume Depletion

Hypotonic hyponatremia in the face of volume depletion is due to sodium loss in excess of water loss, from renal or nonrenal routes. In treating this condition, normal saline (NS) is indicated unless the hyponatremia is symptomatic, necessitating more rapid reversal. Normalization of ECV suppresses ADH secretion and an extremely rapid reversal of the hyponatremia can occur. To avoid extreme overcorrection, it is best to discontinue NS infusion once the blood pressure is stable and sodium begins to rise. The **urine sodium** helps in confirming extrarenal losses of fluid. Extrarenal losses are associated with a low U_{Na}, with the exception of conditions that lead to obligate sodium loss in the urine such as bicarbonate in metabolic alkalosis or ketone bodies in states of ketosis. The urine chloride should still be low (<20 mmol/L) in these situations and helps identify the underlying hypovolemia.

Renal losses demonstrate an elevated U_{Na}, usually in the presence of diuretic use (thiazides or loop diuretics). **Thiazide diuretics** deserve special mention, as they are an extremely common cause of hyponatremia that can be rapid and severe. Thiazides decrease the urine-diluting ability by their distal action but do not affect the countercurrent exchange mechanism for urine concentration, thus predisposing the patient to hyponatremia. The hyponatremia can result from volume depletion and increased ADH activation, but some patients appear to have a primary defect in free water elimination made worse by the administration of thiazides. An additional insult in a patient on chronic, stable thiazide therapy, such as intercurrent illness or a new pharmacologic agent, can sometimes result in new onset hyponatremia. Complete resolution of hyponatremia may take weeks after thiazide withdrawal. Patients who develop severe hyponatremia on a thiazide diuretic are at extreme risk of severe and rapid recurrence and should not receive these agents again.

SIADH

SIADH results from excessive activity of ADH (vasopressin) due to increased release or prolongation of action. Inappropriate ADH response in a patient with hyponatremia is diagnosed when the urine is less than maximally dilute in the presence of relative euvolemia and the absence of certain other conditions (see below). SIADH can be invoked by almost any pulmonary or CNS event in addition to a variety of pharmacologic agents (Table 6-1). To establish a diagnosis of SIADH, other conditions that may mimic the disorder must be ruled out, such as hypothyroidism and cortisol deficiency. Hyponatremia may exist in normal pregnancy, with SIADH-like effects believed to be secondary to effects of human chorionic gonadotropin. The U_{Na} in these conditions varies depending on intake. Hyponatremia that results secondary to hypothyroidism or cortisol deficiency resolves with treatment of the underlying condition. This process can take several weeks, and hyponatremia should be treated, if necessary, in the interim.

In SIADH, sodium handling is intact, and some degree of free water elimination does occur in an apparent override of the ADH system. This is likely due to pressure natriuresis and natriuretic peptides. Approximately one-third of SIADH cases fall into the reset osmostat scenario and do not require treatment for hyponatremia. Free water restriction, loop diuretics, and high oral sodium and protein intake are the mainstays of treatment in the remainder of cases. The degree of free water restriction depends on the U_{osm} present, as this determines the amount of free water that can be excreted with the given osmotic load. For instance, a U_{osm} of 600 mOsm/kg allows a daily dietary intake of 600 mOsm to be excreted in 1 L of urine. Decreasing the U_{osm} to 300 mOsm/kg with loop diuretics allows the same intake to be excreted in 2 L of urine. Sometimes, no underlying cause is evident for SIADH or the reset osmostat variant, but continued surveillance is warranted. SIADH has been known to manifest several years before the onset of a clinically apparent malignancy.

Treatment of Chronic Asymptomatic Hyponatremia

Chronic hyponatremia without acute neurologic events is best treated by fluid restriction. Limiting total fluid intake to 1000 to 1200 mL/day is typically needed, although some patients may need restriction to <1000 mL/day. Fluid restriction can be difficult to maintain as disordered thirst regulation is a feature in some cases of SIADH. Other modalities can be instituted as necessary, but slow correction is of extreme importance. Osmotic demyelination has been reported even with the use of fluid restriction alone and continued laboratory monitoring is necessary to maintain acceptable rates of correction. Chronic treatment of SIADH seldom requires pharmacologic agents and these are usually reserved for cases resistant to the above interventions. Lithium and demeclocycline both induce nephrogenic diabetes insipidus (NDI) and have been used to treat SIADH; however, the former is unpredictable and can have numerous side effects, whereas the latter is expensive and potentially nephrotoxic. Either can cause severe hypernatremia without adequate free water intake. Oral urea is another safe alternative for cases of refractory SIADH. Palatability is probably its biggest drawback, but doses of 30 to 60 g/day reportedly are effective in managing SIADH. A new class of agents that block vasopressin-2 receptors (aquaretics) are being evaluated for use in SIADH and other states of ADH excess. So far, they have only been approved for the short-term management of hyponatremia.

Correction of Acute Symptomatic Hyponatremia

Hyponatremia—acute or chronic—presenting with significant symptoms, may necessitate emergent therapy with hypertonic saline. Loop diuretics are often used in tandem to aid in free water excretion (by lowering the U_{osm}) and to prevent volume overload. Severe CNS symptoms due to hyponatremia usually respond to very modest increases in $[Na^+]$, often a <5% increase in the presenting value. The initial rate of correction generally should be 1 to 2 mmol/L/hour unless persistent symptoms such as continued seizure activity justify a faster reversal rate. Once symptoms have been controlled, the rate of correction is adjusted to no more than a total of 8 mmol/L in the first 24 hours, including the initial rapid correction. Over the next 24 hours, $[Na^+]$ correction should probably not exceed an additional 10 mmol/L. More rapid correction increases the risk of osmotic demyelination, especially in chronic hyponatremia. Acute hyponatremia can be reversed rapidly with less risk, but there is no obvious additional clinical benefit in immediate correction once the acute symptoms have resolved, and osmotic demyelination may occur if the duration of hyponatremia has been underestimated.

As is obvious from the foregoing, correction of symptomatic hyponatremia needs to be very precisely defined. To systematically approach this problem, a simple scheme is presented using a hypothetical obtunded 70-kg male with a $[Na^+]$ of 110 mmol/L. His clinician concludes that the sodium needs to be increased by 4 mmol/L in 2 hours using 3% saline solution without the addition of K^+. The following calculation steps make this estimation clear:

1. Estimate total body water (TBW). This is generally considered 60% of body weight in males and 50% in females, although changes occur with aging and obesity. Thus, in this patient, the TBW is 42 L.
2. Estimate expected change in $[Na^+]$ after infusion of 1 L of saline solution. An approximate estimation for expected correction of $[Na^+]$ after giving 1 L of a saline solution is:

$$\text{Expected change in Na} = \frac{\text{infusate }[Na]*(mmol/L) + \text{infusate }[K]\ (mmol/L) - [sNa]\ (mmol/L)}{\text{estimated TBW (kg)} + 1}$$

Thus, in our patient, the expected correction after 1 L of 3% saline will be

$$\frac{513\ mmol/L - 110\ mmol/L}{42 + 1} = \frac{9.37\ mmol/L \text{ increase expected per}}{1\ L \text{ of 3\% saline}}$$

3. Calculate the total amount of fluid required. Dividing the desired change in $[Na^+]$ by the expected change after infusion of 1 L of solution gives the volume of that solution necessary to reach the desired $[Na^+]$. Thus, in our case
   - Desired change in Na: 4 mmol/L
   - Expected change with 1 L correction fluid: 9.37
   - Amount of fluid required to achieve desired change: 4/9.37 = 0.4 L (400 cc) of 3% saline
4. Calculate the rate of infusion. Dividing the calculated volume by the desired time period gives the rate of infusion. Thus, in our case
   - Amount of fluid required: 400 cc
   - Time of infusion desired: 2 hours
   - Rate of infusion: 400/2 = 200 mL of 3% saline/hour

Therefore, in this obtunded 70-kg man with a $[Na^+]$ of 110 mmol/L, the sodium should increase to approximately 114 mmol/L if 3% saline is infused at 200 mL/hour for 2 hours.

As the dynamics may shift constantly, it is extremely important to closely monitor the $[Na^+]$ for evidence of adequate treatment or for overcorrection. Unless volume depletion is present, loop diuretics are often used to enhance free water excretion and will affect the change in $[Na^+]$. Thus, **calculations only provide a rough estimate to help initiate therapy and do not replace frequent monitoring and adjustment.** Accidental overcorrection may occur if vigilant monitoring is not maintained, with potentially fatal consequences. Treatment of accidental overcorrection may be of benefit, especially if symptoms suggestive of osmotic demyelination appear. Free water or ADH analogs may need to be used to reduce the $[Na^+]$ to levels dictated by correction calculations.

---

* Infusate [Na] in 1 L of 0.9% saline = 154 mmol; 3% saline = 513 mmol.

The above discussion pertains mainly to euvolemic hyponatremia. In patients with hypovolemic hyponatremia, the primary problem is fluid depletion and dehydration. These patients usually respond to 0.9% saline alone, and the [Na$^+$] corrects rapidly once the volume deficit is overcome.

HYPERNATREMIA

Unlike hyponatremia, all cases of hypernatremia are true hyperosmolar states. As sodium is an effective osmole, any increase in the [Na$^+$] to >145 mmol/L automatically increases hypertonicity, leading to intracellular dehydration. Although the [Na$^+$] is elevated, intravascular volume may be low or high, depending on the etiology.

Symptoms

Symptoms are primarily a reflection of CNS involvement and include lethargy, irritability, weakness, confusion, and progression to coma, but they are generally not apparent until the [Na$^+$] has increased to >160 mmol/L. Mortality increases markedly as [Na$^+$] increases to >180 mmol/L. CSF movement into the interstitial areas of brain tissue as well as the increase in intracellular electrolyte and other effective osmoles initially serves to protect from the effects of hypernatremia. As the [Na$^+$] increases, increased cellular volume loss can lead to rupture of cerebral blood vessels with associated morbidity and mortality. Just as with hyponatremia, chronic development of hypernatremia is better tolerated than an equivalent acute change.

Pathogenesis

Hypernatremia develops due to loss of free water or the administration of hypertonic saline solutions as an iatrogenic event. Hypernatremia causes hyperosmolarity that stimulates thirst, protecting against further rise in [Na$^+$] by consumption of free water. A good example of this is the patient with diabetes insipidus, who often has a [Na$^+$] at the upper limits of normal despite urinating many liters a day. The patient is able to maintain a relatively normal [Na$^+$] due to the strong stimulus of thirst, resulting in ingestion of adequate amounts of water. Thus, hypernatremia due to unreplaced losses is a result of the patient's inability to obtain water. This may be seen in elderly, debilitated patients. Rarely, lack of water intake may be due to diminished sensation of thirst (hypodipsia). A significant increase in the [Na$^+$] causes weakness and confusion and decreases the likelihood of adequate water intake. This often makes it difficult to determine whether hypernatremia led to the entire neurologic picture or whether a preceding neurologic deficit initiated the process.

Evaluation and Etiologies of Hypernatremia

The clinical history often makes the underlying etiology obvious. If it is not entirely evident, then the U$_{osm}$ and U$_{Na}$ should be checked (Fig. 6-2). Free water loss leading to hypernatremia and volume depletion should be considered. The degree of volume depletion can initially be masked due to the movement of water from the ICF to the ECF. Isotonic losses, such as a secretory diarrhea, cause volume depletion but do not affect the [Na$^+$], whereas osmotic losses, such as osmotic diarrhea or glucosuria, cause volume depletion as well as hypernatremia. If it is not clear whether free water loss via osmotic diuresis is contributing, calculating the U$_{osm}$ per day [urine volume (L) $\times$ U$_{osm}$ (mOsm/kg)] can be helpful. A total U$_{osm}$ excretion of >1000 mOsm/day is consistent with osmotic diuresis leading to hypernatremia and is often due to glucosuria, diuretics, or a high-protein diet. This situation can also exist in post–acute tubular necrosis and post–obstructive diuresis. The contribution of urea or glucose to osmotic diuresis can be evaluated by measuring the osmolar component of each in the urine. With hypertonic salt administration, often as sodium bicarbonate, the U$_{Na}$ is usually >100 mmol/L.

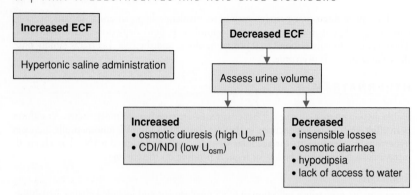

FIGURE 6-2. Etiologies of hypernatremia. CDI, central diabetes insipidus; ECF, extracellular fluid; NDI, nephrogenic diabetes insipidus; U_{osm}, urine osmolality.

Increased *insensible losses* during hot weather in patients at risk (e.g., an elderly patient on loop diuretics) can have a synergistic effect on the development of significant hypernatremia. *Loop diuretics* predispose to hypernatremia due to their interference with the ability to maximally concentrate the urine. Normally, thirst mechanisms prevent hypernatremia from developing, but a significant increase in the $[Na^+]$ may result if access to water is limited.

Diabetes insipidus can be either central (CDI) or nephrogenic (NDI) and can result from congenital or acquired pathology. Both CDI and NDI exist in complete and partial forms, which can sometimes make the diagnosis difficult. As long as water is accessible, clinically significant hypernatremia does not develop. CDI and NDI both benefit from a decreased osmolar load, thus moderation in sodium and protein intake helps decrease the urine volume. Synthetic vasopressin (DDAVP) is used in the treatment of CDI but has no effect in NDI. Mild volume depletion with the use of a thiazide diuretic and, occasionally, the addition of NSAIDs can be used in NDI. Drug-induced NDI is most commonly due to lithium therapy. The use of amiloride is usually quite effective in blocking the access of lithium to the sodium channel in the collecting duct and limiting the NDI, although severe cases can be refractory and may not resolve even with lithium discontinuation. Two other agents that can induce NDI are foscarnet and cidofovir.

Hypercalcemia, usually at levels >11 mg/dL, and hypokalemia, at levels <3 mmol/L, can both cause a form of NDI due to effects on the renal tubules. Treatment of the inappropriate electrolyte level normally resolves the issue, although the effect can remain for many days after correction. Renal failure, acute or chronic, can also predispose to hypernatremia if sodium intake is significantly greater than water intake. Decreased ability to excrete sodium and an inability to retain adequate free water contribute. The renal effects of sickle cell disease, amyloidosis, and Sjögren syndrome are also possible causes of secondary NDI.

Other Causes of Hypernatremia

Rapid shift of water from the ECF to the ICF can occur with prolonged seizures, rhabdomyolysis, or extreme exercise and may result in hypernatremia. As noted above, pregnancy can induce hyponatremia. Interestingly, *pregnancy* may also cause hypernatremia. This is due to the placental release of vasopressinase. Though this phenomenon rarely manifests as significant hypernatremia, certain women may have higher levels of vasopressinase secreted by the placenta, making them more likely to have a pseudo-CDI appearance. DDAVP is not affected by vasopressinase and remains a suitable treatment option. Elderly patients may have a *higher threshold for osmotic ADH release*, but this does not appear to be a true reset osmostat for hypernatremia. Rather, it seems that ADH release in these patients is primarily volume, rather than osmotic dependent. Thus, the U_{osm} can vary greatly depending on the volume status. *Primary aldosteronism* is probably the one true form of reset osmostat for hypernatremia. It appears that the chronic volume excess in this state causes ADH to be released at a higher P_{osm} than usual and mild hypernatremia can be present. *Hypodipsia* due to a CNS insult is uncommon but does exist. Forced intake of water is necessary to avoid hypernatremia.

Correction of Hypernatremia

Hypernatremia corrected too rapidly may have unintended consequences, thus the $[Na^+]$ should be returned to the normal range slowly and with vigilant lab and clinical monitoring. Correction of $[Na^+]$ at a rate of 0.5 mmol/L/hour has been shown to have a low likelihood of complications. Faster correction rates can prevent adequate time for intracellular adjustment of tonicity, leading to cellular swelling. Patients with acute hypernatremia due to hypertonic saline loading can sustain faster corrections of 1 mmol/L/hour. Volume overload is often of primary concern along with the hypernatremia in cases of hypertonic saline administration.

Severe volume depletion or hemodynamic instability merits treatment with NS. Lesser degrees of clinical volume depletion can be treated with 0.2% or 0.45% saline solution (34 and 77 mmol/L $[Na^+]$, respectively). These should be considered as 25% and 50% NS solutions, respectively, with the remaining volume considered to be free water. Once the volume status has been restored satisfactorily, D_5W alone should be used to correct hypernatremia. The dextrose component is metabolized as long as insulin deficiency is not present, leaving free water. Overwhelming the ability to metabolize dextrose is not a concern with the low administration rates used in the slow correction of hypernatremia.

The same scheme presented for hyponatremia can be modified to assess therapy initiation for hypernatremia. The case of a 70-kg female patient presenting from a nursing home with a $[Na^+]$ of 170 mmol/L and stable vital signs is used as an example. The clinician decides to decrease her $[Na^+]$ by 12 mmol/L over the next 24 hours using D_5W. The four-step approach is applied:

1. Assess TBW. TBW tends to be lower by approximately 10% in patients with volume depletion and hypernatremia, and the estimated values most often used are 40% of body weight in women and 50% in men. Thus, the TBW for this patient is 40% of 70 kg, or 28 L.

2. Calculate expected change in $[Na^+]$ after infusion of 1 L of D_5W.

$$\text{Change in sNa} = \frac{[sNa] - \text{infusate } [Na] + \text{infusate } [K]}{\text{TBW} + 1}$$

As D_5W is being used:

$$\text{Change in sNa} = \frac{sNa\,[170] - \text{infusate Na}\,[0] + \text{infusate K}\,[0]}{28 + 1}$$

$$= 5.86 \text{ mmol/L expected decrease per L of } D_5W$$

3. Calculate the amount of fluid required to achieve desired change. Dividing the desired change by expected change per L of infusate gives the amount of fluid required to change the $[Na^+]$ to the desired level:

- Desired change: 12 mmol/L
- Change expected after 1 L D_5W: 5.86 mmol/L
- Total amount of D_5W required: desired change/change expected per L of fluid = 12/5.86 = 2.04 L
4. Calculate infusion rate. Divide the total fluid amount by 24 to give the hourly infusion rate. In this case, it is 2000/24, or approximately 80 mL/hour.

Note that ongoing or insensible losses for the patient have not been taken into account. Using a value of 500 to 1000 mL/day for insensible and ongoing losses in this patient, another 30 to 40 mL/hour may necessary.

Thus, D_5W at a rate of 115 mL/hour should reduce the $[Na^+]$ by approximately 12 mmol/L over a period of 24 hours. Ongoing losses of water should be regularly assessed along with regular monitoring of plasma $[Na^+]$. In addition, potassium should be monitored as there is a potential for hypokalemia with free water repletion.

It has been a common practice to *estimate the total free water deficit*. This can be obtained by dividing the total increase in the $[Na^+]$ above normal by the expected correction from 1 L of D_5W [(170 − 140)/5.86 = 5 L free water deficit]. Estimating the total free water deficit provides no information about isotonic losses, only about the current deficit in relation to the $[Na^+]$, and thus has limited value. To reiterate, calculations are valuable in initiating therapy, but repeated clinical and laboratory evaluation is of primary importance in the ultimate adjustment of fluid administration to ensure an appropriate correction rate.

KEY POINTS TO REMEMBER

- Abnormalities of plasma $[Na^+]$ actually reflect imbalances of water homeostasis.
- Effective plasma osmolality must always be checked in hyponatremia.
- Astute estimation of the volume state is key in making a correct diagnosis.
- Symptomatic sodium disorders need emergent therapy. All asymptomatic cases require gradual and deliberate treatment with frequent monitoring to avoid complications of overcorrection.
- It is best to methodically define treatment goals, speed of correction, and fluid type at the outset. One must be prepared to modify the plan according to ongoing changes and follow-up laboratory values.

REFERENCES AND SUGGESTED READINGS

Adams RD, Victor M, Mancall EL. Central pontine myelinolysis: a hitherto undescribed disease occurring in alcoholic and malnourished patients. *Arch Neurol Psychiatr.* 1959;81:154.

Adrogue HJ, Madias NE. Hypernatremia. *N Engl J Med.* 2000;342:1493.

Arieff Al, Guisado R. Effects on the central nervous system of hypernatremic and hyponatremic states. *Kidney Int.* 1976;10:104.

Brodsky WA, Rapoport S. The mechanism of polyuria of diabetes insipidus in man; the effect of osmotic loading. *J Clin Invest.* 1951;30(3):282–291.

Brunner JE, Redmond JM, Harrar AM, et al. Central pontine myelinolysis and pontine lesions after rapid correction of hoponatremia: a prospective magnetic resonance imaging study. *Ann Neurol.* 1990;27:61–66.

Clark BA, Shannon RP, Rosa RM, et al. Increased susceptibility to thiazide-induced hyponatremia in the elderly. *J Am Soc Nephrol.* 1994;5(4):1106–1111.

Cogan E, Debieve M, Pepersack T, et al. Natriuresis and atrial natriuretic factor secretion during inappropriate antidiuresis. *Am J Med.* 1988;84:409–418.

Davison JM, Sheills E, Philips PR, et al. Metabolic clearance of vasopressin and an analogue resistant to vasopressinase in human pregnancy. *Am J Physiol.* 1993;264: F348–353.

Decaux G, Genette F. Urea for long-term treatment of syndrome of inappropriate secretion of antidiuretic hormone. *Br Med J* (Clin Res Ed). 198l;283:1081–1083.

Ellison DH, Berl T. The syndrome of inappropriate antidiuresis. *N Engl J Med.* 2007;356(20):2064–2072.

Garofeanu CG, Weir M, Rosas-Arellano MP, et al. Causes of reversible nephrogenic diabetes insipidus: a systematic review. *Am J Kidney Dis.* 2005;45(4):626–637.

Ghali JK, Koren M, Taylor JR, et al. Efficacy and safety of oral conivaptan: a V1A/V2 vasopressin receptor antagonist, assessed in a randomized, placebo-controlled trial in patients with euvolemic or hypervolemic hyponatremia. *J Clin Endocrinol Metab.* 2006;91(6):2145–2152.

Goldman MB, Luchins DJ, Robertson GL. Mechanisms of altered water metabolism in psychotic patients with polydipsia and hyponatremia. *N Engl J Med.* 1988;318: 397–403,

Menger H, Jorg J. Outcome of central pontine and extrapontine myelinolysis. *J Neurol.* 1999;246:700–705.

Nguyen MK, Ornekian V, Butch AW, et al. A new method for determining plasma water content: application in pseudohyponatremia. *Am J Physiol Renal Physiol.* 2007; 292(5):F1652–1656.

Renneboog B, Musch W, Vandemergel X. Mild chronic hyponatremia is associated with falls, unsteadiness, and attention deficits. *Am J Med.* 2006;119(71):e1–8.

Sterns RH. Severe symptomatic hyponatremia: treatment and outcome. A study of 64 cases. *Ann Intern Med.* 1987;107(5):656–664.

Soupart A, Ngassa M, Decaux G. Therapeutic relowering of the serum sodium in a patient after excessive correction of hyponatremia. *Clin Nephrol.* 1999;51:383–386.

Disorders of Potassium Balance

Matthew J. Koch

7

OVERVIEW

Hypokalemia and hyperkalemia result from alterations in potassium intake, cellular shifts, or changes in potassium elimination. The body store of potassium consists of approximately 50 mEq/kg; much of which is confined to the intracellular space. Intracellular concentrations (140 mEq/L) are 35 times that normally present in the extracellular (plasma) space (4 mEq/L).

Regulation of Plasma Potassium

The primary regulation of plasma potassium occurs via the influence of aldosterone, mainly in the principal cells of the cortical and medullary collecting ducts. Decreased effective circulating volume (ECV) or an increase in the potassium concentration $[K^+]$ leads to increased aldosterone production and increased potassium secretion in exchange for sodium. Increased ECV or decreased $[K^+]$ leads to decreased aldosterone production. The secretion of potassium is dependent on adequate tubular flow in the distal nephron, providing a system of balances to normalize $[K^+]$ when perturbations to the system are present. Decreased ECV leads not only to increased aldosterone production but also to decreased distal flow rate, allowing plasma $[K^+]$ to remain in a relatively normal range, barring additional factors. Conversely, increased ECV leads to not only a decrease in aldosterone production but also an increased distal flow rate, allowing plasma $[K^+]$ to again remain normal in the absence of additional insults.

Abnormal Plasma Potassium

Deviation from normal plasma $[K^+]$ often occurs when a pharmacologic agent is used that alters potassium balance. The most common example is hypokalemia due to the use of diuretics in a patient with congestive heart failure (CHF) and a decreased ECV. The stimulus to aldosterone production remains intact, but the diuretic-induced increased distal flow rate results in increased potassium secretion. In a similar patient not on a diuretic, the use of a medication such as an ACE inhibitor or spironolactone inhibits the effect of aldosterone and may lead to hyperkalemia. The etiologies, evaluation, and treatment for high or low plasma $[K^+]$ are discussed below.

HYPERKALEMIA

Hyperkalemia is defined as a plasma $[K^+] > 5$ mEq/L. Elevations in the plasma $[K^+]$ can occur in an acute or chronic fashion. Chronic elevation of plasma $[K^+]$ may be better tolerated than an acute increase. As the $[K^+]$ increases, there is an initial increase in cell membrane excitability. Hyperkalemia-induced decrease in cellular sodium transport follows, which leads to a decrease in membrane excitability and causes neuromuscular weakness and cardiac conduction defects.

Clinical Findings in Hyperkalemia

Symptoms

The level at which neuromuscular symptoms or ECG changes occur in a particular patient is highly variable. In addition, the presence of other abnormalities, such as hypocalcemia or hyponatremia, amplifies the effects of hyperkalemia on cardiac conduction. $[K^+]$ levels ≥ 6.5 mEq/L require close clinical and cardiac monitoring and indicate the need for acute treatment. Less severe hyperkalemia in a patient presenting without symptoms or significant ECG changes can usually be treated by correction of the underlying cause and the addition of cation exchange resins [sodium polystyrene sulfonate (SPS)] if necessary. The underlying medical conditions, the presumed rate of rise of the potassium level, and the presence or absence of significant urine output all affect the need, extent, and modality of treatment.

Electrocardiographic Changes

ECG changes classically involve increased amplitude of a narrow T wave and shortening of the QT interval at $[K^+]$ levels >6 mEq/L. As $[K^+]$ increases further to >7 to 8 mEq/L, the PR interval increases, and loss of the P wave can occur along with widening of the QRS. This sine-wave pattern can degenerate rapidly to ventricular fibrillation or asystole if untreated.

Normal Response to Exogenous Potassium Administration

Unless massive amounts of potassium are ingested, the process of intracellular transport mediated by insulin and beta-adrenergic receptors limits the initial rise in $[K^+]$. Insulin and beta$_2$-adrenergic stimulation activate the Na^+/K^+/adenosine triphosphatase (ATPase) transporters in the cell membrane. Insulin release in response to increased $[K^+]$ is the initial defense mechanism to maintain normal plasma potassium levels. The ultimate elimination of the excess potassium occurs via increased urinary excretion due to direct effects of the potassium itself and a secondary potassium-mediated increase in aldosterone release. Adaptation to increased chronic ingestion of potassium allows for large amounts of potassium to be excreted by the kidney each day without a significant increase in the $[K^+]$, as long as adequate urine output is maintained. Acute IV administration of potassium can present an overwhelming load that exceeds cellular uptake capacity. Packed RBCs (pRBCs) stored for >3 weeks can also provide a significant IV load of potassium due to potassium leakage out of the cells. Washing the pRBCs before infusion attenuates this problem.

Causes of Hyperkalemia

Decreased Cellular Uptake

Several processes can limit the intracellular shift of potassium and result in an elevated $[K^+]$ (Table 7-1). Insulin deficiency and nonselective beta blockade both affect the ability to acutely handle a potassium load due to the importance of insulin and beta$_2$-adrenergic stimulation on Na^+/K^+/ATPase transport. Selective beta blockers, such as metoprolol and atenolol, do not have this effect at normal doses. Digitalis at high levels can have a similar effect due to inhibition of the Na^+/K^+/ATPase pump and subsequent decreased intracellular movement of potassium.

Movement of Potassium Out of Cells

Large amounts of potassium can move from intracellular to extracellular sites. Trauma, rhabdomyolysis, and tumor lysis syndrome can release intracellular contents in a dramatic fashion. Nonorganic metabolic acidosis causes potassium movement out of the cell in

TABLE 7-1	CAUSES OF HYPERKALEMIA

Increased potassium intake
  Oral (massive ingestion required)
  IV (including stored, unwashed, packed RBCs)

Decreased cellular uptake
  Insulin deficiency
  Beta blockade (nonselective)
  Digitalis toxicity

Movement to extracellular space
  Hyperosmolar states (hyperglycemia, hypernatremia, mannitol administration)
  Metabolic acidosis (nonorganic)
  Tumor lysis syndrome
  Trauma, rhabdomyolysis
  Extreme exercise
  Familial periodic paralysis
  Succinylcholine

Decreased excretion
  Hypoaldosteronism (Table 7-2)
  Chronic renal insufficiency
  Congestive heart failure, liver disease (decreased ECV)
  Type I renal tubular acidosis (hyperkalemic form)
  Chloride shunt
  Selective potassium excretion defect

Pseudohyperkalemia
  Serum sample
  Mechanical trauma
  Increase in platelets or WBCs
  Repeated clinching of fist/tourniquet

exchange for hydrogen; however, organic acidosis does not have the same effect. Hyperosmolar states, such as hyperglycemia, and mannitol administration cause the movement of potassium out of cells both by solvent drag and the resulting increase in intracellular potassium content. Each increase in the plasma glucose of 180 mg/dL above normal raises the $[K^+]$ by approximately 0.6 mEq/L. Both hypernatremia and mannitol administration have similar effects.

Exercise causes an intensity-dependent increase in the $[K^+]$ that may reach 2.0 mEq/L at extreme levels. If combined with an additional aggravating factor, such as the use of a nonselective beta blocker, the potassium level can increase even more dramatically. Other less common causes include the rare syndrome of familial periodic paralysis, which can be induced by exercise or low-carbohydrate meals. The use of succinylcholine in general anesthesia is commonly associated with the acute release of intracellular potassium as well.

Decreased Renal Excretion
With chronic kidney disease, each remaining functioning nephron adapts to increase the amount of potassium excreted. The ability to excrete an acute potassium load is limited, but significant sustained hyperkalemia usually does not result until end-stage kidney disease (GFR <10–15 mL/minute) is reached, as long as dietary intake is modified and a reasonable ECV is maintained. Decreased ECV, as occurs in CHF and liver disease, limits the distal renal flow and, thus, the ability to excrete potassium. Increased aldosterone production

serves to counteract the decreased distal flow, but this effect is often prevented by the use of medications such as ACE inhibitors or spironolactone in these patient groups.

A hyperkalemic form of type I renal tubular acidosis (RTA) due to limited sodium transport in the distal tubule exists and is often secondary to chronic urinary tract obstruction or sickle cell disease. Other distal tubule defects that can cause hyperkalemia include a chloride shunt, which results from the reabsorption of sodium with chloride instead of in exchange for potassium. A selective potassium-channel excretion defect can also occur without other apparent defects. A chloride shunt, a selective potassium-channel defect, and direct inhibition of the renin-angiotensin-aldosterone system may all be induced by cyclosporine (and tacrolimus) and lead to hyperkalemia with the use of these agents.

Hypoaldosteronism

Hypoaldosteronism is a common cause of hyperkalemia and has several etiologies (Table 7-2). Many medications can either directly or indirectly interfere with the production of aldosterone, while others block its effect at the receptor. The most common include ACE inhibitors and NSAIDs. Angiotensin receptor blockers can also increase the $[K^+]$, but may have a slightly decreased propensity for this compared with ACE inhibitors. This may be due to the presence of higher aldosterone levels with the use of angiotensin receptor blockers compared with ACE inhibitors. Heparin decreases aldosterone production and, in the presence of an ACE inhibitor or renal insufficiency, can cause hyperkalemia. This can occur even with the dose of regular- or low-molecular-weight heparin used in the prophylaxis of deep vein thrombosis.

Hyporeninemic hypoaldosteronism (HRHA), also known as **type IV RTA**, is another common cause of hyperkalemia. It is most often associated with diabetic nephropathy or chronic interstitial nephritis, but hyperkalemia does not usually occur without coexistent renal insufficiency. Decreased aldosterone production is also commonly associated with adrenal aldosterone resistance. Although HRHA often responds to higher-than-usual doses of fludrocortisone, the resultant sodium retention and edema often prevent its use in patients with renal insufficiency. Diuretics combined with dietary potassium restriction are the mainstays of treatment. HIV and AIDS are recognized causes of HRHA as well as adrenal insufficiency. Trimethoprim or pentamidine used for the treatment of HIV/AIDS or other conditions can also result in hyperkalemia through epithelial sodium-channel blockade.

TABLE 7-2	CAUSES OF HYPOALDOSTERONISM

Decreased renin (hyporeninemic hypoaldosteronism—type IV renal tubular acidosis)

Medications: NSAIDs, cyclosporine, beta blockers

HIV/AIDS

Diabetes mellitus

Decreased aldosterone

Primary adrenal failure

ACE inhibitors/angiotensin receptor blockers

Adrenal enzyme defects

HIV/AIDS

Heparin

Blockade of aldosterone receptor or epithelial sodium channels

Medications: amiloride, triamterene, trimethoprim, spironolactone, eplerenone

Pseudohyperkalemia

False elevation in the measured $[K^+]$ can result for several reasons. Potassium can leak from cells in the presence of marked elevations in either the WBC or platelet counts regardless of whether the sample is measured from a serum or plasma collection. Mechanical trauma during a blood draw is the most common cause of pseudohyperkalemia. When this is combined with local exercise, in the form of repeated fist clenching, the sample obtained distal to the tourniquet can have an artificial $[K^+]$ elevation of up to 2 mEq/L. If significant hyperkalemia is detected on a lab draw in an asymptomatic patient without ECG changes, pseudohyperkalemia should be suspected. Repeating the draw as a plasma sample without fist clenching by the patient and in the absence of a tourniquet, if possible, often clarifies the issue.

Evaluation of Hyperkalemia

History and Physical Exam

Evaluate the need for acute treatment in a patient presenting with hyperkalemia; check ECG for peaked T waves, shortened QT, widened QRS, and prolonged PR and perform a neuromuscular exam. Review medications, with particular attention to ACE inhibitors, angiotensin receptor blockers, NSAIDs, potassium-sparing diuretics, potassium supplements, trimethoprim, pentamidine, and heparin. Estimate chronic and current renal function and monitor urine output. The presence of diabetes may suggest HRHA. Assess the patient's dietary history. In particular, the use of salt substitutes should be reviewed, as many of these contain large amounts of potassium salts. If there is no evidence for hyperkalemia due to massive ingestion, massive cellular release, or pseudohyperkalemia, then an evaluation of urinary potassium excretion should follow.

Evaluation of Urinary Potassium Excretion

A spot urine potassium level alone is generally not helpful due to variation with urine concentration. Calculation of the *transtubular potassium gradient (TTKG)* can be quite useful in evaluating hyperkalemia when the cause is not apparent by history and hypoaldosteronism is suspected. Before evaluation, any medication that can potentially affect the potassium level should be discontinued.

$$\text{TTKG} = \frac{(\text{urine potassium/plasma potassium})}{(\text{urine osmolality/plasma osmolality})}$$

The normal value of a TTKG is approximately 8 to 9 but varies with potassium intake. The TTKG should increase to >11 in the presence of hyperkalemia and adequate aldosterone. A value <7 in the presence of hyperkalemia is suggestive of hypoaldosteronism or aldosterone receptor blockade. Two caveats for a valid TTKG assessment are that the urine osmolality should be greater than the plasma osmolality (to ensure that water is being reabsorbed in the collecting duct) and that the urine sodium is >25 mEq/L (to ensure that potassium excretion is not limited by decreased sodium delivery).

Further Evaluation of Suspected Hypoaldosteronism

If the TTKG suggests hypoaldosteronism in the presence of hyperkalemia, plasma renin, aldosterone, and cortisol levels can be obtained. These should be obtained from a morning sample after the patient has been ambulating for ≥3 hrs or after the administration of furosemide the previous evening and again in the morning. The renin level should be low or, occasionally, within the normal range in cases of HRHA but elevated in adrenal insufficiency or pseudohypoaldosteronism (aldosterone resistance). The aldosterone level should be low in cases other than pseudohypoaldosteronism or with the use of medications that block the aldosterone receptor site. The cortisol level is low in primary adrenal insufficiency or in cases of adrenal enzyme deficiency affecting cortisol production (Table 7-3).

TABLE 7-3	RENIN AND ALDOSTERONE LEVELS WITH HYPERKALEMIA AND A LOW TRANSTUBULAR POTASSIUM GRADIENT		
Disorder		Renin	Aldosterone
Primary or secondary hypoaldosteronism		↑	↓
Aldosterone receptor blockade, pseudohypoaldosteronism		↑	↑
Hyporeninemic hypoaldosteronism, chloride shunt		↓	↓

↓, decreased; ↑, increased.

Treatment of Hyperkalemia

As described previously, the treatment of hyperkalemia must be initiated **in the context of the $[K^+]$ and the presence or absence of neuromuscular symptoms and ECG changes.** A significant elevation in the absence of symptoms or ECG changes is most likely due to pseudohyperkalemia or chronic hyperkalemia. Acute treatment with multiple modalities is dangerous in the former circumstance and usually unnecessary in the latter. Correction of contributing factors such as acidemia, hypocalcemia, and hyponatremia decreases the hyperkalemic effects on the cell membrane. Other modalities involve stabilizing the cell membrane with calcium, driving potassium into the cells, and, ultimately, removing excess potassium (Table 7-4). Methods to stabilize the cell membrane or move potassium inside the cell are only temporizing measures, and potassium needs to be removed to resolve the total body excess.

Calcium, as **calcium gluconate,** should only be given in cases of hyperkalemia associated with severe weakness or marked ECG changes. The usual dose is 1 g (10 mL of a 10% solution) IV over 2 minutes. The action of calcium in stabilizing the cell membrane begins shortly after the infusion is complete. A repeat dose may be given after several minutes if ECG changes or severe symptoms persist.

Insulin is usually given as a dose of 10 U regular insulin IV along with 25 to 50 g of dextrose (1–2 ampules of D_5W). If the patient already has hyperglycemia, insulin can be given alone. Patients who are normoglycemic often become hypoglycemic when 10 U of regular insulin is administered with only 25 g of dextrose. The effect of insulin to lower the $[K^+]$ is usually evident within 30 minutes to 1 hour, with an expected decrease of 1 to 1.5 mEq/L lasting up to several hours.

Beta$_2$-adrenergic agents have a similar effect on intracellular transport of potassium. Albuterol is classically given in a dose of 10 to 20 mg by nebulizer or 0.5 mg IV. With IV administration, the onset of action is similar to insulin, but the effect is slightly delayed when given by nebulizer. The magnitude and duration of effect is similar to that of insulin administration. Due to the risk of precipitating coronary events secondary to

TABLE 7-4	AGENTS USED IN TREATING HYPERKALEMIA
Agent	Dosage
Calcium gluconate 10%	10 mL IV over 2 min
Insulin combined with dextrose	10 U regular IV with 50 g dextrose
Albuterol	10–20 mg via nebulizer or 0.5 mg IV
Sodium bicarbonate	50 mEq IV over 2 min
Sodium polystyrene sulfonate	15 g in sorbitol PO; 50 g in sorbitol and tap water rectally

beta-agonist–induced tachycardia, alternate agents are preferred in patients with known or suspected cardiac disease.

Sodium bicarbonate has also been used in the treatment of hyperkalemia, though in the absence of significant acidosis its effects may result primarily from kaliuresis after volume administration. Some studies demonstrate a very limited effect, at least part of which is due solely to dilution. Despite this, it appears that in patients with acidemia, sodium bicarbonate is a viable agent for the treatment of hyperkalemia; however, there may be an extremely limited effect in patients with end-stage kidney disease. Administration is often limited by the complications of sodium loading in patients with CHF or chronic kidney disease. One ampule of sodium bicarbonate (50 mEq) is usually given over several minutes and repeated as necessary. If a significant bicarbonate deficit is present, it can be administered as a continuous IV infusion.

The above measures are **temporizing steps**, shifting $[K^+]$ from the extracellular to the intracellular compartment. Reduction of the total body $[K^+]$ is the necessary for resolution: This can be done by forced excretion (GI or renal) or by removal by hemodialysis.

Renal elimination is preferred when possible and is often the only measure necessary for mild to moderate hyperkalemia. The patient with hyperkalemia and volume depletion may respond readily to fluid administration alone. The apparently euvolemic patient may be treated with simultaneous fluid administration and loop diuretics to enhance kaliuresis. Likewise, the volume-overloaded patient may respond to diuresis. If these measures are unsuccessful or inappropriate based on the clinical scenario, additional measures are necessary to decrease the potassium stores.

Cation-exchange resins like sodium polystyrene sulfonate (SPS) are used to eliminate excess potassium by exchanging potassium for sodium in the GI tract. They can be given orally or rectally. The rectal preparation has a faster onset of action than the oral preparation. Sorbitol is added to the preparations to prevent constipation or intestinal blockage. The added sorbitol is likely an underrecognized cause of upper GI ulcerations and intestinal necrosis sometimes caused by administration of SPS. This is more likely to occur in a patient with decreased GI motility due to opiates, severe illness, or the postoperative state. The normal dose is 15 g PO in 20% sorbitol given q6h as needed. The rectal form is given as 50 g in 70% sorbitol and tap water and should be kept in place for 2 to 3 hours if possible. These can be repeated q4h as needed. Colonic irrigation with tap water between each enema should be used to help reduce the risk of bowel injury, but the sorbitol moiety should not be used in postoperative patients due to the risk of colonic perforation. Each gram of SPS removes up to 1 mEq of potassium. In exchange, 1 to 2 mEq of sodium is absorbed.

Hemodialysis is used when hyperkalemia is not responsive to the usual measures or when an extremely high $[K^+]$ associated with significant ECG changes or severe weakness is present. Peritoneal dialysis can lower $[K^+]$ as well but not nearly as rapidly as hemodialysis. When using a low potassium dialysis bath (0 or 1 mEq/L) to quickly lower a life-threatening plasma potassium concentration, it is vital to repeat the plasma value after approximately 30 minutes of dialysis and adjust as necessary to avoid severe hypokalemia. Extensive prior treatment with agents that drive potassium into the cell can limit the amount of potassium that can be removed during dialysis; predialysis treatment of severe hyperkalemia should probably be limited to a dose of calcium gluconate (if indicated) and a single agent, such as insulin. This should provide adequate protection until hemodialysis can be initiated. If a $[K^+]$ level is checked immediately after the completion of dialysis, it is important to remember that this represents a nadir, and the $[K^+]$ will subsequently shift to the extracellular space (called "rebound"). Thus, potassium supplementation for a $[K^+]$ that appears to have overcorrected after dialysis is seldom appropriate.

Chronic Hyperkalemia

Chronic hyperkalemia is often associated with diabetic-associated HRHA, renal failure, or CHF. The serum potassium in this setting is usually stable and ≤ 6 mEq/L. Many of these patients are appropriately maintained on medications to treat the underlying condition(s), such as ACE inhibitors or spironolactone. Not infrequently these medications are discontinued due to mild elevations in the $[K^+]$. In almost all cases, a moderate reduction in potassium intake, the use of diuretics as indicated, and a tolerance for stable mild to moderate hyperkalemia allows successful continuation.

HYPOKALEMIA

Hypokalemia is defined as a plasma potassium level <3.5 mEq/L. Decreased $[K^+]$ levels usually result from increased potassium elimination via the kidney or GI tract. Intracellular potassium shifts also occur and cause hypokalemia without altering total body stores. Decreased intake can lead to hypokalemia when it occurs over a prolonged period but is generally only a contributing factor to other causes.

Clinical Features

Mild hypokalemia (3.0–3.5 mEq/L) is generally asymptomatic, although it does pose an increased risk of mortality for patients who also have cardiovascular disease or who are on digitalis. This is likely due to a further decrease in $[K^+]$ levels that can occur with sympathetic stimulation, as during myocardial ischemia or arrhythmias. As with hyperkalemia, there is clinical variance regarding the $[K^+]$ at which symptoms of hypokalemia develop. Weakness and muscle pain, usually initially involving the lower extremities, can develop as the $[K^+]$ drops below 3 mEq/L. Further decreases to below 2.5 mEq/L can lead to paralysis, including involvement of the muscles of respiration. Some patients can present with an ileus due to hypokalemic effects on smooth muscle. **Rhabdomyolysis** can occur with severe hypokalemia. This elevates the $[K^+]$ and prevents further decrements but can also serve to mask the underlying etiology. Checking a serum creatine phosphokinase level may aid in the diagnosis of suspected hypokalemic-induced rhabdomyolysis.

ECG changes due to hypokalemia include prominent U waves, diminished or inverted T waves, and ST-segment depression. The ECG changes do not correlate well with the degree of hypokalemia, but with extremely low $[K^+]$ levels the PR and QRS intervals can lengthen and lead to ventricular fibrillation. Hypokalemia can cause nephrogenic diabetes insipidus. Prolonged hypokalemia can cause interstitial nephritis that may not be reversible on correction of the hypokalemia. Chronic, mild hypokalemia may be associated with increased BP and/or glucose intolerance. Increased renal ammonia synthesis occurs in the presence of hypokalemia due to intracellular acidosis. This ammoniagenesis can potentially lead to hepatic coma in an individual with advanced liver disease; thus, hypokalemia should be treated in patients presenting with hepatic encephalopathy.

Causes of Hypokalemia

Decreased Intake
Decreased intake is rarely the primary cause of hypokalemia, although it may contribute to another etiology (Table 7-5). Prolonged malnutrition is required to induce hypokalemia without another cause, such as concomitant diuretic use.

Increased Cellular Uptake
Endogenous or exogenous insulin causes **movement of potassium into cells via the Na^+/K^+/ATPase pump.** This effect is also seen in refeeding syndrome. Sympathetic stimulation (e.g., that occurring with myocardial ischemia or arrhythmia, delirium tremens, or a variety of other situations in which beta$_2$-adrenergic activity is enhanced) can likewise cause significant potassium movement into cells. Patients on chronic beta$_2$-agonists for lung disease are at risk of hypokalemia if they are started on diuretics. Alkalosis causes an unpredictable shift of potassium into cells.

TABLE 7-5	CAUSES OF HYPOKALEMIA

Decreased intake

Increased cellular uptake
  Insulin
  Beta$_2$ stimulation
  New RBC or WBC production
  Hypokalemic periodic paralysis
  Alkalosis
  Hyperthyroidism (selected cases)

Renal losses
  Increased distal flow
  Nonabsorbed anions
  Increased or apparent increased aldosterone (Table 7-6)
  Types I and II renal tubular acidosis
  Amphotericin, cisplatinum, aminoglycosides
  Diuretics
  Hypomagnesemia

Nonrenal losses
  GI
  Sweat

The **treatment of anemia** due to vitamin B$_{12}$ or folic acid deficiency can cause hypokalemia due to the incorporation of potassium into a large number of rapidly forming cells. The use of **granulocyte colony–stimulating factor** in neutropenia can have the same effect. As discussed in the section on hyperkalemia, stored pRBCs lose a large amount of potassium. Washing the pRBCs before transfusion removes this extracellular potassium load, but the cells are then able to take up plasma potassium after administration, and hypokalemia can result.

Hypokalemic periodic paralysis, similar to its hyperkalemic counterpart, is due to sudden shifts of potassium. It is diagnosed by the absence of another etiology and usually by a strong family history. **Hyperthyroidism,** in some cases, is associated with a hypokalemic periodic paralysis, the so-called thyrotoxic periodic paralysis. This is most often found in males of Asian descent. **Hypothermia and barium toxicity** (not seen when barium is used in diagnostic procedures) are other causes of hypokalemia due to intracellular movement. An **in vitro potassium shift** can occur and cause pseudohypokalemia. This has been reported with leukocytosis associated with acute myelogenous leukemia and is due to potassium movement into the myelogenous cells when the drawn sample is allowed to stand for some time before testing.

Increased Renal Excretion

Increased renal excretion is probably the most common scenario for hypokalemia: Increased excretion may result due to increased tubular flow rate or excessive tubular [K$^+$] secretion. Increased flow is often due to **osmotic diuresis,** as with glucosuria. It also occurs with diuretic use and sodium-wasting nephropathies. Increased secretion can occur in the presence of any nonabsorbed anion in the distal tubule, such as bicarbonate in metabolic alkalosis or proximal RTA, penicillin derivatives, toluene in glue sniffing, or beta-hydroxybutyrate in ketoacidosis. Increased secretion also results from excess aldosterone or syndromes of apparent aldosterone excess (Table 7-6). Apparent **aldosterone excess** results from the production of mineralocorticoids that are able to produce the same effects as aldosterone. This can result from excess production of steroids normally metabolized by 11-beta hydroxysteroid

TABLE 7-6	PRIMARY OR APPARENT EXCESS ALDOSTERONE

Primary hyperaldosteronism (low renin, high aldosterone)

Adrenal adenoma, hyperplasia, carcinoma, glucocorticoid-remediable hyperaldosteronism, congenital adrenal hyperplasia

Secondary hyperaldosteronism (high renin, high aldosterone)

Renal artery stenosis, malignant HTN, renin-secreting tumors, low ECV

Increased alternate mineralocorticoids (low renin, low aldosterone)

11-beta HSD-2 deficiency (real licorice, chewing tobacco), overwhelmed 11-beta HSD-2 (Cushing syndrome)

AME (low renin, low aldosterone)

Decreased 11-beta HSD-2 activity due to gene mutation

AME, apparent mineralocorticoid excess; HSD-2, hydroxysteroid dehydrogenase-2.

dehydrogenase, as with Cushing syndrome, or due to inhibition of the enzyme by glyceritinic acid (e.g., real licorice). Rarely, apparent mineralocorticoid excess can occur due to mutations in the gene for 11-beta hydroxysteroid dehydrogenase-2 on chromosome 16. Increased potassium secretion is also present in the classic type I RTA.

Amphotericin causes tubular damage and increased excretion of $[K^+]$. **Cisplatin and aminoglycosides** also cause potassium wasting. Thiazide and loop diuretics as well as acetazolamide cause hypokalemia. Increased distal flow, increased aldosterone production due to decreased ECV, and bicarbonaturia all can contribute to increased potassium elimination with these agents. **Thiazide agents** normally cause a greater decrease in $[K^+]$ than do other diuretics, likely due to the prolonged duration of action. The decrease in potassium on a thiazide reaches a new steady state by 2 weeks, with an average decrease of approximately 0.5 mEq/L on a 50-mg/day dose of hydrochlorothiazide. Smaller daily doses of hydrochlorothiazide (12.5–25 mg) usually have an equal effect on lowering BP, with less of an effect on the $[K^+]$. Gitelman syndrome (pseudothiazide) and Bartter syndrome (pseudofurosemide) also lead to potassium wasting.

Hypomagnesemia can be a significant contributing factor in hypokalemia by causing renal potassium wasting. Adequate potassium retention often cannot take place until the magnesium deficit is replaced, even if large doses of potassium are given. Hypomagnesemia is often associated with diuretics, diarrhea, poor nutrition, aminoglycoside, and cisplatin use.

Extrarenal Losses

Extrarenal losses due to increased losses in the **stool** or through **sweat** can also cause hypokalemia. Lower GI losses from diarrhea, often self-induced by laxatives, or due to a villous adenoma can cause significant potassium loss. Upper GI losses do not contain a significant amount of potassium, but the resultant alkalosis and bicarbonaturia combined with a decreased ECV-induced increase in aldosterone production can also cause hypokalemia from increased renal potassium excretion.

Evaluation of Hypokalemia

The clinical history, including the list of medications, is often sufficient to diagnose the cause of hypokalemia (Fig. 7-1). When the cause is not apparent, **covert ingestion of diuretics or laxatives** should be suspected, and specific tests to evaluate for their presence may be indicated. Obtaining a **24-hr urine collection** for potassium is quite useful, as the total excretion per day should be <15 to 25 mmol of potassium in the presence of

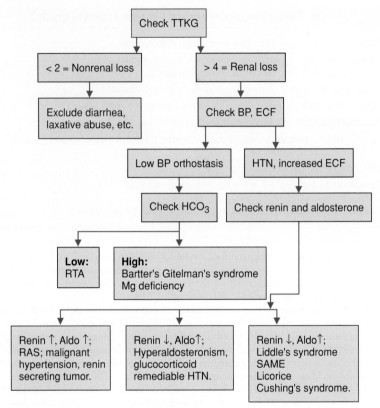

FIGURE 7-1. Simplified approach to hypokalemia. ↓, decreased; ↑, increased; Aldo, aldosterone; ECF, extracellular fluid; RAS, renal artery stenosis; RTA, renal tubular acidosis; SAME, syndrome of apparent mineralocorticoid excess; TTKG, transtubular potassium gradient.

hypokalemia. Random urine potassium may be misleading, especially if the urine is dilute. The TTKG can be checked as well, and the value should be <4 if potassium is being conserved appropriately. The caveats regarding urine sodium and urine and plasma osmolality hold true for TTKG evaluation with hypokalemia as well.

Other evaluations should include the acid/base status and urine pH, as well as noting the presence of hypotension or hypertension. Remote vomiting or diuretic use can present with the expected alkalosis but low potassium excretion. Rarely, chronic laxative use may present with alkalosis rather than acidosis. Renin and aldosterone levels may also aid in the evaluation of possible apparent or true aldosterone excess.

Treatment of Hypokalemia

The approximate **potassium deficit** as the plasma level decreases from 4 to 3 mEq/L may be in the range of 200 to 400 mEq depending on the size of the patient. As the plasma level decreases to <3 mEq/L, the deficit can be >600 mEq, but is unpredictable due to the potential release of potassium from cellular necrosis that maintains, and may even increase, the [K^+]. Thus, cellular shifts can mask a serious potassium deficit, and levels should be checked frequently to ensure adequacy of replacement. This is classically seen in hyperglycemic states in which the combination of hyperglycemia, glucosuria, ketonuria, and insulin treatment all affect the $[K^+]$, and levels can change dramatically during the course of treatment.

Potassium replacement should be given PO whenever possible due to the potential for cardiac arrhythmias with rapid IV administration of potassium, vein sclerosis, and the increased cost in using this route. Oral doses of 40 mEq of potassium are generally well tolerated and can be given q4h. Potassium chloride is usually administered, as the chloride component helps correct the often-coinciding alkalosis and bicarbonaturia. Potassium citrate can be given if hypokalemia associated with acidemia is present. For routine, chronic administration, potassium citrate may be preferable to potassium chloride. The chloride component may contribute to an increase in BP despite being administered with potassium rather than with sodium. IV potassium can be administered in concentrations of 40 mEq/L via a peripheral line or 60 mEq/L via a central line. The rate of infusion should generally not be >10 mEq/hr unless the clinical situation dictates otherwise, in which case, solutions at concentrations up to 200 mEq/L have been administered at 40 to 100 mEq/hr via a central line. The rate of administration should be reduced once the clinical situation necessitating such rapid infusion resolves. Intravenous potassium should be administered in a saline solution rather than with dextrose. The endogenous release of insulin in response to the dextrose can further decrease the $[K^+]$. As hypokalemia often exists in the presence of hyperosmolar states, potassium should generally be mixed in 0.45% saline. Adding potassium to 0.9% saline creates a hyperosmolar solution that may add to the underlying problem.

In the **treatment of chronic hypokalemia,** the use of potassium-sparing diuretics can drastically reduce or eliminate the need to give oral potassium supplements. Spironolactone is commonly used in patients with liver disease and ascites as well as in patients with CHF. Another potassium-sparing agent that can be used is amiloride. Amiloride is favored over the alternate agent triamterene, due to a significant risk of nephrolithiasis and potential renal insufficiency with the latter. In states of aldosterone excess, doses of 20 to 40 mg/day PO of amiloride should be used; otherwise, doses of 5 to 10 mg/day PO are quite useful in combination with loop or thiazide diuretics. Amiloride also has the added benefit of decreasing urinary magnesium excretion.

KEY POINTS TO REMEMBER

- Traumatic blood draw is a common cause of otherwise unexpected hyperkalemia: Repeat potassium drawn with care will be within normal range, and unnecessary treatment can be avoided.
- Acute severe hyperkalemia is a medical emergency and requires prompt attention.
- When treating severe hyperkalemia, maneuvers to shift potassium into the cells (e.g., insulin/dextrose) and to stabilize membranes (e.g., calcium) should be used as soon as possible, with frequent rechecks of potassium level to ensure response to therapy and to detect a rebound, until the potassium can be conclusively lowered with dialysis or enteral (SPS) or renal (fluids/diuretics) loss.
- When treating hypokalemia, one must be careful with the amount of potassium being given IV. Too rapid a correction rate may cause problems.
- Patients in a high-aldosterone state (CHF, cirrhosis) requiring diuretics may develop significant hypokalemia. Use of potassium-sparing diuretics alone or in combination (when more significant diuresis is required) may decrease or eliminate the need for supplemental potassium.

REFERENCES AND SUGGESTED READINGS

Allon M, Shanklin N. Effect of bicarbonate administration on plasma potassium in dialysis patients: interactions with insulin and albuterol. *Am J Kidney Dis.* 1996;28:508.

Blake J, Devereux RB. Differential effects of direct antagonism of AII compared to ACE inhibitors on serum potassium and azotemia in patients with severe congestive heart failure. *Congest Heart Fail.* 2000;6:193.

Cely CM, Contreras G. Approach to the patient with hypertension, unexplained hypokalemia, and metabolic alkalosis. *Am J Kidney Dis.* 2001;37(3):24.

Clausen T, Flatman JA. Effects of insulin and epinephrine on sodium/potassium and glucose transport in soleus muscle. *Am J Physiol.* 1987;252[4 Pt 1]:E492.

Crook MA, Hally V, Panteli JV. The importance of the refeeding syndrome. *Nutrition.* 2001;17:632.

Don B, Sebastian A, Cheitlin M, et al. Pseudohyperkalemia caused by fist clenching during phlebotomy. *N Engl J Med.* 1990;322:1290.

Gardiner GW. Kayexalate (sodium polystyrene sulphonate) in sorbitol associated with intestinal necrosis in uremic patients. *Can J Gastroenterol.* 1997;11:573.

Gennari FJ. Hypokalemia. *N Engl J Med.* 1998;339:451.

Giebisch G. Renal potassium channels: function, regulation, and structure. *Kidney Int.* 2001;60:436.

Halperin ML, Kamel KS. Potassium. *Lancet.* 1998;352:135.

Heering P, Degenhardt S, Grabensee B. Tubular dysfunction following kidney transplantation. *Nephron.* 1996;74:501.

Junco E, Perez R, Jofre R, et al. Renal ammoniagenesis in acute hypokalemia in vivo in the dog. *Contrib Nephrol.* 1988;63:125.

Kaplan JL, Braitman LE, Dalsey WC, et al. Alkalinization is ineffective for severe hyperkalemia in nonnephrectomized dogs. Hyperkalemia Research Group. *Acad Emerg Med.* 1997;4:93.

Knichwitz G, Zahl M, Van Aken H, et al. Intraoperative washing of long-stored packed red blood cells by using an autotransfusion device prevents hyperkalemia. *Anesth Analg.* 2002;95:324.

Kochlatyi S, Mattana J. Triggering of sudden death from cardiac causes by vigorous exertion. *N Engl J Med.* 2000;343:1355.

Ljutic D, Rumboldt Z. Should glucose be administered before, with, or after insulin, in the management of hyperkalemia? *Ren Fail.* 1993;15:73.

Markewitz BA, Elstad MR. Succinylcholine-induced hyperkalemia following prolonged pharmacologic neuromuscular blockade. *Chest.* 1997;111:248.

Naparstek Y, Gutman A. Case report: spurious hypokalemia in myeloproliferative disorders. *Am J Med Sci.* 1984;288:175.

Palmer LG, Frindt G. Aldosterone and potassium secretion by the cortical collecting duct. *Kidney Int.* 2000;57:1324.

Perez G, Oster J, Vaamonde C. Serum potassium concentration in acidemic states. *Nephron.* 1981;27:233.

Roden DM, Iansmith DH. Effects of low potassium or magnesium concentrations on isolated cardiac tissue. *Am J Med.* 1987;82:18.

Roy LF, Villeneuve JP, Dumont A, et al. Irreversible renal failure associated with triamterene. *Am J Nephrol.* 1991;11:486.

Rutledge R, Sheldon GF, Collins ML. Massive transfusion. *Crit Care Clin.* 1986;2:791.

Scheinman SJ, Guay-Woodford LM, Thakker RV, et al. Mechanisms of disease: genetic disorders of renal electrolyte transport. *N Engl J Med.* 1999;340:1177–1187.

Siegel D, Hulley SB, Black DM, et al. Diuretics, serum and intracellular electrolyte levels, and ventricular arrhythmias in hypertensive men. *JAMA.* 1992;267:1083.

Silva P, Spokes K. Sympathetic system in potassium homeostasis. *Am J Physiol.* 1981;241:F151.

Tanaka M, Schmidlin O, Olson JL, et al. Chloride-sensitive renal microangiopathy in the stroke-prone spontaneously hypertensive rat. *Kidney Int.* 2001;59:1066.

Viberti GC. Glucose-induced hyperkalemia: a hazard for diabetics? *Lancet.* 1978;1:690.

West ML, Marsden PA, Richardson RM, et al. New clinical approach to evaluate disorders of potassium excretion. *Miner Electrolyte Metab.* 1986;12:234.

Wiggam MI, Beringer TR. Effect of low-molecular-weight heparin on serum concentrations of potassium. *Lancet.* 1997;349:1447.

Disorders of Calcium Metabolism

8

Jawad Munir

INTRODUCTION

Calcium is the most abundant cation in the body. It plays a critical role in neuromuscular function, bone formation, blood coagulation, and various endocrine functions. The adult human body contains approximately 1.2 to 1.4 kg of elemental calcium, 99% of which is found in the bone, complexed as hydroxyapatite crystals. Less than 1% of total body calcium is found in the extracellular fluid (ECF). Of this small amount, 50% is ionized, and 10% is complexed to anions like citrate, sulfate, and phosphate but is still filterable by the kidney. The remaining 40% is bound to albumin and is not filterable. The normal range is 8.6 to 10.3 mg/dL. The ionized fraction is physiologically active and therefore tightly regulated in a narrow range (4.5–5.1 mg/dL). Decreased total plasma calcium concentration is found in hypoalbuminemia without changes in the ionized calcium level. In general, for every 1.0 g/dL decrement in plasma albumin, there is a 0.8 mg/dL decline in the reported total plasma calcium level. If plasma albumin is abnormal, clinical decisions should be based on ionized calcium level or total calcium level corrected for albumin.

CALCIUM HOMEOSTASIS

The average diet contains 1000 to 1200 mg of calcium, mainly from dairy products. Of this, 20% to 40% is absorbed in the small intestine (Fig. 8-1). A small amount of calcium is also secreted back into the colon (200 mg/day). Hence, the total daily fecal loss of calcium is around 800 mg. Every day, 200 to 500 mg of calcium enters the ECF from the skeleton and the same amount is deposited back as a result of ongoing skeletal remodeling. The amount of calcium entering the ECF from the gut (~200 mg) is excreted by the kidney, keeping the body in a net equal balance.

REGULATION

Plasma-ionized calcium is regulated by an interplay of parathyroid hormone (PTH) and calcitriol $[1,25(OH)_2D_3]$ in intestine, bone, and kidney. The parathyroid gland senses the ECF-ionized calcium concentration via a calcium-sensing receptor (CaSR). High levels of ECF calcium stimulate the receptor and cause a transient rise in intracellular calcium concentration that inhibits the release of PTH. Low concentrations of ECF calcium stimulate PTH production and secretion.

PTH, in the presence of calcitriol, stimulates bone resorption by increasing osteoclast number and activity. In the intestine, PTH stimulates calcium and phosphorus absorption indirectly by promoting calcitriol formation. In the kidney, it enhances tubular reabsorption

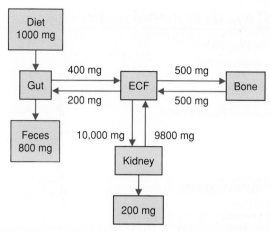

FIGURE 8-1. Daily calcium fluxes in a healthy adult in zero mineral ion balance. Values are expressed in mg/day. ECF, extracellular fluid.

of calcium, stimulates the generation of calcitriol in the proximal tubule, and decreases proximal tubular reabsorption of phosphate.

Calcitriol [1,25(OH)$_2$D3] is formed in the proximal tubule from 1-alpha hydroxylation of calcidiol [25(OH) D]. The main role of calcitriol is to improve the availability of calcium and phosphate. In the intestine and kidney, calcitriol stimulates calcium absorption. In bone, calcitriol complements the actions of PTH, stimulating osteoclastic bone resorption. Calcitriol acts directly on the parathyroid gland to inhibit both PTH synthesis and secretion.

HYPERCALCEMIA

Etiology

Clinically significant hypercalcemia is invariably caused by both an increase in entry of calcium into the ECF from bone resorption or intestinal absorption and a decrease in renal clearance of calcium. Primary hyperparathyroidism (>50%) and malignancy (~40%) account for the majority (>90%) of cases (Table 8-1).

Increased Bone Resorption
This is the most common and most important mechanism of hypercalcemia.

Primary Hyperparathyroidism. Primary hyperparathyroidism is the most common cause of hypercalcemia in *ambulatory* patients. An adenoma of a single gland is found in 85% and 15% of cases are due to hyperplasia of all four glands. Parathyroid carcinoma is responsible in <1% of the cases. Most patients are asymptomatic, and the hypercalcemia, usually modest, is discovered incidentally. These patients remain at risk for long-term consequences of hyperparathyroidism (i.e., nephrolithiasis and osteopenia).

Malignancy. Malignancy is responsible for most cases of hypercalcemia among *hospitalized* patients. There are three mechanisms of malignant hypercalcemia:

- *Osteolytic hypercalcemia* is caused by cytokines produced by the tumor cells that act locally to stimulate osteoclastic bone resorption. This form of malignant hypercalcemia is responsible for the majority of malignancy-associated cases and occurs only with

TABLE 8-1	CAUSES OF HYPERCALCEMIA

Increased Bone Resorption

Primary hyperparathyroidism
Malignancy
Post–renal transplant
Immobilization
Familial hypocalciuric hypercalcemia
Thyrotoxicosis
Paget disease
Vitamin A intoxication
Lithium

Increased Intestinal Absorption

Milk-alkali syndrome
Granulomatous disease
Vitamin D intoxication

Decreased Renal Excretion

Thiazide diuretics

extensive bone involvement by tumor, most often due to breast carcinoma, non–small-cell lung cancer, myeloma, and lymphoma.

- *Humoral hypercalcemia of malignancy* results from tumor products acting systemically to stimulate bone resorption and decrease renal calcium excretion. PTH-related peptide (**PTHrP**) is an important mediator of this syndrome. Humoral hypercalcemia of malignancy is caused most often by squamous carcinoma of the lung, head and neck, or esophagus, or by renal, bladder, or ovarian carcinoma.
- *Tumoral calcitriol production* may occasionally occur in Hodgkin and non-Hodgkin lymphomas.

Post–renal Transplant. Long-term dialysis patients may develop parathyroid hyperplasia and an autonomous secretion of PTH (**tertiary hyperparathyroidism**). Persistent PTH secretion after a successful transplant may lead to hypercalcemia. This is usually mild and tends to decrease over 6 to 12 months.

Immobilization. Sustained bed rest leads to an increase in bone resorption and may lead to hypercalcemia. This is usually seen in patients with renal disease, young patients with spinal cord injuries, or those in full body casts.

Familial Hypocalciuric Hypercalcemia. A mutation in the calcium-sensing receptor causes decreased receptor activity in this autosomal-dominant disorder. Hypercalcemia is mild, and renal calcium excretion is reduced. Patients have hypophosphatemia and normal or mildly elevated PTH levels. Parathyroidectomy is not indicated.

Thyrotoxicosis. Thyrotoxicosis may stimulate osteoclastic bone resorption, causing a mild hypercalcemia. Concurrent hyperparathyroidism should be excluded.

Increased Intestinal Absorption

This is a less frequent cause of hypercalcemia but assumes greater importance in the setting of chronic renal failure.

Milk-alkali Syndrome. Ingestion of large quantities of calcium carbonate–based antacids can lead to this condition, characterized by hypercalcemia, alkalemia, nephrocalcinosis, and renal failure.

Granulomatous Disease. Sarcoidosis, TB, and leprosy cause hypercalcemia due to the conversion of 25(OH)D to 1,25(OH)$_2$D$_3$ by the 1-α hydroxylase present in macrophages contained in the granulomas. Treatment of the underlying disease corrects the hypercalcemia.

Vitamin D Intoxication. Vitamin D intoxication may be observed in dialysis patients overtreated with vitamin D analogs. Hypercalcemia is usually mild and improves with dose adjustment or discontinuation of the drug.

Decreased Renal Excretion

Thiazide Diuretics. Thiazide diuretics are often associated with a mild hypercalcemia due to increased renal calcium reabsorption in the distal convoluted tubule. The hypercalcemia is usually mild.

Clinical Features

Symptoms and signs of hypercalcemia are related to the severity and rapidity of the rise in plasma-ionized calcium concentration. Mild hypercalcemia is often asymptomatic and incidentally discovered on routine blood tests. In contrast, severe hypercalcemia is often associated with neurologic and GI symptoms. **GI symptoms** include anorexia, nausea, vomiting, and constipation. **Neurologic symptoms** include weakness, fatigue, confusion, stupor, and coma. **Renal manifestations** include polyuria and nephrolithiasis. Polyuria combined with nausea and vomiting causes volume depletion resulting in impaired calcium excretion and worsening of hypercalcemia.

Laboratory Studies

- **Calcium** should be interpreted in context of the plasma albumin concentration (corrected calcium), or an ionized calcium should be measured.
- **Phosphorus** may be low in settings of elevated PTH (primary hyperparathyroidism) or PTHrP (e.g., humoral hypercalcemia of malignancy). Phosphorus may be high in vitamin D toxicity or increased bone resorption without hyperparathyroidism (Paget disease).
- **Intact PTH** levels are elevated or inappropriately normal in primary hyperparathyroidism. The PTH is almost always suppressed in patients with hypercalcemia due to other causes, except familial hypocalciuric hypercalcemia, tertiary hyperparathyroidism, and lithium use.
- **PTHrP** can be measured to confirm the diagnosis of humoral hypercalcemia of malignancy.
- **1,25(OH)$_2$D$_3$** levels are elevated in granulomatous disorders and calcitriol overdose.
- **25(OH)D** levels are elevated with noncalcitriol vitamin D intoxication (rare).
- **Urinary calcium.** Patients with familial hypocalciuric hypercalcemia can be distinguished from primary hyperparathyroidism by a low **urinary calcium** (<200 mg calcium/24 hours) or fractional excretion of calcium (<1%).

Management

Acute Hypercalcemia

Total calcium concentrations of >12 mg/dL are usually symptomatic and warrant aggressive therapy. Severely hypercalcemic patients are volume depleted, which prevents renal excretion of calcium. The initial step in therapy is volume repletion.

Volume Repletion. Correction of hypovolemia is the initial goal and often requires at least 3 to 4 L of 0.9% saline in the first 24 hours. Continuing maintenance IV fluids after restoring ECF volume promotes further calcium excretion. The patient should be monitored closely for signs of volume overload. Electrolyte concentrations should be monitored every 8 to 12 hours during induction and maintenance of diuresis.

Diuretics. Although loop diuretics impair tubular reabsorption of calcium, they are generally not used for acute hypercalcemia as they may result in further volume depletion.

They are useful however if evidence of volume overload develops. Thiazide diuretics should be avoided as they enhance calcium reabsorption by the kidney.

Bisphosphonates. Intravenous bisphosphonates inhibit bone resorption and should be administered early because their effect is delayed. **Pamidronate** 60 to 90 mg is infused over 2 to 4 hours. A hypocalcemic response is seen within 2 days, peaks at 7 days, and may persist for 2 weeks or longer. Treatment can be repeated after 7 days if hypercalcemia recurs. **Zoledronate** is a more potent bisphosphonate that is given as a 4 mg dose infused over at least 15 minutes. During treatment with bisphosphonates, renal dysfunction can occur from the precipitation of calcium bisphosphonate. Hydration should precede their use and renal insufficiency is a relative contraindication. Side effects include hypocalcemia, hypomagnesemia, hypophosphatemia, and renal dysfunction. Advanced CKD is a relative contraindication to the use of IV bisphosphonates.

Calcitonin. Calcitonin inhibits bone resorption and increases renal calcium excretion. Salmon calcitonin, 4 to 8 IU/kg IM or SC q6–12h, lowers plasma calcium 1 to 2 mg/dL within several hours in 60% to 70% of patients. The hypocalcemic effect wanes after several days because of tachyphylaxis. Calcitonin is less potent than other inhibitors of bone resorption but has no serious toxicity, is safe in renal failure, and may have an analgesic effect in patients with skeletal metastases. It can be used early in the treatment of severe hypercalcemia to achieve a rapid response. Side effects include flushing, nausea, and, rarely, allergic reactions.

Glucocorticoids. Glucocorticoids lower calcium concentrations by inhibiting cytokine release, by direct cytolytic effects on some tumor cells, by inhibiting intestinal calcium absorption, and by increasing urinary calcium excretion. They are effective in hypercalcemia due to hematologic malignancies including myeloma, tumoral or granulomatous production of calcitriol, and vitamin D and A intoxication. The initial dose is 20 to 60 mg/day of prednisone. Plasma calcium may take 5 to 10 days to fall. After plasma calcium stabilizes, the dose should be gradually reduced to the minimum needed to control symptoms of hypercalcemia.

Gallium Nitrate. Gallium nitrate also inhibits bone resorption as effectively as the IV bisphosphonates and has a similar delayed onset of 2 days. It is given as a 100 to 200 mg/m^2/day continuous infusion for up to 5 days, unless normocalcemia is achieved sooner. There is, however, a significant risk of nephrotoxicity and it is contraindicated if the plasma creatinine is >2.5 mg/dL.

Dialysis. Both **hemodialysis** and **peritoneal dialysis** using dialysate with low calcium are very effective means of treating hypercalcemia. This modality is particularly helpful for patients with very severe hypercalcemia and CHF or kidney disease prohibiting aggressive hydration. Very low calcium dialysis baths should be used with caution as rapid development of hypocalcemia can occur.

Chronic Hypercalcemia
Chronic elevation in plasma calcium is generally asymptomatic and from benign causes. The natural history of mild asymptomatic **primary hyperparathyroidism** is not fully known, but in many patients the disorder has a benign course, with little change in clinical findings or plasma calcium concentration. The possibility of progressive loss of bone mass and increased fracture risk are the main concerns, but the likelihood of these outcomes appears to be low. Deterioration of renal function is unlikely in the absence of nephrolithiasis. The **indications for parathyroidectomy** are as follows:

- Corrected plasma calcium >1 mg/dL above upper limit of normal
- Hypercalciuria >400 mg/day
- Renal insufficiency
- Reduced bone mass (T score <−2.5 by DEXA)
- Age <50 years
- Nephrolithiasis
- Lack of feasibility of long-term follow-up

Surgery is a reasonable choice in healthy patients even if they do not meet these criteria because of a high success rate (95%), with low morbidity and mortality. Often a brief, 1- to 2-day period of mild, asymptomatic hypocalcemia ensues. In rare patients with overt bone disease, hypocalcemia may be severe and prolonged (**hungry bone syndrome**).

Medical therapy may be a reasonable option in asymptomatic patients who can have follow-up, and in patients who are not surgical candidates. Management consists of oral hydration, daily physical activity, avoidance of thiazide diuretics and extremes of calcium intake. Drugs that are useful in reducing bone loss in this setting include estrogen replacement therapy or raloxifene, vitamin D, and oral bisphosphonates. **Cinacalcet** is a calcimimetic (a noncalcium activator of the calcium-sensing receptor) and may hold promise in reducing PTH and calcium levels in this setting.

Malignant Hypercalcemia

Because patients usually have extensive, unresectable disease, with a median survival of <3 months, the approach should be balanced with expected outcome. Repeated doses of IV bisphosphonate can be given. Prednisone usually controls hypercalcemia in multiple myeloma and other hematologic malignancies. A calcium-restricted diet (<400 mg/d) and oral phosphate, which inhibits intestinal calcium absorption, can be tried if the plasma phosphorus level is <3 mg/dL and renal function is normal. Doses of 0.5 to 1.0 g elemental phosphorus PO tid can be used but the dose should be reduced if plasma phosphorus exceeds 4.5 mg/dL or if the product of the plasma calcium and phosphorus exceeds 60.

HYPOCALCEMIA

Hypocalcemia is the result of decreased calcium absorption from the GI tract or decreased calcium resorption from bone. Persistent hypocalcemia does not occur without an abnormality of PTH or calcitriol action on bone, as 99% of total body calcium is contained within the skeleton. True hypocalcemia is present only when the ionized calcium concentration is reduced. Whenever a low total plasma calcium concentration is measured, this value must be compared with the plasma albumin concentration. The binding of calcium to albumin is affected by extracellular pH. Acidemia increases and alkalemia decreases the ionized calcium concentration.

Etiology

True hypocalcemia is caused by decreased PTH secretion, end-organ resistance to PTH, or disorders of vitamin D metabolism. Less commonly, hypocalcemia occurs as a result of either extravascular deposition or intravascular chelation of calcium (Table 8-2).

Decreased PTH Level or Effect

Hypomagnesemia. Severe magnesium deficiency results in decreased PTH secretion from the gland. Patients with hypocalcemia due to hypomagnesemia do not respond to calcium or vitamin D replacement until the magnesium deficit has been replaced.

Hypoparathyroidism. Hypoparathyroidism can be associated with acquired and inherited diseases that result from either impaired synthesis or release of PTH. The most common cause of idiopathic hypoparathyroidism is polyglandular autoimmune syndrome type I, associated with chronic mucocutaneous candidiasis and primary adrenal insufficiency. Occasionally, pernicious anemia, diabetes mellitus, vitiligo, and autoimmune thyroid disease are also associated with hypoparathyroidism. Hypoparathyroidism may be iatrogenic after thyroidectomy.

Familial Hypocalcemia. Familial hypocalcemia results from activating mutations in the calcium-sensing receptor. The receptor behaves as though calcium levels are normal, down-regulating PTH transcription. Thus, hypocalcemia results from inappropriately low PTH levels due to receptor malfunction.

TABLE 8-2	CAUSES OF HYPOCALCEMIA

Decreased PTH Level or Effect

Hypomagnesemia
Hypoparathyroidism (surgical or autoimmune)
Familial hypocalcemia
Pseudohypoparathyroidism

Disorders of Vitamin D Metabolism

Vitamin D deficiency
Drugs (anticonvulsants)
Renal disease
Vitamin D–dependent rickets

Extravascular Deposition/Intravascular Chelation

Hungry bone syndrome
Rhabdomyolysis
Tumor lysis syndrome
Acute pancreatitis
Citrate-containing blood products

Miscellaneous

Septic shock

Pseudohypoparathyroidism. Pseudohypoparathyroidism (Albright hereditary osteo-dystrophy) is a hereditary disorder in which the target cell response to PTH is decreased. Renal calcium excretion is increased and the PTH level is increased. Phenotypic characteristics include short stature, obesity, shortened metacarpals and metatarsals, and heterotopic calcification.

Disorders of Vitamin D Metabolism

Vitamin D Deficiency. Vitamin D (calcidiol) deficiency is a very common problem. Limited exposure to sunlight is the leading cause. Nutritional deficiency of vitamin D can lead to rickets and osteomalacia. As vitamin D is fat soluble, the deficiency can be seen in malabsorption syndromes. **Anticonvulsants** can result in vitamin D deficiency by stimulating the hepatic metabolism of calcidiol.

Chronic Kidney Disease. Decreased glomerular filtration rate lowers renal phosphorus excretion, resulting in hyperphosphatemia. This down-regulates the 1-α hydroxylase enzyme responsible for renal conversion of 25(OH)D to 1,25(OH)$_2$D$_3$. With decreasing levels of calcitriol, patients with chronic kidney disease are prone to develop hypocalcemia. However, the balance is partly maintained by increasing levels of PTH as GFR declines.

Vitamin D–dependent Rickets. This condition is the result of either impaired hydroxylation of calcidiol to calcitriol (type I) or end-organ resistance to calcitriol (type II). Type I patients respond to physiologic doses of calcitriol. Patients with type II disease have mutations in the vitamin D receptor. They tend to have dramatically increased concentrations of calcitriol and respond poorly to calcitriol therapy.

Extravascular Deposition/Intravascular Chelation

Hungry Bone Syndrome. A profound reduction in calcium concentration can occur after surgical removal of parathyroid tissue for secondary or tertiary hyperparathyroidism.

This "hungry bone syndrome" is due to a rapid bone mineralization in the absence of PTH. Symptoms can occur soon after surgery, and patients' calcium levels should be carefully monitored (q4–6h). Hypocalcemia also occurs after thyroid surgery (5% of cases).

Rhabdomyolysis. Crush injuries causing cellular damage initiate a rapid release of intracellular phosphorus that complexes with extracellular calcium, resulting in hypocalcemia.

Tumor Lysis Syndrome (TLS). Same mechanism as rhabdomyolysis.

Acute Pancreatitis. The release of pancreatic lipase digests retroperitoneal and omental fat. The fatty acids, once released, bind to the calcium. The hypocalcemia is aggravated by the hypoalbuminuria and hypomagnesemia associated with acute pancreatitis.

Citrate-containing Blood Products. Massive transfusions of citrate-containing blood products can cause intravascular chelation of calcium, leading to hypocalcemia.

Miscellaneous

Septic Shock. Endotoxic shock has been associated with hypocalcemia through unclear mechanisms. Hypocalcemia may be partially responsible for the hypotension, as myocardial function correlates with ionized calcium levels.

Clinical Features

Symptoms depend not only on the degree of hypocalcemia, but also on the rate of decline of the plasma calcium concentration. Precipitation of symptoms is also influenced by plasma pH and the presence or absence of concomitant hypomagnesemia, hypokalemia, or hyponatremia. **Neuromuscular excitability** symptoms are the most common. The patient may experience circumoral and distal extremity paresthesias or carpopedal spasm. Other manifestations include mental status changes, irritability, and seizures.

On **physical exam**, hypotension, bradycardia, laryngeal spasm, and bronchospasm may be present. The presence of **Chvostek sign** (facial twitch elicited by tapping on the facial nerve just below the zygomatic arch with the mouth slightly open) and **Trousseau sign** (development of wrist flexion, metacarpophalangeal joint flexion, hyperextended fingers, and thumb flexion after a BP cuff has been inflated to 20 mm Hg above systolic pressure for a duration of 3 minutes) should be checked.

Laboratory Studies

- **Plasma albumin** should always be checked to interpret calcium levels.
- **Magnesium** deficiency should be ruled out.
- **Phosphorus** will be low in conditions associated with low vitamin D activity, except for kidney failure where there is decreased renal clearance of phosphorus. The plasma phosphorus will be increased in rhabdomyolysis or TLS.
- **PTH** that is low or inappropriately normal in the setting of hypocalcemia is indicative of hypoparathyroidism. A high PTH is often found with vitamin D–deficiency states, CKD and pseudohypoparathyroidism.
- **25(OH)D** and **1,25(OH)$_2$D$_3$** levels are useful in assessing for vitamin D deficiency and vitamin D–dependent rickets, respectively.

Management

Acute Symptomatic Hypocalcemia

In an emergency situation with seizures, tetany, hypotension, or cardiac arrhythmias, **IV calcium gluconate** should be administered (100–300 mg, or 1–3 mL of 10% calcium gluconate solution, over 10–15 minutes). Patients with symptomatic hypocalcemia or a total plasma calcium concentration corrected for albumin of <7.5 mg/dL should be treated with IV calcium. The first ampule can be administered over several minutes followed by a constant infusion at a rate of 0.5 to 1.0 mg/kg/hr. Adjustments in the rate should be based on serial plasma calcium determinations. Treatment of hypocalcemia is ineffective without adequate treatment of hypomagnesemia. In the setting of metabolic acidosis, hypocalcemia should be corrected before the acidosis.

Chronic Hypocalcemia

Chronic, mild hypocalcemia, seen in the outpatient setting, can be treated with **oral calcium supplements** with or without vitamin D. Patients with hypoparathyroidism generally need both calcium and vitamin D supplementation. The plasma calcium level should be maintained at the lower limit of normal. Oral supplementation of elemental calcium, 1 to 3 g/day, is usually sufficient. Calcium is best absorbed when taken between meals.

Calcitriol is the most potent of the **vitamin D** preparations and has the fastest onset and shortest duration of action. A dose of 0.5 to 1.0 mcg/day is usually required in patients with hypoparathyroidism. Cholecalciferol and ergocalciferol are less potent but inexpensive.

Patients with hypoparathyroidism have decreased distal tubular calcium reabsorption as a result of a lack of PTH. Therefore, the increase in the filtered load of calcium that results from calcium and vitamin D replacement therapy can lead to hypercalciuria, nephrolithiasis, and nephrocalcinosis. If urinary calcium excretion exceeds 350 mg/day, despite plasma calcium concentration in the low-to-normal range, sodium intake should be restricted; if this is not effective, a thiazide diuretic should be added.

KEY POINTS TO REMEMBER

- Primary hyperparathyroidism is the most common cause of hypercalcemia. However, hypercalcemia related to malignancy is the most common cause of hypercalcemia in hospitalized patients.
- The most important step in the initial treatment of hypercalcemia is aggressive volume replacement.
- Severe and persistent hypocalcemia can result after parathyroidectomy (hungry bone syndrome). Active surveillance and aggressive repletion with calcium infusions help to avoid dangerous complications.

REFERENCES AND SUGGESTED READINGS

Bilezikian JP, Silverberg SJ. Asymptomatic primary hyperparathyroidism. *N Engl J Med.* 2004;350:1746–1751.

Bushinsky DA. Disorders of calcium and phosphorus homeostasis. In: Greenberg A, ed. *Primer on Kidney Diseases.* 4th ed. Philadelphia: Elsevier; 2005.

Marx SJ. Medical progress: hyperparathyroid and hypoparathyroid disorders. *N Engl J Med.* 2000;343:1863–1875.

Ziegler R. Hypercalcemic crisis. *J Am Soc Nephrol.* 2001;12:S3–S9.

Disorders of Phosphorus Metabolism

9

Jawad Munir

INTRODUCTION

Phosphorus has several important biologic functions. It is involved in a variety of metabolic and enzymatic processes vital to cellular energy metabolism. Along with calcium, it is a major mineral component of the bone and is necessary for adequate mineralization. The human body, on average, contains 700 g of phosphorus with 85% in the skeleton and 15% in soft tissues. Extracellular fluid (ECF) contains <1% of total body phosphorus. Of the total circulating plasma phosphorus, two-thirds is in the organic form (e.g., phospholipids) and one-third in the inorganic form. Only the inorganic form is measured by the laboratory. The normal range is 2.5 to 4.5 mg/dL. This inorganic form of phosphorus is mostly free in ionic form (75%) as HPO_4 or H_2PO_4 and hence, readily filterable. The rest is protein-bound or complexed with calcium, magnesium, or sodium.

PHOSPHORUS HOMEOSTASIS

The average diet contains 1000 to 1400 mg of phosphorus, mainly from meat, cereals, and dairy products. Of this, 80% is absorbed in the small intestine. The absorption is mostly through passive diffusion but an active component exists and is mediated by vitamin D. A small amount of phosphorus is also secreted back in the colon (200 mg/day). Hence, the total daily fecal loss of phosphorus is 400 to 500 mg. As a result of ongoing skeletal remodeling, 200 to 350 mg of phosphorus enters the ECF from the skeleton and the same amount is deposited back. The amount of phosphorus entering the ECF from the gut (~900 mg) is excreted by the kidney, keeping the body in a net equal balance (Fig. 9-1).

REGULATION

Several factors govern the ECF phosphate concentration.

Parathyroid Hormone (PTH). In the kidney, phosphate is reabsorbed primarily in the proximal tubule (80%), where it is co-transported across the luminal membrane with sodium. PTH inhibits this reabsorption, lowering the plasma phosphate level. PTH acts directly on bone to increase phosphate entry into the ECF and indirectly on the intestine by stimulating the synthesis of calcitriol.

Calcitriol. Vitamin D increases plasma phosphate due to enhanced intestinal phosphorus absorption by increasing sodium-phosphate co-transport across the apical bush border membrane.

Plasma Phosphate Concentration. Elevated phosphorus level itself decreases proximal reabsorption in the renal tubule.

Insulin. Insulin lowers plasma phosphorus levels by shifting phosphate into cells.

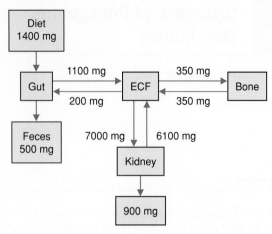

FIGURE 9-1. Normal phosphate homeostasis.

Fibroblast Growth Factor-23 (FGF-23). This molecule belongs to a group of substances called *phosphatonins*. Their main effect is to promote renal excretion of phosphate and lower plasma phosphorus levels.

HYPERPHOSPHATEMIA

Etiology

The three main mechanisms that lead to hyperphosphatemia are impaired renal excretion, transcellular shift into the ECF, and increased phosphate intake (Table 9-1).

Impaired Renal Excretion
Reduced renal excretion of the daily phosphate load is the most common cause of hyperphosphatemia. Renal phosphate clearance can be reduced in the following settings:

- **Acute and Chronic GFR Decrease.** With declining GFR, the fractional excretion of phosphate begins to increase and reabsorption is suppressed. Once GFR reaches around 25 mL/minute or lower, it can no longer keep up with the dietary intake and the plasma phosphorus level begins to rise. Hence, hyperphosphatemia is a frequent finding in advanced CKD.
- **Hypoparathyroidism.** Because PTH decreases proximal tubular reabsorption of phosphate, deficiency of this hormone leads to increased tubular transport of phosphate, resulting in hyperphosphatemia.
- **Pseudohypoparathyroidism** (resistance to the actions of PTH), leads to hyperphosphatemia via the same mechanism as hypoparathyroidism.
- **Acromegaly.** Elevated levels of insulin-like growth factor-1 (IGF-1) found in this disorder directly stimulate phosphate transport in the proximal tubule.
- **Tumoral Calcinosis.** Patients with this disorder also have increased proximal tubular reabsorption of phosphate, leading to hyperphosphatemia.
- **Bisphosphonates.** These drugs directly stimulate phosphate reabsorption by the kidney but this effect is usually negated by the concomitant decrease in plasma calcium, which, in turn, leads to a secondary hyperparathyroidism.

Transcellular Shift
Release of intracellular phosphorus into the ECF can occur when there is a rapid and large-scale cell lysis.

TABLE 9-1	CAUSES OF HYPERPHOSPHATEMIA

Impaired Renal Excretion

Renal failure (acute and chronic)
Hypoparathyroidism
Pseudohypoparathyroidism
Acromegaly
Tumoral calcinosis
Drugs (bisphosphonates)

Transcellular Shift

Rhabdomyolysis
Tumor lysis syndrome
Massive hemolysis
Acidosis
Hypoinsulinemia

Increased Phosphate Intake or Absorption

High phosphate diet (in the setting of CKD)
Fleet® enemas
Vitamin D intoxication

- **Rhabdomyolysis.** Can cause severe hyperphosphatemia acutely, which may then precipitate life-threatening hypocalcemia.
- **Tumor lysis syndrome** usually follows chemotherapy for hematologic malignancies or rapidly growing solid tumors.
- **Massive hemolysis**
- **Acidosis** inhibits phosphate entry into the cells, leading to mild elevation in plasma phosphorus levels.
- **Hypoinsulinemia** (same mechanism as acidosis)

Increased Phosphate Intake

Hyperphosphatemia from an increased exogenous phosphorus load generally occurs only in the setting of CKD.

- **Dietary indiscretion** by the patient.
- **Iatrogenic** when a patient with CKD is given **Fleet® enemas**.
- **Vitamin D intoxication** can result in increased intestinal absorption of phosphorus.

Clinical Features

Symptoms of acute hyperphosphatemia are generally attributable to accompanying hypocalcemia. Hypocalcemia is thought to result from tissue deposition of calcium once calcium $\times$ phosphate product reaches >55 and suppression of 1-α hydroxylase by hyperphosphatemia. Tissue deposition of calcium can occur in blood vessels, skin, kidneys, and other organs. **Calciphylaxis** is the term used for tissue ischemia that may result from the calcification and subsequent thrombosis of small blood vessels. Chronic hyperphosphatemia contributes to renal osteodystrophy.

Laboratory Studies

The laboratory evaluation for hyperphosphatemia is directed at evaluating renal function, potential sources of intrinsic tissue damage and the assessment of endocrine factors involved with phosphate regulation.

- **Plasma creatinine** helps assess renal function.
- **Intact parathyroid hormone (iPTH)** is elevated in CKD but is low in the setting of hypoparathyroidism.
- **Creatine kinase (CK)** is markedly elevated in rhabdomyolysis.
- **Uric acid** levels are often markedly elevated in tumor lysis syndrome in addition to hyperphosphatemia.
- **Markers of hemolysis** (LDH, haptoglobin, bilirubin, etc.) are helpful in the appropriate setting.
- **Calcium** levels are usually low in acute hyperphosphatemia and may need to be treated acutely to avoid hypocalcemia complications.

Management

Acute hyperphosphatemia in patients who do not have renal insufficiency can be managed by correcting the underlying cause and by **saline diuresis**. **Acetazolamide** (15 mg/kg q4h) may be used to enhance phosphaturia.

Chronic hyperphosphatemia is almost always a result of CKD and the treatment is aimed at reducing the intestinal absorption of phosphate.

- *Dietary restriction of phosphate.* The first step is to institute dietary restriction of phosphate to 600 to 900 mg/day. Instruction from a trained dietician is the best method as many food sources contain phosphorus. Dietary restrictions alone are usually not sufficient, and therapy with oral phosphate binders is needed.
- *Calcium-based phosphate binders.* Calcium carbonate starting at 500 mg (200 mg elemental calcium) t.i.d. with meals to a maximum of 3750 mg/day (1500 mg elemental calcium) and calcium acetate starting at 667 mg (167 mg elemental calcium) t.i.d. with meals to a maximum of 6000 mg/day (1500 mg elemental calcium) are effective but carry the risk of increasing calcium and phosphorus product, leading to metastatic calcification.
- *Non–calcium-based phosphate binders.* Use of non–calcium-based binders like sevelamer HCl (starting at 800 mg t.i.d. with meals; max. 7200 mg/day) and lanthanum carbonate (starting at 250 mg t.i.d. with meals; max. 3000 mg/day), are more expensive but do not pose the risk of increasing the calcium-phosphate product. Sevelamer HCl should be used *only* in patients who are on dialysis due to the risk of worsening metabolic acidosis in predialysis CKD.
- *Intermittent hemodialysis* (three times a week) rapidly clears ECF phosphate but this is predominantly an intracellular ion and mobilization of intracellular stores lags behind.
- For this reason, *nocturnal hemodialysis* and CVVHD are much more effective for phosphate clearance because of longer duration of therapy.

HYPOPHOSPHATEMIA

Etiology

Three main mechanisms for hypophosphatemia are redistribution of extracellular phosphate into the intracellular space, decrease in intestinal absorption of phosphate, or increase in renal excretion of phosphate (Table 9-2).

Redistribution of Extracellular Phosphate
This is one of the most important mechanisms of hypophosphatemia in the hospital setting.

- **Respiratory alkalosis** leads to a rise in intracellular pH, which in turn, stimulates glycolysis and phosphate is incorporated into ATP.

TABLE 9-2   CAUSES OF HYPERPHOSPHATEMIA

Cellular Redistribution

Respiratory alkalosis
Refeeding syndrome
Treatment of DKA
Hungry bone syndrome
Sepsis

Decreased Intestinal Absorption

Malabsorption syndromes
Oral phosphate binders
Vitamin D deficiency
Alcoholism

Increased Renal Excretion

Primary hyperparathyroidism
Vitamin D deficiency (secondary hyperparathyroidism)
After renal transplant
Osmotic diuresis (DKA, recovering ATN)
Familial X-linked hypophosphatemic rickets
Autosomal-dominant hypophosphatemic rickets
Fanconi syndrome
Oncogenic osteomalacia

- **Refeeding syndrome** can occur in chronically malnourished individuals, typically 2 to 5 days after they are started on enteral or parenteral feeding. Caloric replacement increases insulin secretion that stimulates cell growth and enhances cellular uptake of phosphate for various molecular pathways.
- **Treatment of diabetic ketoacidosis (DKA)** with IV insulin leads to rapid flux of phosphorus into the cells.
- **Hungry bone syndrome** after partial parathyroidectomy causes movement of phosphate into the cells, leading to hypophosphatemia.

Decreased Intestinal Absorption
This is a relatively uncommon cause of hypophosphatemia, unless combined with diarrhea or the use of phosphate binders.

- **Malabsorption syndromes.** In addition to poor intake and absorption of phosphorus and vitamin D, the accompanying diarrhea also contributes to significant GI losses.
- **Oral phosphate binders.** Indiscriminate use of phosphate binders in ESRD patients who may not be eating very well may lead to low phosphorus levels.
- **Vitamin D deficiency.** Because vitamin D is important in GI absorption of phosphate, severe deficiency of this vitamin can lead to hypophosphatemia. The secondary hyperparathyroidism resulting from vitamin D deficiency contributes further to hypophosphatemia through increasing renal phosphate excretion.
- **Alcoholism.** Alcoholics often have poor intake of both phosphate and vitamin D, resulting in total body phosphorus depletion. Use of dextrose-containing IV fluids leads to insulin secretion, which further lowers plasma phosphate by intracellular redistribution as discussed above.

Increased Renal Excretion

Urinary losses of phosphate may increase in several disease states.

- **Primary hyperparathyroidism.** PTH causes urinary phosphate loss but hypophosphatemia is usually mild because PTH also stimulates calcitriol synthesis resulting in increased intestinal absorption of phosphate.
- **Secondary hyperparathyroidism from vitamin D deficiency.** In this disorder, lack of substrate to allow for compensatory rise in calcitriol level does not occur, leading to severe hypophosphatemia.
- **After renal transplant.** Renal phosphate wasting is common after successful renal transplant due to persistently elevated PTH
- **Osmotic diuresis.** In DKA or recovering ATN, excessive phosphate losses occur in urine, along with other solutes.
- **Familial X-linked hypophosphatemic rickets (XLH).** XLH is caused by mutations in the PHEX gene. The condition is characterized by growth retardation, renal phosphate wasting, hypophosphatemia, and rickets. Plasma concentrations of calcitriol are low.
- **Autosomal-dominant hypophosphatemic rickets (ADHR).** ADHR has a similar phenotype to XLH but is inherited in an autosomal-dominant fashion. Mutations in the FGF-23 are responsible for the disease.
- **Oncogenic osteomalacia.** Paraneoplastic production of FGF-23 by mesenchymal tumors is responsible for phosphaturia in cases of oncogenic osteomalacia.

Clinical Features

Signs and symptoms occur only if total body phosphate depletion is present and the plasma phosphorus level is <1 mg/dL. These are due to the inability to form ATP and to impaired tissue oxygen delivery. **Neuromuscular abnormalities** include weakness, rhabdomyolysis, impaired diaphragmatic function, paresthesias, dysarthria, confusion, seizures, and coma. **Hematologic manifestations** are rare but may include hemolysis and platelet dysfunction. Chronic hypophosphatemia causes **rickets** in children and **osteomalacia** in adults.

Laboratory Studies

The etiology of hypophosphatemia is usually apparent from the clinical scenario. If not, measuring urine phosphate excretion helps to clarify the mechanism.

- **Fractional excretion of phosphorus and 24-hour urine phosphorus.** Fractional excretion of phosphorus $>5\%$ or a urine phosphate excretion of >100 mg/24 hours in the setting of hypophosphatemia indicates excessive renal loss. Excretion rates are lower in states of impaired intestinal absorption or hypophosphatemia from transcellular shifts. One exception is vitamin D deficiency, which causes phosphaturia from secondary hyperparathyroidism.
- **Plasma calcium.** Plasma calcium is typically low in secondary hyperparathyroidism from vitamin D deficiency but high or normal in primary hyperparathyroidism.
- **25(OH)D.** Low levels suggest vitamin D deficiency.
- **PTH** is elevated in primary or secondary hyperparathyroidism.
- **Hypomagnesemia** and **hypokalemia** accompany hypophosphatemia in the setting of refeeding syndrome.

Management

Moderate Hypophosphatemia (1–2.5 mg/dL)

The degree of lowered phosphate levels is usually asymptomatic. Treatment of the underlying cause is very important to correct hypophosphatemia. Persistent hypophosphatemia may be treated with oral phosphate supplements. These include Neutra-Phos (250 mg phosphorus and 7 mEq each sodium and potassium/capsule), Neutra-Phos K (250 mg phosphorus and 14 mEq potassium/capsule) and K-Phos Neutral (250 mg phosphorus, 13 mEq of sodium and 1 mEq of potassium/tablet).

Severe Hypophosphatemia (<1 mg/dL)
This is a serious medical condition and requires IV phosphate therapy, especially when associated with serious clinical manifestations. Intravenous preparations include potassium phosphate (1.5 mEq potassium/mmol phosphate) and sodium phosphate (1.3 mEq sodium/mmol phosphate). An infusion of phosphate, 0.08 to 0.16 mmol/kg (elemental phosphorus, 2.5–5.0 mg/kg) in 500 mL 0.45% saline, is given IV over 6 hours. If hypotension occurs, hypocalcemia should be suspected and the infusion rate slowed. Plasma calcium, phosphate, and other electrolytes should be monitored frequently, as hypophosphatemia is often accompanied by hypomagnesemia and hypokalemia. IV infusion should be stopped when the plasma phosphorus level is >1.5 mg/dL or when PO therapy is possible. Because of the need to replenish intracellular stores, 24 to 36 hours of phosphate infusion may be required. Hyperphosphatemia must be avoided, as it can cause hypocalcemia and ectopic calcification. IV phosphate should be given cautiously in renal failure.

KEY POINTS TO REMEMBER

- Renal failure is the most common cause of hyperphosphatemia.
- Severe hyperphosphatemia leads to hypocalcemia, which can result in acute complications.
- Respiratory alkalosis, refeeding syndrome, and treatment of DKA are the leading causes of hypophosphatemia
- Treatment of hypophosphatemia is important to optimize diaphragmatic function in the setting of respiratory failure.

REFERENCES AND SELECTED READINGS

Bushinsky DA. Disorders of calcium and phosphorus homeostasis. In: Greenberg A, ed. *Primer on Kidney Diseases.* 4th ed. Philadelphia: Elsevier; 2005.

Goodman WG, Quarles LD. Mineral homeostasis and bone physiology. In: Olgaard K, ed. *Clinical Guide to Bone and Mineral Metabolism in CKD.* National Kidney Foundation; 2006.

Hruska KA. Hypophosphatemia and hyperphosphatemia. In: Dubose TD, Hamm LL, eds. *Acid–Base and Electrolyte Disorders.* Philadelphia: Elsevier; 2002.

Kraft MD, Btaiche IF, Sacks GS. Review of the refeeding syndrome. *Nutr Clin Pract.* 2005;20(6):625–633.

Acid-Base Disorders

Bala P. Sankarapandian

10

GENERAL APPROACH TO ACID-BASE DISORDERS

Acid-base disorders are commonly encountered in clinical medicine. Maintenance of acid-base status is essential for normal cellular function as proteins can change configuration and function with abnormal hydrogen ion concentrations [H^+]. The effective diagnosis and management of clinical acid-base disorders are best accomplished with a **stepwise approach** based on pathophysiology. A simple, six-step method can be used to identify and treat acid-base disturbances:

- **Step 1:** Identify the acid-base disorder (acidemia or alkalemia) from the pH in the arterial blood.
- **Step 2:** Examine the direction of change of the partial pressure of CO_2 (PCO_2) and the concentration of bicarbonate (HCO_3^-) from expected normal values.
- **Step 3:** Determine the anion gap (AG) and the expected HCO_3^- to help in the differential diagnosis of metabolic acidosis. By studying the relationship between AG and change in HCO_3^-, mixed disorders can be identified.
- **Step 4:** Differentiate whether the disorder is simple or mixed based on the compensatory responses of the PCO_2 or HCO_3^-.
- **Step 5:** Generate a differential diagnosis for the specific acid-base disorder to identify an etiology.

PHYSIOLOGY OF ACID-BASE BALANCE

Definitions

An **acid** is a substance that donates H^+ ions and a **base** is a substance that accepts H^+ ions. These properties are independent of charge. Acids and bases may be **strong** or **weak.** Strong acids and bases (i.e., hydrochloric acid or sodium hydroxide) are those that are almost completely ionized in the body.

Blood pH is the mathematic expression of the [H^+] of the blood. The **pH value is inversely related to the [H^+]**, as shown in the equation below. An increase in [H^+] reduces the pH; a decrease in [H^+] elevates the pH. Hydrogen ion concentration is usually expressed in nmol/L. The normal extracellular [H^+] is 40 nmol/L, correlating to a pH of 7.4. In general, the **range** of H^+ concentrations compatible with life is 16 to 160 nmol/L, or a blood pH between 7.80 and 6.80.

$$pH = -\log [H^+]$$

The relationship between arterial pH and [H^+] in the physiologic range is shown in Table 10-1. Within the physiologic range of pH, the [H^+] is estimated accurately as 80 minus the decimal of pH (e.g., at pH 7.30, the [H^+] = 80 − 30 or 50 nmol/L). **Acidemia** is an

TABLE 10-1	RELATIONSHIP BETWEEN PH AND [H+] IN THE PHYSIOLOGIC RANGE								
pH	7.80	7.70	7.60	7.50	7.40	7.30	7.20	7.10	6.90	6.80
[H+] (nmol/L)	16	20	26	32	40	50	63	80	125	160

increase in the [H+] or a decrease in the blood pH. **Alkalemia** is a decrease in the [H+] or an increase in the blood pH.

Measurement of blood pH using an arterial blood gas (ABG) is optimally determined on blood drawn anaerobically in a heparinized syringe. The blood pH should be measured rapidly.

Acid-Base Balance and Regulation

Based on a normal Western diet, the kidney must excrete approximately 1 mEq of acid/kg/day. The majority of the acid load is derived from sulfur-containing amino acids. Acid-base homeostasis or **maintenance of pH** occurs in three stages:

1. Chemical buffering by extracellular and intracellular buffers
2. Changes in alveolar ventilation to control the PCO_2
3. Alteration in net acid excretion (NAE) and HCO_3^- reabsorption to regulate plasma HCO_3^- concentration

Physiologic Buffer Systems

Buffering is the ability of a solution containing a weak or poorly dissociated acid and its base to resist change in pH when a strong acid or alkali is added. Buffers are located in the extracellular space, intracellular space, and in the bone. The HCO_3^-/CO_2 pool is the most important physiologic buffering system in the extracellular space. A portion of CO_2 is dissolved in arterial blood and combines with H_2O to form H_2CO_3, which dissociates into H^+ and HCO_3^-. These reactions require carbonic anhydrase to maintain the reactions in equilibrium. This system is able to buffer effectively because the PCO_2 can be regulated by alveolar ventilation.

$$CO_2 + H_2O \leftrightarrow H_2CO_3 \leftrightarrow H^+ + HCO_3^-$$

The **Henderson-Hasselbach equation** shows the pH as a mathematical relationship between HCO_3^- (derived from metabolic processes) and PCO_2 (derived from respiratory processes).

$$pH = 6.1 + \log [HCO_3^-]/(0.03 \times PCO_2)$$

Intracellular buffers are primarily proteins, organic and inorganic phosphates, and hemoglobin. The bone is an important site of buffering for acids and bases. As much as 40% of an acute acid load is buffered in bone. The acid load leads to the uptake of H^+ ions by bone, which causes the dissolution of bone mineral and the release of buffer compounds (e.g., calcium carbonate and calcium bicarbonate).

Regulation of Acid-Base Balance

- PCO_2 represents the **respiratory component** in the acid-base equation. Alveolar ventilation provides the oxygen necessary for oxidative metabolism and eliminates the CO_2 produced by these metabolic processes. Chemoreceptors in the brainstem and the carotid bulb regulate PCO_2 ventilation in response to changes in the pH.

The Pco_2 is normally set at 40 mm Hg. The level falls with increased ventilation and increases with decreased ventilation.

- **Bicarbonate** is the **metabolic component** of the acid-base equation, serving as the proton acceptor. The kidney regulates $[HCO_3^-]$ at approximately 24 mM, which is determined by the buffering state, NAE, and HCO_3^- reabsorption at the tubules. NAE is the net amount of H^+ eliminated from the body. This is accomplished through the elimination of titratable acids (dihydrogen phosphate) and nontitratable acids [ammonium ion (NH_4^+)]. The extracellular pH is the main regulator of NAE. However, under pathophysiologic conditions, effective circulatory volume, aldosterone, and plasma K^+ may affect acid excretion independent of pH. Humans can acidify their urine to a pH as low as 4.4.
- **Bicarbonate reabsorption** must be maximized to excrete the daily acid load. The majority (90%) of reabsorption occurs at the proximal tubule with each HCO_3^- ion reclaimed requiring the secretion of one H^+ ion. Bicarbonate reabsorption is regulated by plasma HCO_3^- levels and effective circulatory volume.
- Serum potassium is linked to acid-base metabolism at the level of cellular distribution, renal tubular handling, and GI transport. In metabolic acidosis, >50% of excess hydrogen ions are buffered in the cells in exchange for intracellular potassium transported to the extracellular fluid. On average, the **plasma potassium concentration rises by 0.6 mEq/L for every 0.1 unit reduction in pH.**

TABLE 10-2	EXPECTED COMPENSATORY RESPONSES FOR PRIMARY ACID-BASE DISTURBANCES	
Disorder	Primary Change	Compensatory Response
Metabolic acidosis	Decreased HCO_3^-	1.2-mm Hg decrease in Pco_2 for every 1-mEq/L fall in HCO_3^-
Metabolic alkalosis	Increased HCO_3^-	0.7-mm Hg increase in Pco_2 for every 1-mEq/L rise in HCO_3^-
Respiratory acidosis	Increased Pco_2	Increase in HCO_3^-
Acute	0.08 decrease in pH for every 10-mm Hg rise in Pco_2	1-mEq/L increase in HCO_3^- for every 10-mm Hg rise in Pco_2
Chronic	0.03 decrease in pH for every 10-mm Hg rise in Pco_2	3.5-mEq/L increase in HCO_3^- for every 10-mm Hg rise in Pco_2
Respiratory alkalosis	Decreased Pco_2	Decrease in HCO_3^-
Acute	0.08 increase in pH for every 10-mm Hg fall in Pco_2	2-mEq/L decrease in HCO_3^- for every 10-mm Hg fall in Pco_2
Chronic	0.03 increase in pH for every 10-mm Hg fall in Pco_2	4-mEq/L decrease in HCO_3^- for every 10-mm Hg fall in Pco_2

HCO_3^-, bicarbonate; Pco_2, partial pressure of CO_2.

Compensatory Responses for Primary Acid-Base Disturbances

A good understanding of expected compensatory responses to acid-base perturbations is critical to properly diagnosing acid-base disorders. Compensatory renal or respiratory responses (Table 10-2) minimize the change in pH by minimizing the alteration in the $[HCO_3^-]$ to $[PCO_2]$ ratio. For example, a high PCO_2 in respiratory acidosis leads to increased NAE and a compensatory elevation in plasma HCO_3^-. On the other hand, a low HCO_3^- in metabolic acidosis stimulates CNS chemoreceptors to induce increased ventilation. This leads to a compensatory reduction in PCO_2. **Note that compensations are never complete.** In other words, blood pH will not return to its initial value before the primary disturbance occurred, although the pH value, at times, can reach the normal range.

EVALUATION OF ACID-BASE DISORDERS

When an acid-base disorder is suspected, an **ABG** (pH, PCO_2, PO_2, and calculated HCO_3^-) and a venous serum **chemistry panel** (serum Na^+, K^+, Cl^-, and HCO_3^-) should be obtained. Assume normal pH of 7.4, PCO_2 of 40 mm Hg, and HCO_3^- of 24 mmol.

Primary Acid-Base Disorders

- Changes in pH and $[H^+]$ can be induced by alterations in HCO_3^- or PCO_2. Because PCO_2 is regulated by respiration, primary abnormalities in the PCO_2 are called **respiratory acidosis** (high PCO_2) and **respiratory alkalosis** (low PCO_2). In contrast, primary changes in plasma HCO_3^- are called **metabolic acidosis** (low HCO_3^-) and **metabolic alkalosis** (high HCO_3^-) (Table 10-3).
- The acid-base map (Fig. 10-1) describes the relationship between the arterial pH, H^+, plasma HCO_3^-, and PCO_2. The center area represents the range of normal values for these parameters. The stippled areas represent the different simple acid-base disturbances. Values between the stippled areas represent mixed acid-base disturbances, which are discussed below.
- The primary event in metabolic acidosis is a fall in HCO_3^- and the expected compensation is a fall in the PCO_2 through hyperventilation. *For example,* if pH = 7.10 and $HCO_3^- = 6$ (falls by 18 from normal value of 24 mmol/L), the PCO_2 would be expected to fall by 1.2 times as much, or 21 mm Hg (40 − 21), to a PCO_2 value of 19 mm Hg. Ultimate restoration of pH depends on the renal excretion of excess acid, a process that takes several days.
- The primary event in metabolic alkalosis is a rise in HCO_3^-. The expected compensation is a rise in the PCO_2 through hypoventilation. *For example,* if pH = 7.49 and $HCO_3^- = 40$ (rises by 16 from 24 mmol/L), the PCO_2 should rise by 0.7 times as much, or 11 mm Hg (40 + 11), to a PCO_2 value of 51 mm Hg. This compensation is limited by the body's response to the concomitant hypoxemia resulting from hypoventilation.

TABLE 10-3	SIMPLE ACID-BASE DISORDERS		
Type of Disorder	pH	Partial Pressure of CO_2	Bicarbonate
Metabolic acidosis	Decreased	Decreased	Decreased
Metabolic alkalosis	Increased	Increased	Increased
Respiratory acidosis	Decreased	Increased	Increased
Respiratory alkalosis	Increased	Decreased	Decreased

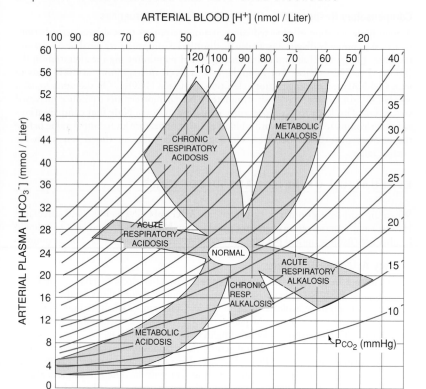

FIGURE 10-1. Acid-base map (see text). HCO_3^-, bicarbonate; PCO_2, partial pressure of CO_2; resp., respiratory. (From DuBose TD, Cogan MG, Rector FC Jr. Acid-base disorders. In: Brenner BM, ed. *Brenner and Rector's The Kidney*. 5th ed. Philadelphia: WB Saunders; 1996:949, with permission.)

- The primary event in respiratory acidosis is a rise in PCO_2. In the first 24 hours, only buffering contributes to the compensatory response. Thus, in acute respiratory acidosis, there may be a dramatic fall in pH. For example, in acute respiratory acidosis there is a simultaneous 0.08 fall in pH and 1 mEq/L rise in the bicarbonate level for every 10-mm Hg increase of PCO_2.
- After 3 to 5 days, the renal acid excretion reaches maximum compensatory response. In chronic respiratory acidosis, the values reach a new steady state (although not back to normal). Consequently there is only a 0.03 drop in pH, due to the kidney's ability to compensate with a 3.5-mEq increase in the bicarbonate level for every 10-mm Hg increase of PCO_2.
- The primary event in respiratory alkalosis is a fall in PCO_2. In acute respiratory alkalosis, there is a dramatic rise in pH given that buffering alone is contributing to compensatory response. There is a simultaneous 0.08 rise in pH and 2-mEq drop in HCO_3^- for every 10-mm Hg decrease in the PCO_2. However, in 3 to 5 days, the renal HCO_3^- dumping reaches maximum compensatory response. There is only a 0.03 rise in pH associated with a 4-mEq drop in HCO_3^- for every 10-mm Hg decrease in PCO_2.

METABOLIC ACIDOSIS

Metabolic acidosis is a clinical disorder characterized by low pH, low HCO_3^-, and compensatory hyperventilation resulting in low P_{CO_2}. Metabolic acidosis can be induced by three mechanisms: addition of a strong acid buffered by HCO_3^-, loss of HCO_3^- from body fluid, or the rapid addition of non-HCO_3^- solution to the extracellular fluid.

Initial Evaluation of Metabolic Acidosis: Anion Gap versus Nongap Acidosis

Calculation of the anion gap (AG) is very helpful in the differential diagnosis of metabolic acidosis (Table 10-4). The AG is equal to the difference between the plasma concentrations of the major cation (Na^+) and the major measured anions (Cl^- and HCO_3^-).

$$AG = [Na^+] - ([Cl^-] + [HCO_3^-])$$

Therefore, the AG is equal to the difference between the *measured* anions and cations. The normal AG is between 10 ± 3 mEq/L. Most of the missing anions are from the negative charges of plasma albumin. A fall in serum albumin of 1 g/dL from normal of 4 g/dL decreases the AG by 2.5 mEq/L. An increase in the AG is usually caused by an elevation in amounts of unmeasured anions. It can also be produced by a fall in unmeasured cations (hypocalcemia, hypokalemia, or hypomagnesemia). *Hyperchloremic metabolic acidosis* results if there is HCO_3^- loss, there is an associated increase in plasma chloride, and the AG is unchanged.

Anion Gap Metabolic Acidosis

AG metabolic acidosis encompasses disorders of organic acidosis resulting from increased acid production. In many cases, the recognition and treatment of these disorders is critical to patient care.

- *Lactic acidosis* is the best example of clinical organic acidosis. Under normal conditions, humans produce relatively small amounts of lactate, the final production of

TABLE 10-4	DIFFERENTIAL DIAGNOSIS OF METABOLIC ACIDOSIS
Normal Anion Gap (hyperchloremic)	**Increased Anion Gap (organic)**
GI loss of HCO_3^-	Increased acid production
Diarrhea	Lactic acidosis
Intestinal fistula or drainage	Ketoacidosis
Ureterosigmoidostomy	Failure of acid excretion
Anion exchange resins	5-Oxoprolinemia
Ingestion of calcium chloride or magnesium chloride	Renal failure
	Toxic alcohol ingestion
Renal loss of HCO_3^-	Ethanol
Renal tubular acidosis	Methanol
Carbonic anhydrase inhibitor	Propylene glycol
Hypoaldosteronism	Ethylene glycol
Potassium-sparing diuretics	Other ingestions
Miscellaneous	Salicylate
Recovery from ketoacidosis	Paraldehyde
Dilutional acidosis	Isoniazid
Addition of hydrochloric acid	
Parenteral alimentation	

HCO_3^-, bicarbonate.

anaerobic metabolism of pyruvate. The key causes of lactic acidosis are decrease in tissue oxygenation (e.g., hypoxemia, septic shock), excessive energy expenditures (e.g., seizures, hyperthermia), deranged oxidative metabolism (e.g., intoxications, malignancy), impaired lactate clearance (e.g., liver failure), or D-lactic acidosis production by D-lactic acid–producing organisms. A separate assay for D-lactate should be ordered if clinical suspicion is high (e.g., blind loop syndromes) as the standard lactate assay does not detect this isomer. Treatment of lactic acidosis must be directed at the underlying cause. Therapy with HCO_3^- has not been found to be effective clinically and may even have deleterious effects.

- *Diabetic ketoacidosis (DKA)* results from a lack of sufficient insulin to metabolize glucose and short-chain fatty acids. Fatty acids are instead oxidized to the ketoacids (beta-hydroxybutyric and acetoacetic acid), resulting in acid-base disturbance. Ketoacids are relatively strong acids and dissociate almost completely, causing a metabolic acidosis with an elevated AG. Initially, the AG may parallel the decrease in HCO_3^- level. With therapy, dissociation between the AG and the decrease in HCO_3^- concentration develops. DKA evolves to a mixed high-gap and hyperchloremic acidosis due to renal elimination of the ketoacid anions as renal perfusion improves with volume restoration. The diagnosis of DKA is made by the combination of AG metabolic acidosis, hyperglycemia, and the presence of serum or urine ketones. The diagnostic test to detect ketones uses a nitroprusside reagent that reacts with acetoacetate only. In DKA, the ratio of beta-hydroxybutyric acid to acetoacetic acid is 5:2. During treatment of DKA, the formation of acetoacetate is favored, so the nitroprusside test may falsely demonstrate a rise in ketones as this ratio varies. The mainstays of therapy for DKA are insulin, volume repletion, and the management of electrolyte abnormalities. Bicarbonate therapy has not been found to improve outcome in limited clinical trials. In addition, there is a significant chance of overshoot alkalemia if HCO_3^- therapy is administered while metabolism of ketoacids leads to HCO_3^- generation.

- *Alcohol or starvation ketoacidosis* should be suspected in patients with a history of alcohol abuse with an unexplained high-AG metabolic acidosis and, often, with a superimposed metabolic alkalosis and respiratory alkalosis. The combination of alcohol ingestion and poor dietary intake is the cause of the ketoacidosis. The ratio of beta-hydroxybutyric acid to acetoacetic acid is up to 20:1. Therefore, the nitroprusside test may grossly underestimate the degree of ketoacidemia in these patients. Therapy consists of vigorous volume, glucose, and electrolyte repletion.

- *Toxic alcohol ingestions* that lead to high-AG acidosis include **methanol** and **ethylene glycol**. Delay in the diagnosis may be associated with considerable mortality and morbidity so early diagnosis is critical for successful therapy. Methanol and ethylene glycol are low-molecular-weight alcohols that readily enter cells. The metabolites are formate (with methanol) or glycolate (with ethylene glycol) and are responsible for the high AG. Initial acid-base status may be normal soon after ingestion. A clue to this early stage is an increased *osmolar gap*. This is defined as the difference between the measured serum osmolality and the calculated osmolality:

$$\text{Calculated serum osmolality} = 2[Na^+] + [glucose]/18 + [urea]/2.8$$

A difference of >15 to 20 mOsm/kg suggests toxic alcohol ingestion. An osmolar gap can also be due to other conditions that are not associated with a high-AG acidosis, including ethanol and isopropyl alcohol. Patients with methanol poisoning present with abdominal pain, vomiting, headache, and visual disturbances (optic neuritis). Ethylene glycol intoxication is similar to that of methanol but does not produce optic neuritis. Calcium oxalate crystals (metabolite of ethylene glycol) in the urine also suggest ethylene glycol intoxication. Most morbidity of methanol and ethylene glycol results from damage mediated by metabolites. Thus, blocking the metabolism is of prime importance to treat these ingestions. This can be done by use of fomepizole (4-methylpyrazole). Fomepizole blocks alcohol dehydrogenase, thereby retarding metabolism of methanol and ethylene glycol. Hemodialysis may also be required to correct severe metabolic abnormalities and to enhance toxic metabolite elimination.

- *Salicylate overdose* can lead to serious and complex acid-base disturbances. Symptoms include nausea, vomiting, tinnitus, altered mental status, coma, and death; these symptoms correlate poorly with plasma levels but almost always are present with very high levels (>50 mg/dL). Treatment includes HCO_3^- infusion to alkalinize the urine to reduce symptoms and promote renal excretion. Hemodialysis should be considered for patients with extremely high levels, severe symptoms, significant renal failure, or refractory acidosis. Acetaminophen ingestion is sometimes associated with an increased AG acidosis due to the accumulation of **5-oxoproline (pyroglytamic acid)**. Glutathione metabolism is thought to be the mechanism. Cessation of the drug leads to resolution of the problem.

- *Acute or chronic renal failure* may lead to high-AG acidosis. Failure to excrete the daily acid load by retention of anions (e.g., phosphates, sulfates) is the pathogenesis of metabolic acidosis. For both acute and chronic renal failure, the AG rises more slowly than the HCO_3^- level drops. In acute renal failure, the HCO_3^- level falls by approximately 0.5 mEq/L/day unless hypercatabolism increases daily acid production. In chronic renal failure, the AG rises by approximately 0.5 mEq/L for each 1-mg/dL rise in serum creatinine.

Nongap (Hyperchloremic) Metabolic Acidosis

- Nongap (hyperchloremic) metabolic acidosis can be caused by three groups of disorders: GI HCO_3^- loss, renal HCO_3^- loss, and miscellaneous causes (inorganic acid intake or dilutional acidosis).

- *Urine anion gap* analysis may help differentiate causes of normal-AG metabolic acidosis. The urine AG is the difference between the measured cations (Na and K) and anions (Cl) in the urine. The value is calculated with the following formula:

$$Urine\ AG = [Na^+] + [K^+] - [Cl^-]$$

As with the plasma anion gap, the urine contains other unmeasured cations and anions. The critical unmeasured cation in the urine is ammonium ion (NH_4^+). In physiologic states with normal acid-base handling, the urine AG has a slightly positive value (0 to approximately 30). In states of acidosis, the kidney normally increases ammonia production to allow enhanced excretion of the acid load. Higher urine ammonium concentration is balanced by higher Cl levels. Thus, with an appropriately high ammonium in the urine, the urine AG becomes negative because the chloride concentration exceeds Na + K. If urinary acidification is inadequate due to renal tubular acidosis (RTA), the urine ammonium levels remain low and the urine AG remains positive. GI loss of HCO_3^- typically results in a negative urine AG. Diarrhea and fistulas are the most common causes of hyperchloremic metabolic acidosis. The intestinal fluid below the stomach is relatively alkaline; the intestinal lining absorbs chloride and secretes HCO_3^-.

- *Renal tubular acidosis (RTA)* is a heterogeneous group of disorders defined by the presence of metabolic acidosis due to diminished net acid excretion by the kidney *despite a normal glomerular filtration rate.* Non-AG acidosis associated with decreased kidney function is not included in this classification system and not called RTA. The problems that lead to RTA center on an inability to secrete H^+ and/or impaired

TABLE 10-5	CHARACTERISTICS OF RENAL TUBULAR ACIDOSIS		
	Type I (classic distal)	Type II (proximal)	Type IV (distal hyperkalemic)
Basic defect	Decreased distal acidification	Diminished proximal HCO_3^- reabsorption	Aldosterone resistance or deficiency
Urine pH	>5.3	Variable: >5.3 if above reabsorptive threshold; <5.3 if below	Usually <5.3
Plasma HCO_3^-	<10 mEq/L	14–20 mEq/L	>15 mEq/L
Plasma K^+	Usually reduced or normal	Usually reduced or normal	Elevated
Diagnosis	Response to $NaHCO_3$ or ammonium chloride	Response to $NaHCO_3$	Measure aldosterone
Nonelectrolyte abnormalities	Nephrocalcinosis, rickets, renal stones	Osteomalacia	Associated with diabetes mellitus

HCO_3^-, bicarbonate; $NaHCO_3$, sodium hydrogen carbonate.

HCO_3 reabsorption. Based on pathophysiologic mechanisms, RTA can be classified as follows (Table 10-5):

- **Type I (classic distal) RTA** is characterized by defects in secretion, permeability, or voltage gradients resulting in the inability of the kidney to excrete hydrogen. Except for the voltage-type defects, in all other forms of type I RTA, potassium becomes the preferred cation for excretion, leading to hypokalemia. The main causes of type I RTA are hypercalcemia, nephrocalcinosis, autoimmune diseases (especially Sjögren syndrome), drugs (amphotericin B, lithium, and ifosphamide), and toxins like toluene. It can also occur as a primary disorder in children and can be hereditary. The diagnosis is based on the inability to lower the urine pH to <5.4 and the response to $NaHCO_3$ treatment. When bicarbonate therapy is given, the urine pH and fractional excretion of HCO_3^- remain constant as the plasma HCO_3^- increases. Treatment for type I RTA is indicated to correct the acidosis and minimize stone formation and nephrocalcinosis. In adults, 1 to 2 mEq/kg/day of alkali is usually necessary.
- **Type II (proximal) RTA** is an uncommon disorder due to the impairment of proximal tubular reabsorption of HCO_3^-. Increased delivery of bicarbonate to the distal nephron leads to substantial potassium and sodium loss as well. Type II RTA is a self-limiting disorder because the reabsorptive capacity of HCO_3^- in the distal nephron remains intact. Therefore, the plasma HCO_3^- concentration will drop to between 14 and 20 mEq/L resulting in a lowered filtered load that will not exceed reabsorption capacity. At this point, acidification will return to normal in the distal nephron. Therefore, the urine pH is variable depending on whether bicarbonate escapes proximal reabsorption. Infusion of bicarbonate should raise the plasma HCO_3^- level, urinary pH, and the fractional excretion of HCO_3^- thereby establishing the diagnosis. The main causes include hereditary causes (e.g., Wilson disease, cystinosis), metal

toxicity (lead, cadmium, mercury), and multiple myeloma or amyloidosis. **Fanconi syndrome** refers to type II RTA in the setting of more global proximal tubule dysfunction with impairment of glucose, amino acid, and phosphate reabsorption. In children, treatment may require large amounts of alkali (10–25 mEq/kg/day) to avoid growth retardation and osteopenia from the acidosis.

- **Type IV (distal hyperkalemic) RTA** refers to metabolic acidosis from aldosterone deficiency or resistance. Hypoaldosteronism (e.g., primary or secondary to diabetes mellitus) impairs distal hydrogen and potassium secretion leading to hyperkalemic metabolic acidosis. Hyperkalemia may also suppress NH_4^+ synthesis in the proximal tubule further worsening the kidneys' ability to excrete an acid load. Generalized tubular defects like obstructive uropathy, cyclosporine, or lupus may also result in type IV RTA by affecting H^+ secretion at the cortical collecting duct. Treatment options for patients with hyperkalemia and metabolic acidosis include a low-potassium diet, sodium bicarbonate replacement, and loop diuretics. Patients with hypoaldosteronism often require mineralcorticoid replacement. Patients with general tubular defects usually do not have a significant degree of acidosis but may require treatment for the hyperkalemia.

- *Other causes. Dilutional acidosis* is due to the rapid expansion of extracellular space with non-HCO_3^- fluid. The fall in HCO_3^- level is usually small and quickly corrected by renal generation of HCO_3^-. *Parenteral alimentation of amino acids* without concomitant administration of alkali may produce hyperchloremic metabolic acidosis. This can be avoided by replacing the chloride salt of amino acids with acetate salt. The acetate is then metabolized to HCO_3^- and replaces that which was consumed in amino acid metabolism. *Ingestion of sulfur* or other inorganic acids can cause profound hyperchloremic metabolic acidosis.

Treatment of Metabolic Acidosis

Treatment of metabolic acidosis is usually best accomplished by treating the underlying disease. In certain situations (e.g., lactic acidosis or DKA), alkali therapy is not beneficial and may be deleterious. However, in patients with severe acidosis, rapid administration of HCO_3^- may be necessary for cardiovascular stability. With severe acidemia, the initial goal is to raise the pH to >7.20. The amount of HCO_3^- required to correct the acidemia can be estimated by the HCO_3^- deficit:

$$HCO_3^- \text{ deficit} = HCO_3^- \text{ space (L)} \times (\text{desired } HCO_3^- - \text{actual } HCO_3^-)$$

where HCO_3^- space (theoretic volume of HCO_3^- distribution) = $0.5-0.8 \times$ body weight in kg.

The HCO_3^- space is not constant but increases with increasing severity of the acidosis. In normal state, this space is 50% of body weight but increases to as high as 80% in severe acidosis (bicarbonate <10 mEq/L). This results from greater use of nonbicarbonate buffers as acidosis worsens. In acute settings, IV sodium HCO_3^- (50 mEq in 50-mL ampules) can be given as a bolus or continuous infusion (2–3 ampules mixed in D_5W). In chronic metabolic acidosis, oral alkali can be given as sodium bicarbonate tablets, or as sodium or potassium citrate solution. Typical starting doses would be sodium bicarbonate 650 mg 2 to 3 times daily (16–24 mEq/day) with the dose increased if necessary.

METABOLIC ALKALOSIS

Initiation and Maintenance of Metabolic Alkalosis

Metabolic alkalosis is a clinical disorder characterized by elevated pH due to an increase in HCO_3^-. Compensatory hypoventilation results in a rise of PCO_2. Metabolic alkalosis can be generated by three mechanisms: net loss of H^+, net addition of HCO_3^-, or the external loss of fluid containing chloride (contraction alkalosis). The kidney has the ability to ultimately correct metabolic alkalosis by the excretion of excess HCO_3^-. Therefore, the perpetuation of metabolic alkalosis requires impairment of renal HCO_3^- excretion. Factors that act to maintain metabolic alkalosis include decreased effective circulatory volume, hyperaldosteronism, hypokalemia, chloride depletion, and hypercapnia.

Differential Diagnosis of Metabolic Alkalosis

Disorders of metabolic alkalosis can be divided into *chloride-responsive* (chloride depletion acts as a maintenance factor), *chloride-resistant* (chloride depletion does not act as a maintenance factor), and *unclassified* categories (Table 10-6).

Chloride-Responsive Metabolic Alkalosis
Chloride-responsive metabolic alkalosis occurs in volume-depleted states with low urine chloride levels (<25 mEq). In metabolic alkalosis, urine chloride levels may be a more accurate determination of volume state than are urine sodium levels. *Vomiting or gastric drainage* is a common cause of metabolic alkalosis. Gastric secretions contain as much as 100 mmol/L of acid. Gastric parietal cells generate one HCO_3^- molecule for each H^+ secreted. *Diuretics* that exert their effect at the thick, ascending limb of the loop of Henle (loop diuretics) or at the distal tubule (thiazide diuretics) stimulate H^+ secretion through renin/aldosterone to initiate metabolic alkalosis. Also, these diuretics maintain metabolic alkalosis by volume depletion. The urinary chloride level may be elevated if it is obtained while the diuretic is still in effect. However, more than 24 to 48 hours after the last diuretic dose, the urine chloride is appropriately low, reflecting volume depletion. In the *posthypercapnic state*, the renal compensation to chronic hypercapnia is an elevation in HCO_3^-. When hypercapnia is corrected too quickly, the patient has an elevated level of HCO_3^- until renal readjustment can occur.

Chloride-Resistant Metabolic Alkalosis
Chloride-resistant metabolic alkalosis occurs in euvolemic states and is associated with elevated urine chloride levels (>40 mEq/L). *Primary hyperaldosteronism* leads to hypokalemic metabolic alkalosis secondary to aldosterone stimulation of distal H^+ secretion. This occurs often in concert with hypertension and volume expansion. *Cushing syndrome* is characterized by an increase in corticosteroid synthesis. Many of these corticosteroids have considerable mineralocorticoid effects to produce hypokalemic metabolic alkalosis. *Black licorice* contains *glycyrrhizic acid* that up-regulates renal mineralocorticoid receptors to mimic primary hyperaldosteronism. *Bartter syndrome* is a rare condition presenting in children with increased renin levels and hyperaldosteronism without hypertension or sodium

TABLE 10-6	TYPES OF METABOLIC ALKALOSIS	
Chloride Responsive	**Chloride Resistant**	**Unclassified**
Vomiting	Hyperaldosteronism	Alkali administration
Gastric drainage	Cushing syndrome	Milk-alkali syndrome
Villous adenoma	Bartter/Gitelman syndrome	Massive transfusion of
Chloride diarrhea		blood products
Diuretics	Black licorice	Hypercalcemia
Posthypercapnia Cystic	Profound potassium	Refeeding syndrome
fibrosis Cation-exchange	depletion	
resins (e.g., antacids)		

retention. The disease occurs due to mutations in the $Na^+/K^+/2Cl^-$ channel in the thick ascending limb of the loop of Henle, leading to Na^+, K^+, and Cl^- wasting. Bartter syndrome may be difficult to distinguish from surreptitious diuretic use and may require screening urine for presence of diuretics.

Unclassified Metabolic Alkalosis

Administration of HCO_3^- or organic anions that metabolize into HCO_3^- (citrate or acetate) can lead to metabolic alkalosis, especially in patients with renal insufficiency. *Milk-alkali syndrome* is seen in patients who consume a large amount of antacids containing calcium and alkali (e.g., calcium carbonate). Hypercalcemia decreases PTH-mediated HCO_3^- loss and also causes alkalosis through contraction. This may be supported by decreased glomerular filtration rate. In addition, the alkalosis acts to reduce calcium excretion and enhances the effect of hypercalcemia. *Massive transfusion* of blood products (>10 U packed RBCs) can produce moderate metabolic alkalosis secondary to elevated citrate that metabolizes into HCO_3^-. Similarly, metabolic alkalosis may be seen in patients undergoing plasmapheresis, as replacement plasma has citrate.

Treatment of Metabolic Alkalosis

- Treatment should be directed at the underlying disease. However, when the pH elevation becomes life threatening (>7.60), rapid reduction in pH can be achieved by hemodialysis. In these acute settings, administration of hydrochloric acid or other acids is not advocated due to significant potential complications. For nonurgent cases, therapy is based on whether the case is chloride responsive or chloride resistant.
- Chloride-responsive metabolic alkalosis responds to the administration of oral or IV sodium chloride in 0.9% or 0.45% solution with potassium supplements. This lowers the plasma HCO_3^- level by reversing the contraction alkalosis, decreasing sodium retention, and promoting HCO_3^- excretion. The optimal rate of fluid replacement is approximately 50 to 100 mL/hour in excess of the sum of all sensible and insensible losses. In addition, for gastric causes, the use of H_2-blockers or proton-pump inhibitors minimizes the gastric acid loss. For diuretic-induced metabolic alkalosis, the use of potassium-sparing diuretics can reduce the degree of the acid-base disturbance.
- Chloride-resistant metabolic alkalosis does not respond to the administration of volume. In edematous states (e.g., patient with heart failure on diuretics), the administration of saline may not be an option. Carbonic anhydrase may be required to decrease the severity of the contraction alkalosis. Acetazolamide (250–375 mg PO daily or b.i.d.) is a carbonic anhydrase inhibitor that increases the renal excretion of HCO_3^-. The effect can be assessed by monitoring urine pH, which should increase to >7.0. For mineralocorticoid excess states, successful treatment requires restoration of normal mineralocorticoid activity, including surgical removal of an adrenal adenoma or by the use of potassium-sparing diuretics in addition to potassium supplements. Bartter syndrome may respond to NSAIDs, potassium-sparing diuretics, and potassium supplements.

RESPIRATORY ACIDOSIS

Respiratory acidosis is a disorder caused by processes that increase Pco_2, resulting in a decrease in pH and a compensatory increase in HCO_3^-. The increase in Pco_2 is due to decreased alveolar ventilation. The physiologic buffer systems generate the immediate response to the low pH during the acute phase. Over the next several days, renal compensation is initiated through an increase in NAE termed the *chronic phase*. The third response to respiratory acidosis is the restoration of effective ventilation.

Acute Respiratory Acidosis

Acute respiratory acidosis results from acute alveolar hypoventilation when only the buffering defense is available. Patients may present with tachypnea, restlessness, stupor, and even coma. Causes of respiratory acidosis include neuromuscular abnormalities, airway obstruction, thoracic-pulmonary disorders, vascular disease, and mechanical ventilation. The key to treatment is restoration of effective ventilation.

Chronic Respiratory Acidosis

Chronic respiratory acidosis is caused by chronic decreased effective alveolar ventilation. Over time, the renal compensatory mechanisms operate at maximal capacity. Most common causes are thoracic-pulmonary disorders (e.g., COPD) and neuromuscular abnormalities. Treatment is difficult, but maximizing pulmonary function may lead to significant improvement. When a patient in a steady state of chronic hypercapnia suffers a new insult, the P_{CO_2} acutely rises. This is termed *acute respiratory acidosis superimposed on chronic respiratory acidosis.*

RESPIRATORY ALKALOSIS

Respiratory alkalosis is a disorder caused by processes that decrease P_{CO_2}, resulting in an increase in pH and a compensatory decrease in HCO_3^-. The decrease in P_{CO_2} is due to increased alveolar ventilation. The buffering response constitutes the acute phase, and the renal response defines the chronic stage of respiratory alkalosis. The third response to respiratory alkalosis is the restoration of appropriate ventilation. Respiratory alkalosis is the most common acid-base disorder in seriously ill patients.

Acute Respiratory Alkalosis

Acute respiratory alkalosis results from acute alveolar hyperventilation when only the buffering defense is available. Patients may present with paresthesias, muscle cramps, tinnitus, and even seizures. Causes of respiratory alkalosis include central stimulation of respiration (e.g., fever, anxiety, and head trauma), peripheral stimulation of respiration (e.g., pulmonary embolism, pneumonia), liver insufficiency, sepsis, and mechanical ventilation. The key to therapy is treating the underlying cause. Correcting significant hypoxemia may be more important than the acid-base disturbance.

Chronic Respiratory Alkalosis

Chronic respiratory alkalosis is caused by chronic increased effective alveolar ventilation. During this period, the renal compensatory mechanisms are fully exerted.

SOME EXAMPLES OF MIXED ACID-BASE DISTURBANCES AND THEIR EVALUATION

A Simple Change in Medicines

A patient with chronic lung disease with edema received diuretics. An ABG done a week previous was pH, 7.38; P_{CO_2}, 50 mm Hg; and HCO_3^-, 29 mmol/L. He presents now with weakness, dizziness, and a low blood pressure. His ABG is pH, 7.46; P_{CO_2}, 56 mm Hg; and HCO_3^-, 39 mmol/L. A review of his baseline laboratory values reveals a mild respiratory acidosis with adequate metabolic compensation. The change was introduction of diuretics.

- **Step 1:** pH is elevated, indicating alkalemia.
- **Step 2:** HCO_3^- is elevated, indicating metabolic alkalosis. The P_{CO_2} is elevated as well, but this signifies an acidosis of respiratory origin. As the pH is alkalemic, the

primary change in this acid-base disorder is a metabolic alkalosis, and the elevated P_{CO_2} (above baseline) is an attempt at compensation.

- **Step 3:** Information for calculation of AG is not given, so it is assumed to be within normal limits.
- **Step 4:** The next step is to gauge the appropriateness of the compensatory response: Acutely, if the HCO_3^- changed 10 mmol/L, the expected change in the P_{CO_2} would be to 57 mm Hg (Table 10-2), which is quite close to this patient's value.
- **Step 5:** It appears that this patient with chronic compensated respiratory acidosis developed an acute metabolic alkalosis. Given the clinical circumstances, it is clear that the diuretic therapy caused hypovolemia and a contraction alkalosis, making the pH alkalemic.
- **Step 6:** Appropriate therapy is withdrawal of diuretics and volume repletion.

Mind the Gaps

A 25-year-old female with acute respiratory distress syndrome in the medical ICU requires inverse ratio ventilation to maintain adequate oxygenation. Two days after initiation of this therapy, her morning ABG reads pH, 7.12; P_{CO_2}, 38 mm Hg; HCO_3^-, 12 mmol/L. Other laboratory data: Na, 130 mmol/L; Cl, 93 mmol/L; K, 5.0 mmol/L; BUN, 40 mg/dL; glucose, 100 mg/dL.

- **Step 1:** pH is very low, indicating severe acidemia.
- **Step 2:** HCO_3^- is quite low, suggesting metabolic acidosis.
- **Step 3:** The patient has a significant AG (25). The HCO_3^- level is appropriate for the gap.
- **Step 4:** P_{CO_2} is slightly decreased; however, no evident compensation has occurred.
- **Step 5:** Thus, a formulation is made for severe anion gap metabolic acidosis without compensation.

Her renal function is normal as are lactic acid levels; serum ketones are not detectable. Serum osmolality is noted to be 330 mOsm/L. As her calculated osmolality is 280 mOsm/L, she has an osmolal gap of 50, which is abnormal. However, most of the usual offenders that can cause an elevated osmolal gap (ethanol, methanol, ethylene glycol, and so forth) are unlikely here, as the patient is in an ICU. The offending agent is identified after a careful review of medicines: The patient was started on high-dose infusions of lorazepam to enhance sedation during inverse ratio ventilation. Lorazepam infusions contain propylene glycol, which can cause a metabolic acidosis with AGs and osmolal gaps should sufficiently high doses be used. Such high doses are sometimes required in the ICU, exposing the patient to the risk of propylene glycol toxicity. Propylene glycol levels can be measured and correlate quite strongly with osmolality and osmolal gap.

A Gap in the Gap

A 25-year-old diabetic was admitted to the ICU with profound ketoacidosis, pH of 7.1, and AG of 25. Treatment was started with IV saline and insulin infusion. A few hours later, the following ABG results are received: pH, 7.28; P_{CO_2}, 28 mm Hg; HCO_3^-, 13 mEq/L; and AG, 18.

- **Step 1:** pH is decreased, suggesting acidemia.
- **Step 2:** HCO_3^- is low, suggesting metabolic acidosis. P_{CO_2} is low, reflecting respiratory compensation for the acidemia.
- **Step 3:** The AG is 18. Expected HCO_3^- for this AG is 19 (taking 12 as normal AG and 25 as normal HCO_3^- value). However, the observed HCO_3^- is 13. This suggests the presence of a non-AG metabolic acidosis in addition to an AG metabolic acidosis and respiratory compensation.

- **Step 4:** Expected P_{CO_2} is 28 mm Hg. As observed P_{CO_2} is 28 mm Hg as well, the compensatory response is appropriate.
- **Step 5:** It is clear that the patient who presented with an AG metabolic acidosis now has a non-AG acidosis in addition, with persistent (albeit improved) acidemia and appropriate respiratory compensation. Two fundamentally important factors in addressing a metabolic acidosis are to look for an AG and to decide if the acidosis is entirely due to the gap process or to a combination of a gap acidosis along with a nongap acidosis. Matching the observed HCO_3^- to the expected HCO_3^- for the gap observed helps in detecting a hidden nongap acidosis.

The development of nongap acidoses is common in ketoacidosis due to ketoacid metabolism of and excretion in the urine. Administration of insulin helps metabolize the ketone bodies to HCO_3^-. The HCO_3^- generated is used to buffer intracellular acidosis. Thus, although the AG closes (due to the removal of ketones), the HCO_3^- level and acidemia lag behind, accounting for the nongap acidosis.

When All Is Not What It Seems

At times, mixed acid-base disorders can be difficult to detect if not carefully and systematically scrutinized. A patient in the ICU developed pancreatitis, and nasogastric suction was instituted for 2 to 3 days. The course was complicated by sepsis and shock. The following laboratory values were received: pH, 7.41; P_{CO_2}, 40 mm Hg; HCO_3^-, 25 mEq/L; Na, 140 mmol/L; and Cl, 90 mmol/L. The pH, P_{CO_2}, and HCO_3^- values are in the normal range. Thus, if the casual observer decided to stop here, the fact that there is an AG of 25 would be completely missed.

The presence of an AG is strong evidence of a metabolic acidosis. Expected HCO_3^- for an AG of 25 is 12 mEq/L. The HCO_3^- level in this patient is 25, suggesting a coexisting metabolic alkalosis.

A review of the clinical scenario explains the acid-base abnormalities: The metabolic alkalosis was generated by nasogastric suction. At this point, septic shock developed. The resulting metabolic acidosis counterbalanced the pH and HCO_3^- concentration. This is a good example of a mixed disorder with a metabolic alkalosis and abnormal AG.

Triple acid-base disorders are combinations of metabolic acidosis and alkalosis with either respiratory acidosis or respiratory alkalosis. (The two respiratory disorders cannot coexist; one can either breathe fast or slow!)

KEY POINTS TO REMEMBER

- Acid-base disorders are commonly encountered. A systematic approach makes analysis and management simple.
- In any acid-base disorder, it is important to check the AG as this may be the only indication of an abnormality (see **Some Examples of Mixed Acid-Base Disturbances and Their Evaluation,** above).
- When allocating primary and compensatory responses in mixed acid-base disturbances, it is important to estimate the adequacy of the response.
- Calculating a urine AG helps identify non-AG acidosis.
- In assessing urine electrolytes in cases of metabolic alkalosis, it is not advisable to look at the urine sodium. An obligate loss with the HCO_3^- being filtered may lead to high urine sodium even in the face of volume contraction. Urine chloride is preferred in this case.

REFERENCES AND SUGGESTED READINGS

Adrogué HJ, Madias NE. Medical progress: management of life-threatening acid–base disorders—first of two parts. *N Engl J Med.* 1998;338:26–34.

Adrogué HJ, Madias NE. Medical progress: management of life-threatening acid–base disorders—second of two parts. *N Engl J Med.* 1998;338:107–111.

DuBose T, Hamm L. *Acid-Base and Electrolyte Disorders: A Companion to Brenner and Rector's The Kidney.* Philadelphia: WB Saunders; 2002.

Halperin M, Goldstein M. *Fluid, Electrolyte, and Acid-Base Physiology: A Problem-Based Approach.* 3rd ed. Philadelphia: WB Saunders; 1999.

Rose B, Narins R, Post, T. *Clinical Physiology of Acid-Base and Electrolyte Disorders.* New York: McGraw-Hill, Medical Publishing Division; 2001.

Schrier R. *Renal and Electrolyte Disorders.* 6th ed. Philadelphia: Lippincott Williams & Wilkins; 2003.

Overview and Management of Acute Kidney Injury and Acute Tubular Necrosis

11

Anitha Vijayan

DEFINITION AND STAGING

The term *acute kidney injury* (AKI) denotes the loss of renal function over hours to days, resulting in accumulation of nitrogenous waste products and disruption of volume, electrolyte, and acid-base homeostasis. AKI is synonymous with the historical term *acute renal failure* (ARF) and is increasingly replacing ARF in recent literature. The term AKI was first proposed in 2004, by Acute Dialysis Quality Initiative (ADQI) and experts from other premier nephrology and critical care associations. The newer term reflects the fact that a rise in serum creatinine does not necessarily mean *failure* of the kidneys, but a *dysfunction*, which may or may not lead to failure. The term *kidney* helps with the general public's understanding of the disease, similar to the chronic kidney disease (CKD) nomenclature update in 2002.

An exact definition of AKI or ARF has varied from study to study and this lack of uniformity has hindered the design and conduct of clinical trials in AKI. The recently formed group, Acute Kidney Injury Network (AKIN), has defined AKI as: **An abrupt (within 48 hours) reduction in kidney function—a rise in serum creatinine (SCr) by ≥0.3 mg/dL, a percentage increase in SCr of ≥50% from baseline, or documented oliguria of <0.5 mL/kg/hour for more than 6 hours.** The AKIN group also modified the RIFLE criteria (Risk, Injury, Failure, Loss, and ESRD) proposed by ADQI to include a classification or staging system for AKI (Table 11-1).

ACUTE KIDNEY INJURY

Spectrum and Epidemiology

Loss of renal function can be due to many different pathophysiologic processes. Generally, AKI is a disease of the hospitalized patient with incidence varying from 5% in the overall hospital population up to 25% in patients in the intensive care unit (ICU). The incidence varies significantly according to the various definitions used in the literature. In contrast, only 1% of patients being admitted to the hospital present with AKI. AKI is associated with high mortality, which has not changed significantly in the last 55 years. The average mortality quoted in the literature is anywhere from 45% to 60%. Studies have demonstrated that AKI is an independent factor contributing to the mortality and not just an innocent bystander as previously believed. In a study of hospitalized patients who received intravenous (IV) radiocontrast procedures, the risk of mortality was increased 5.5-fold in those who developed AKI (compared with patients who did not develop renal injury), after accounting for comorbid conditions. Some of the other possible reasons for the persistent poor survival rates include the following:

- Inadequate dialysis prescription. Studies have shown that prescribed dialysis efficiency is rarely achieved in AKI. Also, it is possible that more intensive dialysis is required in the sicker AKI patients compared with more stable chronic dialysis patients.

TABLE 11-1	CLASSIFICATION/STAGING SYSTEM FOR AKI	
Stage	**Serum Creatinine Criteria**	**Urine Output Criteria**
1	Rise in SCr ≥0.3 mg/dL or ≥150–200% from baseline	<0.5 mL/kg/h for >6 h <0.5 mL/kg/h for >12 h
2	Rise in SCr >200–300% from baseline	<0.3 mL/kg/h for >24 h
3	Rise in SCr >300% from baseline, or SCr >4 mg/dL with an acute increase of at least 0.5 mg/dL	or anuria >12 h

From Mehta RL, Kellum JA, Shah SV, Molitoris BA, Ronco C, Warnock DG, Levin A; the Acute Kidney Injury Network. Acute Kidney Injury Network: report of an initiative to improve outcomes in acute kidney injury. *Crit Care.* 2007;11(2):R31 with permission.

- Inability of dialysis to provide actual renal replacement. The endocrine, cytokine, and immunologic functions of the kidney are not being replaced with dialysis.
- Delay in initiation of dialysis. The optimal timing of renal replacement therapy remains a question and limited studies have suggested that early initiation of renal replacement therapy might improve survival.

Diagnostic Approach

Although the terminology has changed, the approach to diagnosing or categorizing AKI has not changed. The initial approach should always focus on delineating whether the AKI is a result of prerenal, intrinsic (renal), or postrenal processes. Prerenal azotemia suggests problems with effective renal perfusion and is the cause of AKI in approximately 50% to 80% of all cases. "Renal" AKI is due to an intrinsic renal disease and accounts for approximately 10% to 30% of AKI cases. As the name suggests, postrenal azotemia results from obstruction to urine flow and is responsible for approximately 5% to 10% of cases. By definition, *prerenal* and *postrenal lesions* impose functional restraints on renal performance; renal function is expected to improve dramatically after removal of such lesions, if achieved in a timely fashion. In contrast, intrinsic AKI is not expected to reverse swiftly and the clinical course and prognosis depend on the underlying cause. Prerenal AKI is the most common cause of AKI in "community-acquired" and non-ICU patients. Postrenal is seen in about 15% of patients coming to the hospital with AKI, but is less likely to be diagnosed in the hospitalized patient. In the ICU, the most common cause is acute tubular necrosis (ATN) from multiple causes—the so-called multifactorial ATN. Prerenal and postrenal AKI are discussed in detail in Chapter 12. The intrinsic causes of AKI can be subclassified under the following etiologies: vascular, glomerular/microvascular, interstitial, or tubular. The most common cause of AKI due to intrinsic renal disease is ATN and is discussed in detail later in this chapter. The other intrinsic etiologies of AKI such as vasculitis, acute glomerulonephritis, thrombotic microangiopathies, interstitial nephritis, and crystalline nephropathies are discussed in other chapters.

Evaluation of the Patient with Acute Kidney Injury

The following questions should be answered by the end of the history and physical exam in a patient with AKI:

- Is this patient volume depleted?
- Could this patient have a urinary tract obstruction?

- Has this patient been exposed to a major nephrotoxin (medications, IV contrast, over-the-counter agents, herbal products)?
- Could this patient have intrinsic renal disease?
- Does the patient have a preexisting condition (e.g., decompensated CHF, liver cirrhosis) increasing vulnerability to renal injury?
- Is there a need for serologic testing and/or renal biopsy?

History

Urine Patterns and Frequency

Establish the amount of urine passed and recent trends. Elicit any history of hematuria, dysuria, or pyuria. Urgency, frequency, dribbling, and incontinence, especially in elderly men, may point toward prostatic disease. Onset of urinary symptoms may also provide a temporal clue to the duration of illness. For hospitalized patients, a careful review of the intake and output charts is essential. However, these are notoriously inaccurate unless the patient is in an ICU setting. A better gauge in such circumstances may be the patient's weight records.

Volume Status

History of dizziness or orthostatic instability may point toward intravascular depletion, whereas weight gain, edema, or periorbital swelling (especially in the mornings) may signify fluid retention. Consider the possible mechanisms of fluid loss—hemorrhage, diarrhea, polyuria, and situations leading to excessive insensitive losses (e.g., fever or diminished intake due to dysphagia)—as they all predispose to volume depletion. Review the patient's records or chart for episodes of blood pressure swings. For postoperative patients, it is essential to review the intra- and postoperative hemodynamic records.

Medications

This includes over-the-counter medicines, herbal products, and health and food supplements. Scout for nephrotoxins (e.g., NSAIDs, ACE inhibitors, aminoglycosides). In hospitalized patients, exclude covert nephrotoxic exposure, such as IV contrast media with radiologic studies and angiograms. Some drugs may precipitate or exacerbate urinary retention and should be considered (e.g., tricyclic antidepressants, carbidopa, and certain antihypertensive agents). Several herbal products and supplements have been implicated in interstitial nephritis and tubular necrosis.

Infections

The source and severity of infection and management undertaken in any patient with AKI must be carefully reviewed. Patients with infections can end up with AKI due to a variety of mechanisms: Some infections directly lead to renal involvement (e.g., *Legionella* infection can cause an interstitial nephritis); other infections involve the kidneys indirectly. For example, bacterial endocarditis or hepatitis C with cryoglobulinemia can cause an immune complex deposition glomerulonephritis leading to renal failure. Severe infections may cause sepsis leading to renal insufficiency. Finally, the many different antibiotics in use today can cause nephrotoxicity, either directly or by causing acute allergic interstitial nephritis.

Other Potential Etiologies

Patients should be carefully questioned for other symptoms of systemic diseases. Arthralgias, arthritis, skin rash, oral ulcers, hair loss, and significant cytopenias in the past may suggest the possibility of a connective tissue disorder (e.g., SLE). Sinusitis, cough, and hemoptysis may suggest diseases such as Wegener granulomatosis or Goodpasture syndrome. A history of recent sore throats or significant skin infections may suggest acute poststreptococcal glomerulonephritis. Bone pain and anemia may suggest underlying multiple myeloma. Also important is a history of chronic liver disease. If cirrhosis is present, assess the severity and degree of compensation of cirrhosis of the liver; hepatorenal syndrome is a devastating complication usually seen with advanced, decompensated liver disease. Patients with ascites are prone to develop spontaneous bacterial peritonitis that can lead to sepsis and ATN. Any history suggestive of purpura must alert the clinician to the possibility of cryoglobulinemia (especially if the patient is hepatitis C positive).

Risk Factors

An attempt must be made to appraise **preexisting conditions** that could adversely affect the patient's ability to exercise maximum autoregulation. For example, recent decompensation of CHF may tip off the clinician to a state of altered autoregulation and higher susceptibility to renal insult. Similarly, the presence of hypertension, diabetes, or significant peripheral vascular disease should also raise the possibility of diminished autoregulatory capacity.

Physical Exam

Determination of the patient's **volume status** by a thorough examination is an absolute prerequisite when dealing with the renal patient. Check the patient's pulse and blood pressure. If blood pressure is normal or high, evaluate for orthostatic hypotension in the sitting and standing positions, paying careful attention to the pulse as well. Assess for jugular venous distention and edema. Mucous membranes and skin turgor need to be checked for assessment of degree of hydration. The **cardiac exam** should focus on the location and character of apical impulse, presence of S_3 (volume overload) or S_4 (pressure overload), and functional regurgitant murmurs suggesting valve ring dilatation because of volume overload. The presence of dyspnea and tachypnea suggest fluid overload. Acidosis may induce Kussmaul respiration, but this deep-sighing character is not to be confused with the dyspnea of pulmonary edema. Inspiratory crackles at the lung bases occur in pulmonary edema.

    Abdominal examination can provide valuable clues in the workup for AKI. Hepatomegaly, splenomegaly, and ascites can occur due to passive congestion in fluid-overload states. The liver may be pulsatile if the volume overload has resulted in severe functional tricuspid regurgitation. Exclude obstruction by assessing bladder distention, performing a prostate exam, and placing a Foley catheter if indicated. **Other systemic signs** such as rash (e.g., vasculitis, atheroemboli, interstitial nephritis, lupus), arthritis (e.g., vasculitis, connective tissue disorders), pulmonary hemorrhage (vasculitis, lupus) can also provide diagnostic clues. A complete and thorough examination is required in addition to the above to elicit possible causes of the AKI, to assess the degree of compensation, and to detect features suggestive of uremic syndrome.

Diagnostic Tests

Examination of Urine

Urinalysis and microscopic examination of the urine sediment is probably the most important test in the evaluation of AKI. The urinalysis should not reveal protein, blood, cells, or casts in prerenal azotemia and in uncomplicated postrenal failure, unless there is underlying CKD. The urinalysis and sediment may help to not only separate renal causes from pre- and postrenal etiologies, but also to differentiate between a tubular, glomerular, or interstitial process (Table 11-2). If the urine dipstick tests strongly positive for blood but no RBCs are seen, hemoglobinuria or myoglobinuria should be suspected, suggesting rhabdomyolysis or severe intravascular hemolysis leading to AKI. It must be kept in mind that in certain diseases that affect the preglomerular blood vessels, such as thrombotic microangiopathies (e.g., thrombotic thrombocytopenic purpura or hemolytic-uremic syndrome), the urine sediment may be bland despite a bona fide renal etiology. The overall clinical presentation must therefore always be kept in mind. Similarly, the urine can be bland in one-third of the patients with ischemic ATN. Details of various types of casts and interpretations can be found in Chapter 1.

TABLE 11-2 · URINALYSIS (UA) IN AKI

	UA Protein	UA Blood	FeNa (%)	Sediment
Prerenal	No	No	<1	Bland; hyaline casts
Acute tubular necrosis	+	+	>1	Muddy brown granular casts; epithelial cells and epithelial cell casts
Glomerulonephritis	++	++	<1	Dysmorphic RBCs; RBC casts
Acute interstitial nephritis	+	+	>1	Eosinophils; WBCs and WBC casts; rarely, RBC casts
Postrenal	Maybe	Maybe	>1	Monomorphic RBCs and WBCs or crystals may be seen

Urinary Indices

In oliguric AKI, the differentiation of prerenal failure from ATN is critical in guiding appropriate management. Various parameters in the urine have been evaluated to make such a differentiation. The basic principle of these parameters is fairly uniform: In the face of diminished perfusion, the intact renal parenchyma tries to conserve as much salt as possible to restore extracellular fluid volume and, hence, renal perfusion. Thus, the urine is very concentrated and allows excretion of very little sodium. However, once the renal parenchyma is damaged, the tubules lose their ability to concentrate the urine and to conserve sodium. It must be kept in mind that these indices are usually not useful in nonoliguric states. Some of these indices are presented in Table 11-3.

$$FENa = [(\text{urine Na/plasma Na})/(\text{urine creatinine/plasma creatinine})] \times 100$$

$$FEUrea = [(\text{urine urea nitrogen/blood urea nitrogen})/(\text{urine creatinine/} \\ \text{plasma creatinine})] \times 100$$

Although fractional excretion of sodium (FENa) is useful in distinguishing prerenal AKI from ATN, its sensitivity diminishes in the setting of diuretic use. FEUrea has a sensitivity of 85%, specificity of 92%, and the positive predictive value for FEUrea was 98%. FEUrea >50 is consistent with ATN; <35 is consistent with prerenal injury.

TABLE 11-3 · URINE DIAGNOSTIC INDICES IN THE DIFFERENTIATION OF PRERENAL FAILURE FROM ATN

	Typical Findings	
Diagnostic Index	Prerenal Azotemia	Acute Tubular Necrosis
Fractional excretion of sodium (%)	<1	>1
U_{Na}	<20	>20
Urine osmolality	>500	variable
Plasma BUN to PCr ratio	>20	<10–15
Renal failure index	<1	>1

PCr, plasma creatinine; P_{Na}, plasma sodium; UCr, urine creatinine; U_{Na}, urine sodium.

Blood Counts and Coagulation Screen

Review of the blood counts and screening tests for coagulation abnormalities may provide extremely valuable information about underlying disease processes leading to AKI. A peripheral smear must be examined where indicated. The presence of schistocytes in cases of AKI suggests thrombotic thrombocytopenic purpura, hemolytic-uremic syndrome, and disseminated intravascular coagulation as possible etiologies. Rarely, schistocytes can also be seen in conditions with severe renal vasculitis, such as diffuse lupus nephritis.

Chemistry Panel

Review of lab values including electrolytes, BUN, and creatinine and acid-base balance is essential to establishing the previous baseline and trend leading to the current abnormality. If severe metabolic acidosis is present, anion and osmolar gaps should be evaluated so as to not miss a severe metabolic derangement or toxic ingestion causing the AKI. This is further discussed in Chapter 10.

Radiologic Evaluation

Exclusion of obstruction is of paramount importance. **Renal ultrasound** is readily available and extremely accurate in excluding urinary tract obstruction as a cause of AKI. Ultrasonography is useful in delineating renal sizes (a marked difference may suggest renovascular disease) and echo texture. Ultrasonography (or alternative imaging) should be obtained early in the workup of AKI, especially in patients presenting to the emergency room or hospital with an elevated creatinine. However, in the intensive care setting, where obstruction is an unlikely cause of AKI, the yield from ultrasound is very low and it should not be ordered routinely. An ultrasound can provide false negative results in the setting of profound volume depletion (along with obstruction) as well as in cases of retroperitoneal fibrosis, in which dilatation of calyces and ureters may not occur. Computerized tomography and magnetic resonance imaging are alternative modalities to rule out obstruction.

Serologic Profile and Special Tests

In situations suggestive of intrinsic renal disease, various serologic tests (Table 11-4) are indicated to delineate the etiology. These tests are discussed in detail in other chapters covering vasculitis, lupus nephritis, and intrinsic causes of AKI.

Tissue Diagnosis

Renal biopsy is usually not required to establish the diagnosis of or to treat ATN. However, if the cause of AKI is not apparent, or if there is a suspicion of rapidly progressive glomerulonephritis, then renal histology is required to make a diagnosis and aid in management. This must be done in a timely fashion, as certain disease processes irreversibly destroy renal parenchyma if they are not treated expeditiously. In cases of suspected acute interstitial nephritis with a clear inciting agent, discontinuation of the agent and observation of the renal function can be chosen over a kidney biopsy, especially in high-risk patients. In cases of suspected glomerulonephritis (based on historical features, urine abnormalities, and blood and serologic tests), a renal biopsy is necessary before immunosuppressive therapy is instituted. For instance, even when diagnosis of lupus nephritis is obvious, most nephrologists obtain a tissue diagnosis to correctly define and classify the disease and to outline progression and future therapy options.

Newer Biomarkers

There is great interest in the development of newer serum and urine biomarkers for early diagnosis of AKI. Serum creatinine usually rises 24 to 48 hours after injury and by this time the proverbial horse is already out of the barn. Biomarkers than can detect renal injury within hours (similar to troponin for myocardial injury) can go a long way toward early diagnosis and management. If volume resuscitation, optimization of blood pressure

TABLE 11-4	EXAMPLES OF SEROLOGIC OR SPECIAL TESTS SUGGESTING CAUSES OF RENAL FAILURE
Test	**Associated Condition**
ANA, double-stranded DNA	SLE
C-ANCA	Wegener granulomatosis
P-ANCA	Microscopic polyangiitis, Churg-Strauss syndrome
Rheumatoid arthritis factor	Vasculitis, cryoglobulinemia
Cryoglobulins	Cryoglobulinemia-associated MPGN
Anti–glomerular basement membrane antibodies	Goodpasture syndrome
Antistreptolysin-O titer	PSCGN
Complement levels	Low in PSCGN, cryoglobulinemic GN/MPGN I, lupus nephritis, shunt nephritis, GN with subacute bacterial endocarditis
Hepatitis B and C	Hepatitis-associated GN
HIV	Collapsing focal segmental glomerulosclerosis, interstitial nephritis

GN, glomerulonephritis; MPGN, membranoproliferative glomerulonephritis; PSCGN, poststreptococcal glomerulonephritis.

or other therapies can be started in the early stages of AKI (initiation phase), then this can potentially prevent the continued deterioration of renal function. Some of the promising biomarkers include serum and urine neutrophil gelatinase associate lipocalin (NGAL), which has been demonstrated to be elevated as early as 1 hour after coronary artery bypass grafting in patients that later developed AKI, documented by rise in creatinine. Interleukin-18 (IL-18) has also shown similar results, including in the setting of delayed graft function after kidney transplantation. Other molecules of interest include cystatin C and kidney injury molecule -1 (KIM-1). Further studies are underway to determine if any of these markers will replace creatinine as the diagnostic tool for AKI.

ACUTE TUBULAR NECROSIS

ATN refers to AKI resulting from ischemic or toxic damage to the renal tubules. The common etiologies of ATN are listed in Table 11-5.

Pathogenesis of Ischemic Injury

Ischemic ATN is progression or persistence of any prerenal condition to a point where there is compromise and damage to the tubular epithelium. Although 25% of the cardiac output flows into the renal circulation, most of the blood flow is relegated to the cortex, and the medulla is maintained in a relative hypoxic state. The S_3 segment of the proximal tubule is especially vulnerable in ischemic states and most of the damage occurs in this segment. Overwhelming levels of angiotensin II, endothelin-1, and circulating catecholamines cause intense intrarenal vasoconstriction, overcoming the protective effects of prostaglandins and nitric oxide. Other factors also come into play: The ischemic response stimulates release of inflammatory cytokines, which in turn leads to increased expression of adhesion molecules on the leukocytes and their ligands on the

TABLE 11-5	CAUSES OF ATN	
Ischemia	**Toxins**	**Drugs**
• Any prolonged prerenal condition • Sepsis	• Radiocontrast • Myoglobin (rhabdomyolysis) • Hemoglobin (intravascular hemolysis) • Ethylene glycol/methanol • Tumor lysis (uric acid, phosphate) • Miscellaneous (snake venom, paraquat)	• Aminoglycosides • Cisplatin • Amphotericin B • Intravenous bisphosphonates • Crystalline nephropathies (Indinavir, Acyclovir)

epithelium. This mutual arrangement results in increased leukocyte-endothelium adhesion and endothelial injury.

There is congestion and obstruction of capillaries in the outer medulla causing persistent medullary ischemia. The tubular cells suffer damage that is reflected in disruption of the actin cytoskeleton, leading to loss of the brush border; loss of polarity of the cells, leading to failure of the tight junctions; and a loss of cell-matrix interaction, causing detachment from the basement membranes. Thus, although these cells may appear intact on light microscopy, these epithelia lose function and also allow significant tubular back leak leading to loss of GFR. With further injury, these cells undergo apoptosis or, in some cases, frank necrosis.

Pathogeneisis of Nephrotoxic Injury

Various endogenous and exogenous toxins can lead to tubular damage and AKI. A list of some of the important toxins is presented in Table 11-5. Contrast-induced nephropathy is discussed in detail in Chapter 14. A frequently encountered nephrotoxic injury is rhabdomyolysis.

Rhabdomyolysis

Destruction of striated muscles from a variety of insults results in outflow of intracellular contents (potassium, phosphorus, myoglobin, uric acid, creatine kinase) into circulation. The incidence of AKI in rhabdomyolysis is reported to be anywhere from 10% to 50%. In cases of traumatic rhabdomyolysis, the incidence of AKI is as high as 85%. The common causes that are encountered include cocaine use, immobilization (e.g., alcoholic patient or patient with seizures or stroke; patient found at home after a fall; or postsurgery patients with large muscle mass or obesity, or undergoing urological or bariatric surgeries), trauma (gunshot wound with vascular compromise, motor vehicle accidents, crush injury following earthquakes or building collapse), or extreme exertion (exercise in severe heat, new recruits at army camps, etc.).

Pathogenesis. Vasoconstriction plays a major role in nephrotoxicity associated with myoglobin. Hemeproteins also can cause direct cytotoxic effects on tubular epithelial cells; the mechanism remains ill defined. Renal ischemia is believed to result from activation of endothelin receptors as well as scavenging of nitric oxide. Myoglobin is also believed to generate free radicals that can induce oxidative injury to the tubules. This may be inhibited in an alkaline pH.

Clinical Findings. Classical manifestations are severe myalgias, dark urine (with or without decreased urine output), and appropriate clinical scenarios (exercise, crush injury, recent surgery, medications, immobilization, etc). Laboratory data can reveal profound **hyperkalemia** and **hyperphosphatemia** (due to release from damaged myocytes), **hypocalcemia**

(due to calcium-phosphorus binding), and a disproportionate elevation of the creatinine in relation to blood urea nitrogen. Creatinine kinase (CK) elevation happens within 12 hours after the injury and the rise is in proportion to the severity and extent of the muscle injury. Kidney injury has been reported with **CK levels** >5000 IU/L, but is typically seen with values >25,000 IU/L. Urinalysis reveals **positive dipstick for blood** (reagent for hemoglobin crossreacts with myoglobin), **without erythrocytes** on microscopy. **Pigmented granular casts** can be seen, indicating the presence of tubular injury. In contrast to most other etiologies of ATN, fractional excretion of sodium tends to be <1% in early stages, probably reflecting potent vasoconstriction.

Management. **Early, aggressive volume repletion** is absolutely essential in preventing AKI in the setting of rhabdomyolysis. Initial therapy should be with normal saline for volume expansion, at a rate of 1 to 2 L in the first hour and then continued at 150 to 300 mL/hour, depending on the urine output and the patient's volume status. Mannitol and sodium bicarbonate infusion have been recommended in rhabdomyolysis, but there are no studies demonstrating a benefit over normal saline. Sodium bicarbonate infusions can have deleterious effects if acid-base status is not monitored closely—especially in the setting of hypocalcemia, given the risk of increased calcium binding in the setting of alkalosis. Once anuric or oliguric AKI has resulted as a result of tubular injury, aggressive fluid resuscitation should be discontinued and fluids should be administered judiciously or stopped altogether in order to avoid volume overload. **Early initiation of renal replacement therapy** should be considered in anuric or oliguric patients given the risk of life-threatening hyperkalemia with ongoing muscle damage.

Management of Acute Tubular Necrosis

ATN occurs in many different clinical scenarios. Recommendations for therapy in any given case have to be tailored according to the clinical circumstances. Here, we present the basics of therapy for the spectrum of prerenal azotemia and ischemic ATN; the management of other individual causes is presented in relevant sections elsewhere in this text.

Restoration of Effective Circulatory Volume
Restoration of effective circulatory volume is one of the crucial aspects of management in patients with ischemic renal injury. The initial fluid of choice is a crystalloid solution, such as normal saline in most situations, administered until euvolemia is restored. In some cases, use of a colloid solution may seem enticing. Albumin, gelatin, and dextrans have been the most frequently used agents but are plagued with problems such as anaphylactoid reactions, coagulopathy, and precipitation of oliguria and AKI. Fluids must be administered with caution in oliguric AKI in order to avoid volume overload and respiratory failure. If fluid resuscitation is not successful in improving blood pressure, inotropic or pressor agents may be needed.

Withdrawal and Avoidance of Nephrotoxins
It is extremely important to avoid further injury to the suffering kidney. Contrast media should be avoided wherever possible. NSAIDs, ACE inhibitors, and angiotensin receptor blockers should be held. Nonnephrotoxic antibiotics should be prescribed whenever possible. If a potentially toxic antibiotic (e.g., aminoglycoside) has to be used, dosage should be carefully adjusted, and drug levels should be closely monitored.

Diuretics
It has long been believed that diuretics promote urine flow and therefore discourage cellular debris from obstructing the tubules. The diuretic challenge is traditionally used in patients with oliguria in an attempt to convert them to a nonoliguric state. The latter condition is easier to manage but does not improve survival or promote faster renal recovery. Indeed, some recent studies argue that there is no benefit in sustained diuretic use, and there may be some harm associated with the practice. Randomized controlled studies have

not shown an increased risk of adverse events with the use of diuretics. The current recommendation is to attempt diuresis if patients are volume overloaded and have oliguric AKI. If there is no significant diuretic response, then the drug should be discontinued. If diuretics are being administered then it is very important to note that higher-than-standard doses must be utilized for the loop diuretics to be effective. For example, with a glomerular filtration of <30 mL/minute, the dose of furosemide should be approximately 160 to 200 mg IV as a bolus. If there is a diuretic response, then it can be continued as intermittent doses or as a continuous infusion. Studies have not shown a difference in outcome with either method. The use of diuretics to convert from an oliguric to nonoliguric state should not sway the physician away from a nephrology consultation or institution of other appropriate therapy. Also, volume status should be ascertained carefully prior to diuretic administration, as it may exacerbate the volume deficit.

Dopamine and Fenoldopam

Dopamine (DA). DA is the archetype dopaminergic agent. It is nonselective, acting on both DA-1– and DA-2–like receptors and, therefore, does have beneficial effects on renal hemodynamics. It causes renal vasodilatation, increases GFR, and enhances sodium excretion promoting tubular flow. However, these desirable effects are eclipsed by extrarenal actions of dopamine. It is arrhythmogenic and, at higher doses, can lead to systemic and renal vasoconstriction, mediated through adrenergic receptors. To avoid these unwanted effects, the concept of *renal-dose DA* was developed. At a dose of 1 to 3 μg/kg/minute, it was believed that the predominantly dopaminergic renal effects would be achieved and the undesirable adrenergic effects avoided. This concept had support from animal data. However, human studies using renal-dose DA showed no benefit in either preventing or treating AKI. This was demonstrated in multiple studies reviewed elsewhere. At this time, routine use of renal-dose DA either for prevention or treatment of AKI **is not recommended** based on available clinical data.

Fenoldopam. Fenoldopam is highly selective for DA-1 receptor and does not stimulate DA-2 or adrenergic receptors. Even though small, uncontrolled trials have suggested a role for fenoldopam in the prevention of AKI in patients with CHF and cirrhosis and ventilated patients with high positive end-expiratory pressures, randomized trials have not seen a benefit with this agent. Fenoldopam was studied in several clinical settings (ICU, sepsis, prevention of contrast-induced nephropathy, and AKI associated with cardiac surgery). In patients with sepsis in the ICU, fenoldopam was associated with a smaller increase in creatinine compared with placebo, but there was no difference in survival or severe renal failure. Fenoldopam was not superior to placebo in preventing AKI post–IV contrast or after cardiac surgery. There was also no benefit when fenoldopam was given to intensive care patients with early AKI. Although a recent meta-analysis implies that this drug may reduce mortality and need for renal replacement therapy in critically ill patients, the **use of this drug cannot be uniformly recommended** with the data available to date.

Experimental Agents

There is ongoing research to identify agents that might have a prophylactic role in AKI. Studies have looked at molecules such as insulinlike growth factor-1 (IGF-1), anaritide, thyroxine, and urodilatin. A detailed discussion of these agents is beyond the scope of this review. To date, although several proteins and hormones seemed beneficial in animal studies, none have proven to be effective in the treatment of ATN in clinical trials. It must be kept in mind that most of these agents are in preclinical stages of development or have undergone only preliminary human trials.

Other Aspects of Management

Acid-Base and Electrolyte Disturbances. Hyperkalemia and metabolic acidosis are frequently encountered in AKI. The individual management of these conditions is discussed elsewhere. If conservative therapies fail, then renal replacement therapy is initiated.

Nutritional Support. Nutrition is one of the important facets of supportive care. AKI is a stressful, catabolic state. Adequate nutrition is essential; enteral or parenteral support may be necessary. Unlike CKD where protein restriction is recommended, protein requirements in AKI vary from 1.0 g/kg (prior to dialysis initiation or during hemodialysis) to 2.5 g/kg (in continuous renal replacement therapy).

Dose Adjustment of Medications. It is important to scour through the entire medication list and adjust the medications for the patient's renal function. Various guidelines (e.g., Aronoff GA, Berns JS, Briere ME. *Drug Prescribing in Renal Failure: Dosing Guidelines for Adults.* 4th ed.) are available to make recommended dose adjustments. Please see also Appendixes D and E in this textbook. The pharmacist is also a valuable resource in making medication adjustments in renal failure. If the patient requires initiation of hemodialysis or continuous renal replacement therapy, then dose adjustments are again necessary in some cases to ensure adequate drug levels.

Course of ATN

Traditionally, ATN has been described to pass through four phases. **Initiation** refers to an early stage in which ischemia leads to cell injury. **Extension** refers to the phase where cellular polarity is disrupted and results in sloughing of viable and damaged cells causing tubular casts with obstruction and back leak. During the **maintenance** phase, the cells are undergoing dedifferentiation, migration, and some proliferation, and results in fully established renal failure. In the **recovery** phase, cellular redifferentiation and reestablishment of polarity are associated with signs of renal function recovery. All of these phases may not be clinically obvious and one may progress to the next rapidly. In oliguric patients, an osmotic diuresis may be seen in the recovery phase (post-ATN diuresis) and meticulous attention should be paid to fluid balance and electrolyte replacement. ATN can last from days to several weeks in patients with baseline normal renal function, and renal recovery should not be counted out, even after weeks of oliguria. Studies have shown that 90% of patients with ATN can regain sufficient renal function to discontinue dialysis. However, these patients are at a higher risk of developing CKD and ESRD and need to be followed closely.

KEY POINTS TO REMEMBER

- Prerenal azotemia is the most common cause of AKI. Rapid restoration of effective circulatory volume usually leads to prompt and complete resolution of AKI.
- In addition to other aspects of history and exam, a complete exam of the urine, including study of the sediment, is key.
- Drug history includes prescription, over-the-counter medications, herbal products, and health supplements.
- Obstruction must be considered and excluded in all cases of community-acquired AKI.
- Newer biomarkers are necessary for early diagnosis of AKI
- Prevention of AKI remains the mainstay of therapy.
- As the GFR declines, dose adjustment of medications is needed to prevent complications.

REFERENCES AND SUGGESTED READING

Brady HR, Brenner BM. Acute renal failure. In: Braunwald E, Fauci AS, Kasper DL, et al., eds. *Harrison's Principles of Internal Medicine.* 15th ed. New York: McGraw-Hill; 2001:1547.

Brivet FG, Kleinknecht DJ, Loirat P, et al. Acute renal failure in intensive care units—causes, outcome, and prognostic factors of hospital mortality; a prospective, multicenter study. French Study Group on acute renal failure. *Crit Care Med.* 1996;24:192.

Guerin C, Girard R, Selli JM, et al. Intermittent versus continuous renal replacement therapy for acute renal failure in intensive care units: results from a multicenter prospective epidemiological survey. *Intensive Care Med.* 2002;28:1411.

Han WK, Bonventre JV. Biologic markers for the early detection of acute kidney injury. *Curr Opin Crit Care.* 2004;10:476–482.

Hoste EAJ, Lameire NH, Vanholder RC, et al. Acute renal failure in patients with sepsis in a surgical ICU: predictive factors, incidence, comorbidity, and outcome. *J Am Soc Nephrol.* 2003;14:1022.

Hou SH, Bushinsky DA, Wish JB, et al. Hospital acquired renal insufficiency: a prospective study. *Am J Med.* 1983;74:243.

Kellum J, Levin N, Bouman C, et al. Developing a consensus classification system for acute renal failure. *Curr Opin Crit Care.* 2002;8:509.

Klahr S, Miller SB. Current concepts: acute oliguria. *N Engl J Med.* 1998;338:671–675.

Lazarus JM, Brennar BM, eds. *Acute Renal Failure.* 3rd ed. New York: Churchill Livingstone; 1993:133.

Lennon AM, Coleman PL, Brady HR. Management and outcome of acute renal failure. In: Johnson RJ, Feehaly J, eds. *Comprehensive Clinical Nephrology.* London: Harcourt; 2000.

Liano F, Pascual J. Epidemiology of acute renal failure: a prospective, multicenter, community-based study. Madrid Acute Renal Failure Study Group. *Kidney Int.* 1996;50:811.

Mehta RL, Chertow GM. Acute renal failure definitions and classification: time for change? *J Am Soc Nephrol.* 2003;14:2178.

Mehta RL, Kellum JA, Shah SV, et al. Acute kidney injury network: report of an initiative to improve outcomes in acute kidney injury. *Crit Care.* 2007;11:R31.

Mehta RL, McDonald B, Gabbai FB, et al. A randomized clinical trial of continuous versus intermittent dialysis for acute renal failure. *Kidney Int.* 2001;60:1154.

Mehta RL, Pascual MT, Soroko S, et al. (for the PICARD Study Group). Diuretics, mortality, and nonrecovery of renal function in acute renal failure. *JAMA.* 2002;288:2547.

Molitoris BA, Chan L, Shapiro JI, et al. Loss of epithelial polarity: a novel hypothesis for reduced proximal tubule sodium transport following ischemic injury. *J Membr Biol.* 1989;107:119.

Molitoris BA, Falk SA, Dahl RH. Ischemia induced loss of epithelial polarity: role of the tight junction. *J Clin Invest.* 1989;84:1334.

National Kidney Foundation. K/DOQI Clinical practice guidelines for chronic kidney disease: evaluation, classification, and stratification. *Am J Kidney Dis.* 2002;39:S1–S246.

Parfrey PS, Griffiths SM, Barrett BJ, et al. Contrast material–induced renal failure in patients with diabetes mellitus, renal insufficiency, or both: a prospective controlled study. *N Engl J Med.* 1989;320:143.

Ragaller MJR, Theilen H, Koch T. Volume replacement in critically ill patients with acute renal failure. *J Am Soc Nephrol.* 2001;12:S33.

Rose BD. Prerenal disease versus acute tubular necrosis. In: *Pathophysiology of Renal Disease.* 2nd ed. New York: McGraw-Hill; 1987:65–119.

Singer I, Epstein M. Potential of dopamine A-1 agonists in the management of acute renal failure. *Am J Kidney Dis.* 1998;31:743.

Solomon R, Werner C, Mann D, et al. Effects of saline, mannitol, and furosemide to prevent acute decreases in renal function induced by radiocontrast agents. *N Engl J Med.* 1994;331:1416.

Tepel M, van der Giet M, Schwarzfeld C, et al. Prevention of radiographic contrast agent induced reductions in renal function by acetylcysteine. *N Engl J Med.* 2000; 343:180.

Thadhani R, Pascual M, Bonventre JV. Medical progress: acute renal failure. *N Engl J Med.* 1996;334:1448–1460.

Tonelli M, Manns B, Feller-Kopman D. Acute renal failure in the intensive care unit: a systematic review of the impact of dialytic modality on mortality and renal recovery. *Am J Kidney Dis.* 2002;40:875.

Tumlin JA, Wang A, Murray PT, et al. Fenoldopam mesylate blocks reductions in renal plasma flow after radiocontrast dye infusion: a pilot trial in the prevention of contrast nephropathy. *Am Heart J.* 2002;143:894.

Vanholder R, Biesen WV, Lameire N. What is the renal replacement method of first choice for intensive care patients? *J Am Soc Nephrol.* 2001;12:S40.

Vijayan A, Miller SB. Acute renal failure: prevention and non-dialytic therapy. *Semin Nephrol.* 1998;18:523.

Weisbord SD, Palevsky PM. Acute renal failure in the intensive care unit. *Semin Respir Crit Care Med.* 2006;27:262–273.

Prerenal and Postrenal Acute Kidney Injury

12

Alexis Argoudelis and Anitha Vijayan

PRERENAL ACUTE KIDNEY INJURY

Definition

Prerenal kidney injury is characterized by preserved renal parenchymal function responding appropriately to diminished perfusion. Because the integrity of the renal parenchymal tissue is preserved, timely restoration of perfusion and glomerular ultrafiltration pressure should correct GFR. There is a continuum from compensated renal hypoperfusion, without a change in GFR, to prerenal injury with reduced GFR to ischemic acute tubular necrosis (ATN). Prerenal azotemia has been described as the cause of AKI in 30% to 70% of community-associated kidney injury and up to 30% of hospital-associated kidney injury depending on the various patient populations.

Pathogenesis

The most common scenarios leading to prerenal AKI include:

1. Intravascular volume depletion (e.g., gastrointestinal losses)
2. Decreased effective circulating volume (e.g., decreased cardiac output or cirrhosis)
3. Renal vasoconstriction (e.g., sepsis, hypercalcemia, liver disease, and NSAIDs)
4. Efferent arteriolar vasodilatation due to ACE inhibitors or ARBs

The hallmark of the prerenal state is decreased perfusion of the kidney. There are immediate systemic and renal compensatory responses, recruiting multiple neurohumoral systems, directed at maintaining blood flow and GFR.

The **adrenergic system** responds to maintain blood pressure. Increased sympathetic activity results in increased cardiac output and restoration of perfusion pressure. Peripheral resistance is increased to maintain blood pressure. This may act as a double-edged sword, as renal vasoconstriction due to sympathetic drive may cause decreased renal blood flow (RBF). However, other intrarenal mechanisms may help maintain RBF. Sympathetic activity also stimulates release of renin through beta-adrenergic receptors. Hypovolemia is a potent nonosmotic stimulation for release of **antidiuretic hormone** (ADH) from the posterior pituitary. ADH acts to exert maximal water conservation and excretion of concentrated urine. Acting through the V_1-receptors, it also causes vasoconstriction, and increased peripheral resistance and blood pressure.

At the renal level, the first line of defense against fluctuations of arterial blood pressure is **autoregulation**. The afferent arteriole senses the degree of stretch and thus relaxes when the perfusion pressure (and, therefore, stretch) is low. This myogenic reflex can maintain RBF through wide fluctuations of arterial pressure. The second prong of renal autoregulation depends on tubuloglomerular feedback: The macula densa in the cortical collecting duct senses low distal solute delivery and this leads to afferent arteriolar dilatation.

Maintenance of GFR through falling perfusion pressures stems from the ability to independently maneuver the afferent and efferent arterioles. As flow increases because of afferent arteriolar relaxation, glomerular pressure is maintained through efferent arteriolar constriction, mediated through the renin-angiotensin-aldosterone system.

The **renin-angiotensin-aldosterone system** is critical in renal self-defense. With decreased renal perfusion, renin is released from the juxtaglomerular cells and leads ultimately to the formation of angiotensin II (AII). AII increases proximal tubular resorption of solutes. AII also stimulates the adrenal gland affecting aldosterone release, which leads to enhanced distal sodium reabsorption. AII exerts complex effects on glomerular hemodynamics. With modest hypotension or congestive heart failure (CHF), AII can actually preserve GFR by its *preferential* vasoconstrictive action on the efferent arteriole. Efferent arteriolar constriction causes increased intraglomerular pressure and thus maintains the filtration fraction. With increasing AII activity, the afferent arteriole also starts to constrict, leading to decreased filtration. This explains why it is so deleterious to challenge a volume-depleted patient with ACE inhibitors or angiotensin receptor–blocker medications. Generation of prostacyclin and nitric oxide are two important paracrine influences that protect the afferent arteriole from vasoconstrictive influences. For instance, loss of prostacyclin production due to NSAIDs leads to early decompensation of renal function.

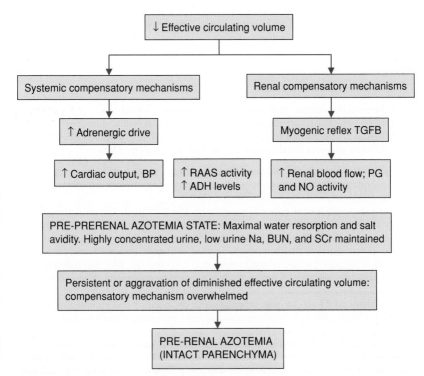

FIGURE 12-1. Algorithm for prerenal azotemia. ADH, antidiuretic hormone; NO, nitric oxide; SCr, serum creatinine; PG, prostaglandin; RAAS, renin-angiotensin-aldosterone system; TGFB, tubuloglomerular feedback.

The above cascades of events are depicted in Figure 12-1. The success of these autoregulatory mechanisms is seen by maintenance of renal function under conditions of diminished effective volume. However, if the decrease in the effective circulatory volume continues or aggravates, the renal compensatory mechanisms are overwhelmed. The afferent arteriolar vasodilatation is no longer enough to maintain flow. Indeed, with overwhelming levels of AII, vasoconstriction in the renal vasculature may commence. The RBF drops, as does the urine output. The state of prerenal azotemia has arrived. The BUN and plasma creatinine start to rise as the kidney is still striving to hold onto water and salt through persistent tubular action. If this sequence is not reversed soon, the parenchyma will no longer remain intact, and the patient may suffer ischemic acute tubular necrosis (ATN).

Causes

The important causes of prerenal AKI are summarized in Table 12-1. It is very important to appreciate factors limiting the ability of renal autoregulation to maintain homeostasis. Under normal circumstances, the kidney may be able to preserve function despite significantly low

TABLE 12-1	MAJOR CAUSES OF PRERENAL AZOTEMIA

Intravascular Volume Depletion

Hemorrhage: traumatic, surgical, gastrointestinal, postpartum
Gastrointestinal losses: vomiting, nasogastric suction, diarrhea
Renal losses: drug-induced or osmotic diuresis, diabetes insipidus, adrenal insufficiency
Skin and mucous membrane losses: burns, hyperthermia, other causes of increased insensible losses
"Third-space" losses: pancreatitis, crush syndrome, hypoalbuminemia

Decreased Cardiac Output

Diseases of myocardium, valves, pericardium, or conducting system
Pulmonary hypertension, pulmonary embolism, positive-pressure mechanical ventilation
Systemic vasodilatation
Drugs: antihypertensives, afterload reduction, anesthetics, drug overdoses
Sepsis, liver failure, anaphylaxis

Renal Vasoconstriction

Norepinephrine, ergotamine, liver disease, sepsis, hypercalcemia

Pharmacologic Agents That Acutely Impair Autoregulation and Glomerular Filtration Rate in Specific Settings

Angiotensin-converting enzyme inhibitors or angiotensin receptor blockers in renal artery stenosis or severe renal hypoperfusion
Inhibition of prostaglandin synthesis by NSAIDs and COX-2 inhibitors during renal hypoperfusion
Calcineurin inhibitors, radiocontrast agents

Adapted from Brenner, BM, ed. *Brenner & Rector's The Kidney.* 7th ed. Philadelphia: WB Saunders; 2004, with permission.

perfusion pressures. However, if the patient has limited ability to maintain afferent arteriolar dilatation due to preexisting large or small vessel disease (e.g., atherosclerosis, diabetes) renal function may decompensate at relatively higher mean arterial pressures. Thus, an elderly patient exposed to ACE inhibitors in a prerenal state could suffer from prerenal azotemia even with relatively modest decreases in blood pressure.

Clinical Findings

Unfortunately, signs and symptoms of prerenal kidney injury are usually very subtle and frequently patients are asymptomatic. The careful monitoring of urine output for oliguria (<400–500 mL/day) is critical in reversing oliguric prerenal kidney injury.

A history of **lightheadedness or orthostatic instability** may point toward intravascular depletion, whereas weight gain, edema, or periorbital swelling (especially in the mornings) may signify fluid retention as in CHF. Hemorrhage, diarrhea, polyuria, and situations leading to excessive insensitive losses (e.g., fever or diminished intake due to dysphagia) all predispose to volume depletion. A review the patient's records should be conducted for **episodes of blood pressure swings**. For postoperative patients, it is essential to review the intra- and postoperative hemodynamic records for hypotension. A thorough review of **medications** should be conducted. Scout for nephrotoxic medications that can induce glomerular hypoperfusion such NSAIDs, cyclooxygenase-2 inhibitors (COX-2 inhibitors), ACEI, ARBs, or calcineurin inhibitors. History and physical examination should focus on symptoms and signs of heart failure or liver disease. If the volume status is not apparent by a thorough examination and history, then additional procedures such as central venous pressure or pulmonary capillary wedge pressure measurement might be required. Ultimately, the diagnosis of prerenal AKI rests on a combination of clinical findings and laboratory testing.

Diagnosis

Urinalysis in prerenal kidney injury is often characterized as "bland" with no protein and no blood seen; typically hyaline casts can be seen under magnification.

Urine indices in the oliguric state, such as the **fractional excretion of sodium (FENa)** and the **fractional excretion of urea (FEUrea)** in patients who have had exposure to diuretics are useful but imperfect tools to help differentiate the prerenal state from ATN. In oliguric AKI, the differentiation of prerenal failure from ATN is critical to guide appropriate management. Various parameters in the urine have been evaluated to make such a differentiation (see Chapter 11).

In prerenal AKI, the FENa is <1%, in the absence of diuretic use. In one study, the FENa was low in only 48% of diuretic-treated patients with prerenal azotemia. Urea reabsorption by the proximal tubule is increased in prerenal states. This leads to a FEUrea of <35 %. Given that most of the diuretics used clinically work at distal sites, FEUrea should not be affected by their use. The positive predictive value of FEUrea is 98%. FEUrea values in CKD have not been standardized, so caution must be used. Interpretations of urinary indices must be made in conjunction with other assessments of the patient because there are clinically important exceptions to these generalizations. For example, patients with certain types of ATN, such as contrast-induced renal injury, may present with all the clinical characteristics of ATN but with FENa rates <1%.

Treatment

The treatment of prerenal AKI should be expeditious to avoid ischemia to the renal tubules and ATN. The basic principles of management are outlined below.

Restoration of Effective Circulatory Volume

As outlined, the fundamental problem in most cases of prerenal azotemia is diminished effective circulatory volume. Prompt and effective restoration relieves this stress, establishes urine flow, and normalizes renal function. The initial fluid of choice is administration of a crystalloid solution to restore the euvolemic state. **Normal saline** is usually the most effective choice. Alternatives include colloid solutions such as albumin, gelatin, and dextrans. However, anaphylactoid reactions, coagulopathy, and precipitation of oliguria and AKI may sometimes be seen with these agents.

Treatment of Underlying Causes
If cardiac output is compromised, then this needs to be corrected aggressively. This may involve preload and afterload reduction and diuresis in CHF or appropriate use of inotropic agents, vasodilators, or other means to maintain blood pressure and perfusion. If the hypoperfusion is a result of sepsis, then antibiotic administration and pressor support will help renal perfusion to some extent. In patients with hepatorenal syndrome the underlying hepatic dysfunction needs to be reversed either with recovery of injured liver (e.g., acetaminophen overdose) or with liver transplant. The cardiorenal and hepatorenal syndromes are discussed below. If medications interfering with the renin-angiotensin pathway or diuretics are being used, they should be discontinued. Other medications that may need discontinuation or dose adjustment include calcineurin inhibitors, NSAIDs, and COX-2 inhibitors.

HEPATORENAL SYNDROME

Introduction and Definition

Hepatorenal syndrome (HRS) is the most frequent cause of renal dysfunction in patients who have cirrhosis. Two types of HRS were originally defined by the International Ascites Club (IAC). **Type 1 HRS** presents as rapid and progressive impairment of renal function defined by a doubling of the initial serum creatinine to a level >2.5 mg/dL (220 μmol/L) or a 50% reduction of the initial 24-hour creatinine clearance to a level <20 mL/minute in <2 weeks. This is associated with a dismal prognosis. **Type 2 HRS** presents as impairment in renal function with serum creatinine levels >1.5 mg/dL (132 μmol/L) that does not meet criteria for type 1 HRS. Type 2 HRS develops gradually over weeks and is associated with a better survival.

Etiology and Pathogenesis

Renal vasoconstriction is the main hemodynamic derangement that defines HRS. The main variable responsible for these hemodynamic changes is portal hypertension in the setting of cirrhosis causing a splanchnic arterial vasodilation. This vasodilation occurs mainly because of the production of nitric oxide as a consequence of endothelial stretching and possibly bacterial translocation. The accumulation of plasma volume in the splanchnic bed causes a compensatory response because of decreased central blood volume with activation of systemic vasoconstrictor and antinatriuretic systems (RAAS, sympathetic system, ADH). This accounts for the sodium and water retention as well as renal vasoconstriction, as the kidney senses a relative hypovolemic state. Recent studies suggest that the development of HRS may also be due, in part, to reduction in cardiac output.

Presentation and Diagnosis

HRS occurs in about 10% of hospitalized patients who have cirrhosis and ascites. In addition, the probability of developing HRS in patients who had cirrhosis and ascites was 18% at 1 year and increased to 39% at 5 years. Individuals who develop HRS most often exhibit clinical features of advanced cirrhosis along with low arterial blood pressure, low urine volume, and severe urinary sodium retention (urine sodium ≤10 mEq/L). Dilutional hyponatremia is almost universally found. Elevated serum creatinine levels define HRS;

however, these levels usually are lower than those seen in noncirrhotic patients who have AKI because of reduced muscle mass and low endogenous production of creatinine in cirrhosis. Suggested **diagnostic criteria** for hepatorenal syndrome are:

1. Low GFR, as indicated by plasma creatinine levels >1.5 mg/dL or 132 μmol/L
2. Absence of shock (sepsis or hypovolemia), volume depletion, and use of nephrotoxic drugs (e.g., NSAIDs)
3. No improvement in creatinine level despite stopping use of diuretics for at least 4 to 5 days and volume repletion with 40 g intravenous albumin
4. Absence of proteinuria or ultrasonographic evidence of urinary tract obstruction or parenchymal renal disease

Treatment

The only definitive cure for HRS is recovery of hepatic function either with liver transplant or spontaneous recovery of the diseased liver. Temporizing measures can provide a bridge to liver transplantation or recovery. The combination of drugs to induce splanchnic vasoconstriction (octreotide) and renal vasodilation (midodrine) has been beneficial in improving renal function in HRS. The effect is augmented by the use of intravenous albumin. Alternatively, vasopressin analogues (e.g., terlipressin), which can also cause splanchnic vasoconstriction along with renal vasodilation, can be used instead of the combination. However, the drug is not available in the United States. Even though intravenous albumin appears to augment the response to these agents, its use remains controversial. The other potential modalities of therapy include **transjugular intrahepatic portosystemic shunt (TIPS)** and Molecular Adsorbent Recirculating System (MARS). In TIPS, a self-expandable metal stent is inserted between the hepatic vein and the intrahepatic portion of the portal vein using a transjugular approach, with a resulting decrease in portal pressure. It is primarily reserved for treatment of variceal bleeding, although small studies have suggested some improvement in renal function. MARS is a modified form of dialysis using albumin-containing dialysate that is recirculated and perfused online through charcoal and anion exchanger columns, and enables the removal of water-soluble and albumin-bound substances. It is believed that this system removes some of the vasoactive substances that mediate the hemodynamic changes that lead to HRS, thereby improving systemic hemodynamics and renal perfusion. Short-term studies suggest survival benefit with MARS in HRS, but larger studies are required before this expensive therapy can be widely recommended. Hemodialysis is extremely controversial in HRS. Generally, hemodialysis is usually offered only if the patient is awaiting liver transplant or there is a chance for liver recovery. In the absence of these possibilities, dialysis adds little to overall survival in this condition.

CARDIORENAL SYNDROME

Renal insufficiency is found in 20% to 40% of patients admitted to the hospital for heart failure and has been termed *cardiorenal syndrome* (CRS). Features of CRS include the presence of renal insufficiency, tendency for hyperkalemia, low systolic blood pressure, diuretic resistance, and anemia. Progressive kidney injury results in a series of abnormalities that include changes in coagulation, fibrinolysis, endothelial dysfunction, anemia, calcium–phosphorous balance, renin-angiotensin-aldosterone system, lipid abnormalities, and arrhythmias. A history of cardiac disease or acute myocardial infarction should prompt evaluation for decreased cardiac output states such as heart failure or cardiogenic shock. Prior hypertension, diabetes mellitus, or significant peripheral vascular disease should also raise the possibility of diminished renal autoregulatory capacity.

Pathogenesis

About 30% to 50% of patients with CHF have an impaired GFR. The interdependence between the kidneys and the heart often makes it challenging to distinguish whether the heart or the kidney is the main player in AKI. Aggressive therapy for CHF will occasionally result in further decrease in renal function, but equally true are cases of improved renal function after therapy for CHF. The survival advantages imparted by both ACE inhibitors and ARBs in both CHF and CKD clearly support the role of AII in the pathogenesis of this end-organ damage. The exact mechanism of renal deterioration associated with cardiac disease remains a mystery and is the basis of ongoing studies. In CKD, aside from the anemia-induced LVH, the hemodynamic interdependence between the heart and the kidneys and the nonhemodynamic association is mediated through endothelial damage associated with microalbuminuria and vascular calcification.

Treatment

Volume status should be ascertained carefully and loop diuretics should be administered intravenously in the setting of overt volume overload. In the setting of renal dysfunction, large doses of diuretics (e.g., furosemide 120–200 mg) may need to be administered to achieve a desirable diuresis. Small studies have shown that nitrates reduce preload and afterload and may allow for decreased doses of diuretics. Inotropic agents have been used successfully in the cardiogenic shock stage but need further evaluation with lesser degrees of cardiac failure. Nesiritide should be used with caution as deterioration of renal function has been seen in some cases. Hemofiltration has been shown beneficial in achieving faster fluid removal in several trials, but is invasive and expensive. A larger multicenter evaluation is needed before its use can be widely recommended. One interesting study demonstrated that hypertonic saline infusion along with furosemide achieved significantly more diuresis than with standard therapy and this approach warrants additional scrutiny.

POSTRENAL ACUTE KIDNEY INJURY

Definition

Obstructive uropathy describes an impediment to urine flow due to structural or functional change anywhere from the renal pelvis to the tip of the urethra. This resistance to flow increases pressure proximal to the point of obstruction. Renal parenchymal damage may or may not be associated. **Obstructive nephropathy** describes any functional or pathologic changes in the kidney that result from urinary tract obstruction (UTO).

Epidemiology

UTO is a common cause of renal failure and leads to approximately 400,000 hospitalizations per year in the United States. The overall prevalence of obstructive uropathy is approximately 3%, with both genders being affected equally. Early identification is critical as the extent to which the renal function recovers with treatment is inversely proportional to the duration and degree of obstruction. Hydronephrosis is found at postmortem examination in 2% to 4% of patients.

Classification

Obstructive uropathy is classified based on the duration, level, and degree of obstruction. The duration is acute or chronic depending on how long-standing it has been (hours to weeks vs. months to years). Obstruction is considered upper tract if it is located above the ureterovesical junction and lower tract if located below it. The degree of obstruction is either complete or partial.

TABLE 12-2	CONGENITAL CAUSES OF OBSTRUCTIVE UROPATHY

Ureter
Ureteropelvic junction obstruction
Ureteroceles
Ectopic ureter
Ureteral valves

Bladder
Myelodysplasias (e.g., meningomyelocele)
Bladder diverticula

Urethra
Prune-belly syndrome
Urethral diverticula
Posterior urethral valves

Etiology

Obstructive uropathy may be the result of anatomic or functional abnormalities anywhere in the urinary tract. These abnormalities are either congenital (Table 12-1) or acquired (Tables 12-2 and 12-3). The etiology varies depending on the age and sex of the patient. In children, ureteropelvic junction obstruction due to an aperistaltic segment or a stricture in the ureter, posterior urethral valves in boys, and neurologic abnormalities are the most common causes. Nephrolithiasis is the most common cause of obstructive uropathy in young men. In women, pregnancy (due to the effects of progesterone and, later, mechanical pressure by the gravid uterus) and gynecologic tumors account for most of the cases. In the older age group, obstructive uropathy is more common in men due to increased incidence of benign prostatic hyperplasia and carcinoma of the prostate.

TABLE 12-3	ACQUIRED INTRINSIC CAUSES OF OBSTRUCTIVE UROPATHY

Intraluminal	**Intramural**
Intrarenal	**Anatomic**
• Tubular precipitation of proteins: Bence-Jones proteins	• Tumors (renal pelvis, ureter, bladder, urethra)
• Tubular precipitation of crystals: uric acid, medications (e.g., acyclovir, indinavir, sulfonamides)	• Strictures (ureteral or urethral)
	• Infections
	• Granulomatous disease
	• Instrumentation or trauma
	• Radiation therapy
Extrarenal	**Functional disorders of the bladder**
• Nephrolithiasis	• Diabetes mellitus
• Blood clots	• Multiple sclerosis
• Papillary necrosis	• Spinal cord injury
• Fungus balls	• Anticholinergic agents

TABLE 12-4	ACQUIRED EXTRINSIC CAUSES OF OBSTRUCTIVE UROPATHY

Reproductive and Urological

• Uterus (pregnancy, prolapse, tumors)
• Ovary (abscess, cysts, tumors)
• Fallopian tubes (pelvic inflammatory disease)
• Prostate (benign hyperplasia, adenocarcinoma)

Gastrointestinal

• Crohn disease
• Appendicitis
• Diverticulitis
• Colorectal carcinoma

Vascular Disorders

• Aneurysms (abdominal aortic, iliac)
• Venous (ovarian vein thrombophlebitis, retrocaval ureter)

Retroperitoneal Disorders

• Fibrosis (idiopathic, drug related, inflammatory)
• Infection
• Radiation therapy
• Tumor (primary or metastatic)
• Iatrogenic complication of surgery

Pathophysiology

Obstruction to the urinary flow affects the kidney through a variety of factors with complex interactions that alter both glomerular hemodynamics and tubular function. The GFR drops after the onset of UTO due to a decrease in net hydrostatic pressure across the glomerular capillary wall. This is caused initially by an increase in intratubular pressure. In later stages of obstruction, this happens mainly due to a fall in intraglomerular pressure. This reduction in the intraglomerular pressure is a manifestation of decreased renal blood flow, caused by AII and thromboxane A_2–mediated vasoconstriction. Obstructive nephropathy is also associated with several abnormalities of tubular function believed to be caused by increased pressure within the tubules, leading to altered transport of sodium, water, and several other ions and solutes. In long-standing obstruction, the parenchyma atrophies, and fibrosis and scarring of the tubulointerstitium follow.

Clinical Findings

Clinical manifestations of UTO vary depending on the duration, site, and severity of obstruction and whether it is unilateral or bilateral.

Pain

Pain is an important initial symptom of acute obstruction. Acute upper tract obstruction causes pain on the affected side due to stretching of the renal capsule, whereas lower tract obstruction presents with lower abdominal pain due to bladder distention. Pain may be deceptively absent in patients with chronic, slowly developing obstruction. In cases of unilateral ureteral obstruction (e.g., because of a stone or clot), typical colicky pain may be described with radiation of pain down to the groin, testes, or labia. Vesicoureteral reflux classically presents with flank pain during micturition. In cases of ureteropelvic junction obstruction, flank pain may develop after ingestion of large amounts of fluids or administration of diuretics.

Palpable Mass
Kidney size may increase due to hydronephrosis and a palpable flank mass may be discerned in long-standing cases. A palpable mass in the suprapubic area may represent a distended bladder.

Change in Urine Output and Pattern
Complete bilateral obstruction (or unilateral obstruction in a patient with a solitary kidney) results in anuria. Partial or intermittent obstruction can result in polyuria or polyuria alternating with oligoanuria. Hesitancy, poor urinary stream, dysuria, and post-void dribbling are frequently associated with lower tract obstruction.

Renal Failure
Obstructive uropathy by itself can lead to renal failure due to pressure atrophy, intrarenal reflux, and ischemia, or it can be superimposed on another renal parenchymal disease and accelerate the rate of its progression. Obstruction should be considered in all patients with renal failure without a history of kidney disease and relatively benign urinary sediment.

Other Complications
Recurrent urinary tract infections without any explanation (and failure of adequate antibiotics to clear them) should always raise the suspicion of stasis and obstruction. **Hypertension** may be seen with both unilateral and bilateral obstruction of any duration. Unilateral obstruction causes elevated renin levels with activation of the renin-angiotensin-aldosterone axis, leading to hypertension. In cases of bilateral obstruction, hypertension is due to increased extracellular fluid volume secondary to impaired sodium excretion.

In addition to being a cause, **nephrolithiasis** can be a result of UTO. Chronic obstruction promotes infection. Infection with urease-producing organisms leads to increased urine pH, precipitating struvite stone formation. Infection in this setting is extremely difficult to eradicate unless the stone is removed. **Hyperkalemic-hyperchloremic acidosis** may sometimes complicate partial obstruction. The etiology of this defect is an acquired "pseudohypoaldosterone" state. Tubules damaged by obstruction cannot respond fully to aldosterone, leading to difficulty in excreting potassium and hydrogen ions. Any elderly, nondiabetic patient who has a chemical picture suggestive of hyperkalemic-hyperchloremic acidosis should be carefully evaluated for obstruction. Renal tubular defects leading to **impaired concentrating ability** of the kidney (nephrogenic diabetes insipidus) result in polyuria and polydipsia. Elderly patients with impaired thirst mechanisms may present with dehydration and hypernatremia. **Polycythemia** has been associated with hydronephrosis and is likely related to increased production of erythropoietin by the obstructed kidney.

Diagnosis
Lab Evaluation
Urinalysis is expected to be bland in uncomplicated UTO. However, clues to underlying etiologies may be provided by abnormalities in the urine. Hematuria suggests the presence of stones or a sloughed papilla. A more ominous possibility is an underlying urothelial neoplasm. Crystals may be seen with metabolic abnormalities leading to production of stones. Thus, the type of crystal seen provides information on not only the presence of a stone but possibly also the type of stone causing obstruction. The presence of infection may change the pace at which relief of obstruction is sought, especially in cases of unilateral obstruction.

Blood counts and chemistries should be checked to assess degree of dysfunction and also to identify metabolic abnormalities of renal failure that may need to be addressed urgently.

Radiologic Evaluation

Imaging is a key diagnostic step in evaluation of urinary tract obstruction. Various imaging modalities are available, and the initial choice is dictated by the results of history, exam, and lab tests.

- *Plain films* (KUB x-ray) of the abdomen can provide a gross estimate of kidney size. It may reveal renal pelvic, ureteral, or bladder calculi (90% of which are radio-opaque).
- *Ultrasound* is noninvasive, is >90% sensitive and specific, does not involve contrast exposure, is inexpensive, and is readily available. It can determine renal size and reveal dilatation of the collecting system. False-positive results can be seen in cases of extrarenal pelvis, congenital megacalices, diuresis, renal cysts, and calyceal diverticula. A dilated collecting system without obstruction can be seen in cases of ileal conduits, vesicoureteral reflux, primary megaureter, and acute pyelonephritis. At times, hydronephrosis is not seen despite the presence of obstruction. This can happen with severe dehydration, retroperitoneal fibrosis, staghorn calculi, or intrarenal pelvis. Figure 12-2 shows an ultrasonographic image of obstruction with preserved renal cortex. Ultrasound should be obtained in all cases of AKI presenting in the emergency room, as obstruction accounts for about 15% of all those cases. In the intensive care unit, the yield from an ultrasound is extremely low, since UTO is extremely rare.
- *Intravenous urography* can be useful to define anatomy and the location of the obstruction if ultrasound shows hydronephrosis. However, this is hardly used given the potential for exacerbation of renal failure with intravenous radiocontrast.
- *Isotope renography* is performed by injection of a radionuclide tracer; images are then obtained with a gamma-scintillation camera. The images reveal delayed excretion of the tracer. Sensitivity of the test is enhanced by administration of furosemide (Lasix renogram). Furosemide administration causes a rapid washout of the tracer in cases of functional obstruction but cannot do so if there is mechanical obstruction to urine flow.

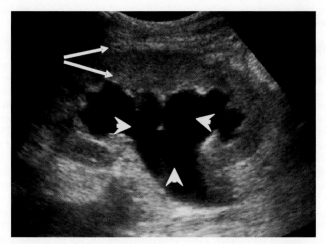

FIGURE 12-2. Ultrasound of the kidney demonstrating the dilated calyces (*arrowheads*) with preserved renal cortex (*between arrows*). (Courtesy of William D. Middleton, MD, Washington University School of Medicine, St. Louis, MO.)

- *Computerized tomography* (CT) has become a very useful tool to assess UTO. Unlike ultrasound, it can also simultaneously evaluate the cause of the obstruction. "Stone protocol" CT scans do not require contrast, but contrast may be needed if other details of abdominal anatomy are to be evaluated. *Magnetic resonance imaging* (MRI) has the advantage of not requiring radiocontrast administration and superior spatial resolution, but it is expensive and more cumbersome than CT or ultrasound.
- *Antegrade pyelography* entails a percutaneous nephrostomy and injection of a contrast medium. This is also used for drainage. *Retrograde pyelography* is done by ureteral catheterization through a cystoscope followed by contrast injection. This carries the risk of introduction of infection to the upper tract from below.
- *Voiding cystourethrography* is the gold standard for the diagnosis of vesicoureteral reflux. It is also used for evaluation of posterior urethral valves and urethral strictures. If obstruction is strongly suspected as the cause of AKI and ultrasound is inconclusive, the physician must strongly consider seeking a urology consultation for cystoscopy.

Management

Therapy is aimed at achieving three main goals:

- *Elimination of any life-threatening complication of obstruction.* This involves rapid restoration of intravascular volume, treatment of severe metabolic complications (e.g., hyperkalemia, acidosis), and initiation of aggressive management of infection.
- *Preservation of renal function.* If the problem is bilateral obstruction, immediate steps to relieve the obstruction are mandated. The longer the obstruction, the higher the risk for irreversible renal parenchymal damage. The location of the obstruction dictates the procedure of choice. For the lower urinary tract, a Foley catheter is all that may be needed. If a transurethral catheter cannot be placed, a urology consultation may be needed to place a suprapubic catheter. For an upper tract obstruction, the placement of percutaneous nephrostomy tubes or ureteral catheters/stents is requested in consultation with interventional radiology or urology.
- *Determination of the cause of obstruction and its definitive treatment.* Definitive diagnosis and therapy can be planned and pursued once the patient has been stabilized and the urinary system decompressed.

Postobstructive Diuresis

Polyuria associated with substantial losses of water and solutes is commonly seen after relief of severe, bilateral obstruction. The factors causing this phenomenon are osmotic diuresis caused by retained urea and other osmoles, volume overload, tubular concentration defects, and accumulation of natriuretic factors (e.g., atrial natriuretic peptide). The first two of these factors are predominant early and cease with excretion of the excess solute and water. However, tubular insensitivity to ADH at times may persist longer. The diuresis can be substantial and volume status and electrolytes need to be monitored to gauge fluid and electrolyte support. However, overzealous fluid replacement will lead to persistent high urine flow rates despite resolution of the osmotic diuresis.

Volume depletion will develop once the obstruction is relieved if urine losses are not replaced. It is reasonable to start with 0.45% saline and replace approximately two-thirds of the urine losses. Volume status, urine output, and chemistry values in blood and urine need to be closely monitored. If signs of hypo- or hypervolemia develop, the replacement rate can be adjusted accordingly. The replacement fluid rate can be gradually decreased over the course of the next few days. Plasma chemistry values may help further adjustment of the type of fluid being used (e.g., hypotonic vs. isotonic fluids, requirement for potassium, magnesium, and phosphorus).

Prognosis

Renal function recovery clearly correlates with the degree of obstruction and its time course. Recovery from complete obstruction can be seen within 1 week if no irreversible renal injury has occurred but may take up to 12 weeks to achieve a new lower baseline if some damage has occurred. Recovery from partial obstruction will typically be seen within 7 to 10 days. Correction of the obstruction may not be necessary if the patient is largely asymptomatic, the plasma creatinine concentration is normal, and there seems to be little or no parenchymal atrophy on renal ultrasonography. In a prospective study in patients with unilateral obstructive uropathy with a normal-functioning contralateral kidney, the preoperative renographic clearance and perfusion of the corresponding kidney were the only predictors of recoverability of unilateral renal obstruction. Kidneys with a renographic GFR <10 mL/minute/1.73 m^2 were irreversibly damaged. Improvement or stabilization of function can be expected after relief of obstruction of kidneys with a renographic GFR ≥10 mL/minute/1.73 m^2.

KEY POINTS TO REMEMBER

Prerenal Kidney Disease
- Prerenal azotemia is the most common cause of AKI. Rapid restoration of effective circulatory volume usually leads to prompt and complete resolution of AKI.
- In addition to other aspects of history and exam, a complete exam of the urine, including study of the sediment, is key.
- Fractional excretion of sodium is useful in the *oliguric state only*.
- Fraction excretion of urea may be a useful marker to distinguish prerenal AKI from ATN in the setting of diuretic use.
- HRS can be temporarily treated with vasopressin analogues, alpha-adrenergic agonists, and albumin.
- CRS management is complicated by the delicate balance between the need for diuresis and the coexistent need to maintain adequate renal perfusion.

Postrenal Kidney Disease
- Ultrasound is a cost-effective and efficient way to evaluate for UTO.
- Degree of obstruction may be underestimated in the severely dehydrated patient; in such cases, repeating the ultrasound after adequate volume replacement may highlight the hydronephrosis.
- Rarely, in cases of retroperitoneal fibrosis or lymphomas, the ureters are encased, and hydronephrosis is not seen despite severe UTO.
- UTO may present with polyuria if the obstruction is incomplete.
- Prompt relief of obstruction is essential to avoid parenchymal destruction.
- Fluid replacement during a postobstructive diuresis (due to retained volume and solutes) should be judicious. It is important not to "chase" the urine output; this may lead to replacement of the postobstructive diuresis by a diuresis due to IV fluids.

REFERENCES AND SUGGESTED READINGS

Badr KF, Ichikawa I. Prerenal failure: a deleterious shift from renal compensation to decompensation. *N Engl J Med.* 1988;319:623.

Beers MH, Porter RS, Jones TV, et al. *The Merck Manual of Diagnosis and Therapy.* 18th ed. Whitehouse Station, NJ: Merck; 2006.

Blantz RC, Konnen KS. The relation of distal tubular delivery and reabsorptive rate to nephron filtration. *Am J Physiol.* 1977;233:F315.

Brenner, BM, ed. *Brenner & Rector's The Kidney.* 7th ed. Philadelphia: WB Saunders; 2004.

Cárdenas A, Gines P. Hepatorenal syndrome. *Clin Liv Dis.* 2006;10(2):371–385.

Carvounis CP, Nisar S, Guro-Razuman S. Significance of the fractional excretion of urea in the differential diagnosis of acute renal failure. *Kidney Int.* 2002;62(6):2223–2229.

De Nicola L, Blantz RC, Gabbai FB. Nitric oxide and angiotensin II. Glomerular and tubular interaction in the rat. *J Clin Invest.* 1992;89:1248.

Fonarow GC. The confounding issue of comorbid renal insufficiency. *Am J Med.* 2006;119(12 Suppl 1); S17–S25.

Gabbai FB, Thomson SC, Peterson O, et al. Glomerular and tubular interactions between renal adrenergic activity and nitric oxide. *Am J Physiol.* 1995;37:F1004.

Goldstein MH, Lenz PR, Levitt MF. Effect of urine flow rate on urea reabsorption in man. Urea as a "tubular marker." *J Appl Physiol.* 1969;26:594–599.

Khalaf IM, Shokeir AA, El-Gyoushi FI, et al. Recoverability of renal function after treatment of adult patients with unilateral obstructive uropathy and normal contralateral kidney: a prospective study. *Urology.* 2004;64:664–668.

Klahr S. New insights into the consequences and mechanisms of renal impairment in obstructive nephropathy. *Am J Kidney Dis.* 1991;18:689.

Klahr S. Obstructive nephropathy. In: Massry SG, Glassock RJ, eds. *Massry & Glassock's Textbook of Nephrology.* 4th ed. Philadelphia: Lippincott Williams & Wilkins; 2001:986.

Klahr S. Obstructive nephropathy: pathophysiology and management. In: Schrier RW, ed. *Renal and Electrolyte Disorders.* 6th ed. Philadelphia: Lippincott Williams & Wilkins; 2003:498.

Klahr S. Urinary tract obstruction. In: Schrier RW, ed. *Diseases of the Kidney and Urinary Tract.* 7th ed. Philadelphia: Lippincott Williams & Wilkins; 2001:757.

Klahr S, Miller SB. Current concepts: acute oliguria. *N Engl J Med.* 1998;338:671–675.

Korbet SM. Obstructive uropathy. In: Greenberg A, ed. *Primer on Kidney Diseases.* 3rd ed. San Diego: Academic Press; 2001:336.

Obialo CI. Cardiorenal consideration as a risk factor for heart failure. *Am J Cardio.* 2007;99(6B):21D–24D.

Ragaller MJR, Theilen H, Koch T. Volume replacement in critically ill patients with acute renal failure. *J Am Soc Nephrol.* 2001;12:S33.

Rose BD. Pre-renal disease versus acute tubular necrosis. In: *Pathophysiology of Renal Disease.* 2nd ed. New York: McGraw-Hill; 1987:65–119.

Steiner RW, Tucker BJ, Blantz RC. Glomerular hemodynamics in rats with chronic sodium depletion: effect of saralasin. *J Clin Invest.* 1979;64:503.

Thadhani R, Pascual M, Bonventre JV. Acute renal failure. *N Engl J Med.* 1996;334:1448.

Zeidel ML, Pirtskhalaishvili G. Urinary tract obstruction. In: Brenner BM, ed. *Brenner & Rector's The Kidney.* 7th ed. Philadelphia: WB Saunders; 2004.

Intrinsic Causes of Acute Kidney Injury

13

Kamalanathan Sambandam

INTRODUCTION

Once hemodynamic and postrenal causes of acute kidney injury (AKI) have been excluded, acute renal dysfunction that is intrinsic to the kidneys must be considered. In the approach to intrinsic AKI, it is helpful to group the etiologies by the site of initial nephron pathology: the supplying microvasculature, the glomerulus, the tubule, or the interstitium (Table 13-1). Although significant clinical overlap exists, a few readily attainable clinical findings might suggest the category to which a particular case of intrinsic AKI belongs:

- *Microvascular:* new or accelerating hypertension with evidence of microangiopathic hemolytic anemia.
- *Glomerular:* new or accelerating hypertension and volume overload, heavy proteinuria, and/or significant hematuria, especially if red blood cell casts are present.
- *Tubular:* urinary sediment containing characteristic tubular cell casts or crystals.
- *Interstitial:* the presence of pyuria or white blood cell casts.

This chapter will focus on the causes of intrinsic AKI that involve the nonglomerular segments of the nephron. Glomerular causes of renal insufficiency found in Table 13-1 are discussed in Chapters 16, 17, and 18.

MICROVASCULAR ACUTE KIDNEY INJURY

Atheroembolic renal disease, malignant hypertension, and *scleroderma renal crisis* may manifest as an acute decline in renal function and each involves injury to the small arteries and arterioles supplying the glomeruli as the primary pathologic event. In *antiphospholipid syndrome* (APS), *hemolytic-uremic syndrome* (HUS), *thrombotic-thrombocytopenic purpura* (TTP), *preeclampsia,* and *HELLP* (hemolysis, elevated liver enzymes, low platelets) *syndrome,* the initial site of injury may be the supplying microvasculature and/or the glomerular capillaries themselves as a result of generalized endothelial dysfunction. Special emphasis is given to atheroembolic renal disease because of its increased incidence compared with others in this category. Malignant hypertension, HUS, TTP, preeclampsia, and HELLP are discussed in detail elsewhere in this manual and will only be briefly touched on here.

ATHEROEMBOLIC RENAL DISEASE

Definition and Pathogenesis
Atheroembolic renal disease refers to AKI that arises from the occlusion of the renal microvasculature by lipid debris and subsequent inflammation. Setting the stage for its

TABLE 13-1	CAUSES OF INTRINSIC ACUTE KIDNEY INJURY ACCORDING TO SITE OF PRIMARY INJURY			
Microvasculature	**Glomerulus**	**Tubule**	**Interstitium**
Atheroembolic renal disease	Rapidly progressive glomerulo-nephritis	Crystalline nephropathy	Acute interstitial nephritis
Malignant hypertension		Myeloma kidney	Infiltrative malignancies
Scleroderma renal crisis		Acute tubular necrosis (toxic or ischemic)	Acute pyelonephritis

Antiphospholipid syndrome
Preeclampsia/ HELLP syndrome
HUS/ TTP

HELLP, hemolysis, elevated liver enzymes, and low platelets; HUS/TTP, hemolytic uremic syndrome/ thrombotic thrombocytopenic purpura.

occurrence is the presence of aortic atherosclerosis upstream of the kidneys. Although spontaneous atheroemboli may occur in approximately 20% of cases, more often there is an inciting event leading to plaque destabilization and distal showering of lipid. In two thirds of provoked cases, plaque destabilization occurs from vascular wall trauma during either vascular surgeries or percutaneous endovascular procedures. In one third of provoked cases, anticoagulation or thrombolytic administration initiates the disease process. The lipid lodges in the small arterioles and incites thrombus formation, causing distal ischemia and infarction. Within days there may be recanalization of the thrombus and restoration of blood flow, but an inflammatory foreign body arteritis then ensues, leading to progressive fibrosis and eventual obliteration of the vessel lumen. Continued nephron ischemia thus occurs.

Epidemiology

Atheroembolic renal disease is most commonly a disease of the elderly white male. The mean age of presentation is 66 to 70 years and men are affected four times as commonly as women, paralleling the prevalence bias of atherosclerotic vascular disease. Clinically significant renal atheroemboli occurs in <0.2% of cardiac catheterizations, though it is certainly underrecognized. It occurs much more commonly with aortography and aortic surgeries; and with the progress of invasive endovascular procedures, the incidence is likely increasing.

Clinical Presentation and Diagnosis

The main manifestations of atheroembolic disease are listed in Table 13-2. Patients usually have multiple cardiac disease risk factors, a history of cerebrovascular accidents, or an abdominal aortic aneurysm. Lipid embolism can occur from 3 days to 3 months after the inciting event. The **typical patient** is noted to have blue or dark red discoloration of the toes associated with increasing creatinine several days after a vascular procedure. The **skin** is the most commonly affected organ, but the reliance on characteristic skin findings for diagnosis may contribute to the underrepresentation of this disease among dark-skinned races. **Other organ systems** such as the gastrointestinal tract and central nervous system may be simultaneously

TABLE 13-2	CLINICAL AND LABORATORY FINDINGS IN PATIENTS WITH RENAL ATHEROEMBOLIC DISEASE

Very Common

New onset, accelerated, or labile hypertension
Skin findings: cyanotic or ulcerated digits or scrotum, livedo reticularis on back or lower extremities, nodules, and/or purpura
Eosinophiluria by Hansel stain
Peripheral blood eosinophilia
Elevated erythrocyte sedimentation rate or c-reactive protein

Common

Gastrointestinal symptoms: nausea, abdominal pain, and/or gastrointestinal bleeding
Microscopic hematuria
Mild proteinuria (rarely in the nephrotic range)
Renal artery stenosis on imaging study
Various markers of ischemic organ injury: elevated creatine kinase, amylase/lipase, and/or transaminases

Uncommon

Fevers
Central nervous system symptoms: focal neurologic deficits and/or progressive dementia
Retinal emboli with Hollenhorst plaque visible on fundoscopy
Hypocomplementemia

involved. The multisystem disease involvement, together with the variable occurrence of eosinophilia and depressed complement levels, may mimic a vasculitis.

Renal biopsy reveals empty clefts in arcuate and interlobular arteries from the dissolution of lipid from these sites by the fixation process. Early lesions display an inflammatory arteritis composed of eosinophils, neutrophils, and macrophages, which is later replaced by a giant cell foreign body reaction with proliferation and fibrosis of the vascular intima. Acutely, the tubules may show signs of acute tubular necrosis (ATN). Late in evolution, patchy glomerular sclerosis and tubular atrophy may be visualized in areas supplied by affected vessels. Similar arteriolar inflammation or fibrosis can be found in other tissues, especially the muscle, gastrointestinal tract, and skin. Biopsy of skin lesions may have an especially high diagnostic yield.

Course and Management

Three patterns of disease evolution may be apparent in atheroembolic renal disease:

- *Acute* (35% of cases): An abrupt deterioration in renal function occurs 3 to 7 days after the inciting event, usually with multisystem organ involvement from a massive embolic shower.
- *Subacute* (56% of cases): Repeated smaller embolic showers or progressive obliterative arteritis in previously involved vessels leads to a stepwise deterioration in renal function with stabilization by 3 to 8 weeks. This is the most common pattern of the disease.
- *Chronic* (9% of cases): Renal insufficiency is slowly progressive and is hard to distinguish from worsening hypertensive nephrosclerosis or ischemic renovascular disease.

Progression to dialysis dependence occurs in approximately one-third of the patients who survive the initial insult, though a mild improvement in glomerular filtration rate can occur. No means of reversing the tissue injury exists. Therefore, therapy consists of aggressive **supportive care** addressing the most common mechanisms of death in the acute multivisceral forms of the disease. These include ongoing cardiac ischemia, decompensated heart failure, stroke, and malnutrition in the setting of gastrointestinal ischemia. With multivisceral involvement, further **anticoagulation or intravascular manipulations should be strictly avoided**, perhaps even in the setting of recurrent cardiac ischemia. Particular attention should be given to the management of hypertension and volume overload. If renal replacement therapy is required, hemodialysis should be performed without anticoagulation. If this is not possible, peritoneal dialysis should be employed. **Nutritional support** should be aggressive, even administered parenterally if needed.

In addition to these basic management principles, several adjunctive therapies may be considered. Though corticosteroids have not been proven to affect renal outcome, low doses (0.3 mg/kg of prednisone) might improve anorexia and abdominal pain from mesenteric involvement. Association data suggests a benefit from statin use, perhaps through atherosclerotic plaque stabilization and reductions in inflammation. Even with the above meticulous therapeutic regimen, the one-year mortality rate with multivisceral disease is 25%. Regarding prevention, a small study evaluated the brachial artery approach during cardiac catheterization in those with extensive aortic atherosclerotic disease and found no improvement in risk. However, high-risk patients might still be benefited by this approach.

OTHER MICROVASCULAR CAUSES OF INTRINSIC AKI

Definitions and Pathogenesis

- *Scleroderma renal crisis* refers to a clinical entity of acute and progressive renal dysfunction with worsening hypertension occurring in scleroderma patients. An incompletely understood endothelial cell dysfunction with vascular hyperresponsiveness underlies its pathogenesis as in the other tissues that scleroderma effects.
- In *APS*, antibodies with specificity for anionic phospholipids or the plasma proteins that bind to them induce activation of platelets and endothelial cells, leading to a procoagulant state. If thrombosis occurs primarily in the microvasculature, this can result in an acute or chronic thrombotic microangiopathy in multiple organs, including the kidney. *Catastrophic APS* is said to be present if an additional procoagulant stimulus (e.g., infection, surgery, or withdrawal of anticoagulation) initiates fulminant, predominantly microvascular thrombosis that clinically involves at least three different organ systems in a span of <1 week. Finally, macroscopic thrombosis may involve the renal arteries in APS and may mimic the microvascular forms of the disease with acute renal failure and accelerating hypertension.
- *HUS* and *TTP* are syndromes of systemic thrombotic microangiopathy and prominent consumptive thrombocytopenia. In HUS, drugs, infections, or toxins initiate endothelial and neutrophil activation or a deficiency in complement regulatory molecules leads to microvascular thrombosis. TTP appears to result from the accumulation of large von Willebrand multimers from reduced ADAMS13 protease activity. The large multimers then initiate platelet aggregation and activation in the small vessels.
- *Preeclampsia* is a syndrome of new or worsening hypertension with proteinuria occurring in the late stages of pregnancy. *HELLP* (hemolysis, elevated liver enzymes, low platelets) is a more severe form of the disease in which microangiopathic anemia is more prominent and there is also evidence of liver dysfunction. In preeclampsia, endothelial dysfunction seems to occur from an imbalance of placenta-derived angiogenic and antiangiogenic factors. These problems are covered further in Chapter 22.

Clinical Presentation and Diagnosis

The vasculopathy in these disorders leads to glomerular ischemia, which prompts a vicious cycle of high renin and angiotensin-induced vasoconstriction, rises in blood pressure and further glomerular ischemia. This is most apparent in scleroderma renal crisis, in which there is fairly prompt reversal of the disease with the initiation of angiotensin-converting enzyme inhibition. Because of this shared pathophysiologic mechanism of ischemic hyper-reninism, the appearance of accelerating hypertension and worsening renal function is common to all of the diseases in this category of AKI. Marked hypertension may lead to signs of decompensated heart failure or angina. Headaches, altered mental status, seizures, or focal neurologic deficits can be evident from hypertensive encephalopathy or cerebral microvascular occlusions. Retinal hemorrhages, exudates, or papilledema may be observed on fundoscopic exam. **Laboratory data** may reveal findings consistent with a microangio-pathic hemolytic anemia (schistocytosis, elevated lactate dehydrogenase, and reduced hap-toglobin). Hematuria, granular casts, and worsening proteinuria may be present in varying degrees on urinalysis.

Renal biopsy findings are remarkably similar amongst the diseases in this category, except that malignant hypertension and scleroderma renal crisis may involve the pre-glomerular vessels more prominently. Early on, fibrinoid necrosis with a paucity of inflam-matory infiltrate is seen in the small arteries and arterioles. Thrombi may be visualized in glomerular capillary loops. Glomerular endotheliosis, or swelling of endothelial cells with subendothelial deposition of hyaline material, may be seen in any of these diseases but is more prominent in preeclampsia. Later, the intima displays myxoid thickening and finally undergoes fibrous proliferation, resulting in the typical concentric onion-skin lesions that may obliterate the lumen of smaller vessels. There is secondary ischemic sclerosis and drop-out of supplied glomeruli and tubules. Some of the clinical features that distinguish the diseases in this category of intrinsic AKI are discussed in Table 13-3. Basic principles of management are also presented there.

TUBULAR ACUTE KIDNEY INJURY

The causes of intrinsic AKI in which the primary site of injury is the renal tubule include *acute tubular necrosis* (ATN), the *crystalline nephropathies*, and *myeloma cast nephropathy* (see Table 13-1). Though not helpful for diagnosing cast nephropathy, clues to the pres-ence of the remaining causes of AKI in this category may be obtained from analysis of the urine sediment: muddy brown casts may be visualized in ATN and characteristic crystals might be seen in the crystalline nephropathies. ATN will not be discussed any further here as it is presented in Chapter 11.

CRYSTALLINE NEPHROPATHIES

Definition and Pathogenesis

The crystalline nephropathies describe the AKI that results from the intratubular pre-cipitation of various compounds. The most common cause of crystalline nephropathy is **tumor lysis syndrome (TLS)**, which includes the entities **acute uric acid nephropathy** and **acute phosphate nephropathy**. Less commonly, crystalline nephropathy may result from the precipitation of **calcium oxalate, acyclovir, sulfonamide, methotrexate, indinavir,** or **triamterene**. Finally, there are rare case reports of its occurrence with the use of ciprofloxacin, foscarnet, and ampicillin, and with plasma cell dyscrasias.

Intratubular crystal formation and deposition is promoted by three mechanisms: high tubular fluid concentration of a substance, prolonged intratubular transit time, and

TABLE 13-3	THE MICROVASCULAR CAUSES OF INTRINSIC ACUTE KIDNEY INJURY (except atheroembolic renal disease)				
	Malignant Hypertension	Scleroderma Renal Crisis	Microvascular APS[b]	HUS/TTP	Preeclampsia/HELLP
Incidence	Most common microvascular cause of AKI at 2.6 per 100,000 patients per year	10% of patients with scleroderma, almost always within first 5 years after diagnosis	25% of patients with primary APS	11 cases per million people per year	5% of pregnancies
Risk Factors	Longstanding hypertension, black race, abrupt interruption of BP medications, secondary causes of HTN	More extensive and rapidly progressive scleroderma skin involvement, cooler temperature environments, black race, initiation of corticosteroids at high dose, use of cyclosporine	Procoagulant states including a recent thrombotic event, withdrawal of anticoagulation, pregnancy, infection, surgery, etc.	• Infection: enteritis with shiga-toxin–producing bacteria, HIV, pneumococcal infection • Drugs: quinine, contraceptives, calcineurin inhibitors, chemotherapeutic medications, thienopyridines • Peripartum	Previous preeclampsia or positive family history, primigravid, age >40 or <18, multifetal gestation, previous hypertension or renal disease, diabetes, obesity
Distinguishing Clinical Features[a]		Signs of scleroderma (sclerodactyly, interstitial lung disease, etc.) are present and usually obvious. Autoantibodies (e.g., anti-Scl-70 or anti-ribonucleic acid polymerase)	Signs of APS (previous thrombosis in an atypical vessel, infarcts in other vascular beds, livedo reticularis, etc.) or SLE is present. Lupus anticoagulant or antiphospholipid	Hemolytic anemia and thrombocytopenia is prominent. Fever may be present. ADAMS13 activity may be low in idiopathic TTP but is variable. Presence of accelerated hypertension is less consistently seen.	Elevation in BP can be relatively mild. Usually occurs after 20th week of pregnancy. Evidence of fetal compromise may be evident. Reduction in GFR is usually mild. Proteinuria often

becomes nephrotic in later stages. Glomerular endotheliosis is prominent early on.

- Prevention: Low-dose aspirin in high-risk patients
- Treatment: Antihypertensive therapy and close mother and fetal monitoring until fetal maturity. Deliver fetus if maturity is reached or severe preeclampsia occurs.

- Treatment:
  —Typical HUS (post-enteritis)-supportive care alone
  —Atypical HUS or TTP-supportive care plus plasma exchange (less desirably, high-dose plasma infusion) +/− corticosteroids

antibody is present. Thrombocytopenia may be significant. Focal renal cortical atrophy may be evident. Course may be chronic, acute, or fulminant (i.e., catastrophic APS).

- Prevention: Avoidance of precipitants (see Risk Factors) +/− aspirin or hydroxychloroquine.
- Treatment: Address underlying precipitant, anticoagulation, +/− antiplatelet therapy, +/− glucocorticoids. If catastrophic APS present, initiate plasma exchange or intravenous immune globulin in addition to above.

may be present. 10% of patients may be normotensive at diagnosis.

- Prevention: Avoidance of renal ischemia from drugs or volume depletion. At-risk patients should monitor BP closely and if a sustained rise occurs, renal function should be assessed.
- Treatment: Initiate ACEI promptly. Renal function may initially worsen, but continued therapy will allow eventual improvement, with >50% of patients able to stop dialysis.

Principles of Management

- Treatment: Reduce BP by 25% within 2–6 hours and toward 160/100 mm Hg by 24–48 hours. Renal function may initially worsen slightly.

---

[a]As all may present with accelerating hypertension and worsening renal function, the clinical features that distinguish the diseases are emphasized.

[b]Antiphospholipid antibody syndrome may also present with large-artery thrombosis that may manifest similarly to the microvascular form of the disease.

ACEI, angiotensin-converting enzyme inhibitor; AKI, acute kidney injury; APS, antiphospholipid syndrome; BP, blood pressure; GFR, glomerular filtration rate; HELLP, hemolysis elevated liver enzymes, low platelets syndrome; HIV, human immunodeficiency virus; HUS, hemolytic uremic syndrome; SLE, systemic lupus erythematosus; TTP, thrombotic thrombocytopenic purpura.

decreased solubility. The first two mechanisms occur in the setting of decreased effective circulating volume, which is a major risk factor for all of the crystalline nephropathies. Decreased effective circulating volume leads to an increase in proximal tubular fluid reabsorption. This results in both high concentrations of the offending compound in the distal tubule and decreased distal flow rates. Underlying chronic kidney disease is also a major risk factor for the crystalline nephropathies because a larger amount of the compound is excreted per functioning nephron and because drugs are frequently overdosed in renal insufficiency. The third mechanism, decreased solubility, is often dependent on the distal tubular fluid pH. Compounds with a pKa <7, such as uric acid, calcium oxalate, sulfonamides, methotrexate, and triamterene, tend to precipitate in acidic urine while compounds with a pKa >7, such as indinavir and calcium phosphate, tend to precipitate in alkaline urine. The clinical contexts in which the more common crystalline nephropathies occur are summarized in Table 13-4. The pathogenesis of crystalline AKI from TLS and ethylene glycol intoxication is discussed further below because of their relevance to their treatment.

Pathophysiology of Tumor Lysis Syndrome

TLS results from the sudden release of normally intracellular compounds to the extracellular space from massive tumor cell death. The **main risk factor** is the presence of a large tumor burden with a rapid doubling time and thus exquisite response to cytolytic therapy. Most cancers associated with TLS are high-grade lymphoproliferative malignancies with up to 6% of these patients developing this complication. It has also been reported with several aggressive solid tumors including lung and breast carcinoma. Though the disease usually arises in the setting of traditional potent chemotherapy directed against nucleic acid processing, it has also been observed with interferon, endocrine therapies such as corticosteroids or tamoxifen, and radiation treatment. Furthermore, spontaneous TLS can occur when aggressive cancers rapidly outstrip their nutrient supply.

The AKI due to TLS has historically been thought of as an acute uric acid nephropathy. Purine nucleosides are released by dying cells and are metabolized to hypoxanthine and xanthine. Xanthine oxidase converts both intermediates to uric acid. At normal plasma pH, 98% of uric acid exists as the more-soluble ionized salt, urate. In the normally acidic tubular fluid, it exists primarily as the less-soluble uric acid and may precipitate in the kidney. Now that hypouricemic therapy is commonly employed for prophylaxis in at-risk patients, acute phosphate nephropathy has become an important cause of AKI in TLS. Significant amounts of phosphate complexed with adenosine exist in the intracellular compartment, especially in metabolically active cancer cells. Once released by cell death, phosphate precipitates in the renal tubules and other tissues as calcium phosphate.

Pathophysiology of Ethylene Glycol Intoxication

Ethylene glycol is metabolized by hepatic alcohol dehydrogenase to four toxic organic compounds: glycoaldehyde, glycolic acid, glyoxylic acid, and oxalic acid. Accumulation of the organic anions glycolate, glyoxylate, and oxalate leads to a severe anion gap metabolic acidosis. These compounds, especially glycolic acid, are direct cell toxins and cause multiorgan dysfunction with heart failure, ATN, and nervous system depression. Oxalate precipitates with calcium in several tissues including the renal tubules causing crystalline nephropathy.

Clinical Presentation and Diagnosis

Extensive crystal deposition in any of the forms of crystalline nephropathy may result in pain from distention of the renal capsule, which is similar to ureteral colic. In some cases (especially with indinavir and sulfonamides), nephrolithiasis may coexist with intratubular crystal deposition. Hypocalcemia due to the coprecipitation of calcium in acute phosphate nephropathy and oxalate nephropathy may result in paresthesias, lethargy, or tetany. High levels of acyclovir accumulating with the onset of renal failure can lead to hallucinations, delirium, and myoclonus. Similarly, toxic levels of methotrexate can also cause neurologic disturbances as well as nausea, rash, and mucositis.

The clinical manifestations of **ethylene glycol** intoxication evolve over time as the alcohol is metabolized. During the first 30 minutes to 12 hours, ethylene glycol causes ine-briation, with progression to seizures or coma. Twelve to 36 hours postingestion, peak concentrations of organic acid intermediates lead to profound acidosis with Kussmaul respirations and cardiopulmonary failure. Twenty-four to 72 hours postingestion, the oxalate end-product accumulates in tissues, resulting in AKI. This time course is prolonged in cases of ethanol co-ingestion due to competitive inhibition of alcohol dehydrogenase.

Urine sediment findings will often reveal hematuria, pyuria, and mild proteinuria. Although the offending substances have unique crystal morphologies on urine microscopy, examining the sediment is not independently diagnostic. Obstructed tubules may not empty urine into the collecting system and therefore the absence of crystals does not exclude crystalline nephropathy. Furthermore, the presence of crystals does not prove their pathogenic role because calcium oxalate, calcium phosphate, and uric acid crystalluria can be seen in normal individuals and because patients receiving typical offending medications can sometimes display crystalluria without AKI.

Renal ultrasound may reveal bilaterally enlarged and echogenic kidneys and can identify concomitant macroscopic lithiasis. Renal biopsy is required to make a definitive diagnosis. Light microscopy reveals crystalline deposits, usually in the distal tubules, with a surrounding interstitial infiltrate that may contain giant cells as part of a foreign body reaction. Evidence of ATN can also be present as many of the inciting agents display direct tubular cell toxicity. Polarized microscopy may demonstrate birefringence depending on the offending agent. A summary of the laboratory findings characteristic for the more common etiologies of crystalline nephropathy is found in Table 13-4.

Course and Management

In most cases of crystalline nephropathy, the chance for full renal recovery is excellent. In the drug-related crystalline nephropathies, recovery of renal function is expected to occur within days to weeks after cessation or even just dose reduction of the drug. Phosphate nephropathy due to phosphate-containing laxatives prior to colonoscopy may have a worse prognosis because the population affected by this entity is older and has a higher prevalence of underlying chronic kidney disease.

The mainstay of **prevention** is avoidance of the two most frequent predisposing factors: volume depletion and drug overdosing by failing to adjust for renal impairment. Establishing a brisk urine output (e.g., $\geq$100–150mL/hour) in high-risk patients is extremely important. For substances with pKa <7 (e.g., uric acid, calcium oxalate, sulfonamides, methotrexate, and triamterene) urinary alkalinization by administering intravenous isotonic bicarbonate solutions or oral citrate can be considered. Urine pH should be periodically followed to ensure an appropriate level of alkalinization. Acetazolamide may be added if a metabolic alkalosis ensues. Attempting to acidify the urine to increase the solubility of weakly basic compounds is dangerous and not recommended. These preventive strategies are based on underlying pathophysiologic mechanisms and evidence for reductions in crystalline nephropathy occurrence is lacking, except perhaps in the case of high-dose methotrexate administration.

Treatment of established AKI consists of discontinuing the offending agent and, if nonoliguric and not volume overloaded, applying the same principles used in prevention: establishing brisk urine flow with volume expansion and the judicious use of diuretics and, for weak acids, urinary alkalinization. Moderate to large doses of diuretics may be required to establish adequate urine flow and care must be taken with bicarbonate loading to avoid

TABLE 13-4	CAUSES OF CRYSTALLINE NEPHROPATHY, THEIR DISTINCTIVE CLINICAL STRATEGIES FOR TREATMENT		
Inciting Agent	Context of Occurrence	Laboratory Findings	Prevention and Treatment
Phosphate Nephropathy	TLS—especially posttreatment form; phosphosoda bowel prep; very rarely in rhabdomyolysis and severe hemolysis	• Crystalluria with weakly birefringent, long prisms often in rosettes • Hyperphosphatemia out of proportion to renal insufficiency; in TLS, rhabdomyolysis, and hemolysis, hyperkalemia out of proportion to renal insufficiency and high LDH • Renal biopsy: von Kossa stain positive crystals	• Prevention:[a] Non-calcium-based phosphate binders; avoid treatment of hypocalcemia unless symptomatic or ECG changes present • Treatment:[a] Non-calcium-based phosphate binders; consider early initiation of renal replacement therapy, especially continuous modalities
Uric Acid Nephropathy	TLS—especially spontaneous form; very rarely in rhabdomyolysis or HGPRT deficiency	• Crystalluria with brownish, strongly birefringent, rhomboid plates, rosettes, or needles • Uric acid >15 mg/dL in absence of prerenal state, urine uric acid: urine creatinine often >1 and almost always >0.75; in TLS and rhabdomyolysis, hyperkalemia out of proportion to renal insufficiency and high LDH	• Prevention:[a] In those at high risk of TLS[b] start hypouricemic therapy, usually allopurinol but may consider rasburicase in patients with multiple high-risk features, especially children. • Treatment:[a] Rasburicase
Oxalate Nephropathy	EG poisoning; primary hyperoxaluria; very rarely with high-dose IV ascorbic acid, xylitol, or sorbitol infusions	• Crystalluria with birefringent monohydrate needles or dyhydrate envelope shapes • Hypocalcemia; in EG poisoning osmolal gap >10 mOsm/L and detectable serum and urine EG early with later disappearance of both and development of severe anion gap acidosis • Renal biopsy: silver nitrate/ rubeanic acid stain positive crystals	• Prevention:[a] Consider urine alkalinization; for high-risk EG ingestion[b] prompt fomepizole or, less desirably, ethanol therapy; consider thiamine, magnesium, and pyridoxine in alcoholics; avoid treatment of hypocalcemia unless symptomatic or ECG changes present. • Treatment:[a] Consider urine alkalinization; begin fomepizole or, less desirably, ethanol if EG level >20 mg/dL; consider early dialysis support, especially if EG >50 mg/dL and renal insufficiency or acidosis is present.
Acyclovir	High-dose IV acyclovir bolus; very rarely with oral acyclovir or with oral valacyclovir	• Crystalluria with birefringent needles, occasionally engulfed by white cells	• Prevention:[a] Increase time of IV acyclovir infusion to ≥1 hour. • Treatment:[a] Lowering dose without stopping the drug may be sufficient in many.

Indinavir	20% on chronic therapy develop AKI, especially with longer treatment and smaller body size.	• Crystalluria with birefringent plates, fans, or starbursts • Isosthenuria common • Contrast computed tomography with wedge-shaped perfusion defects in up to 50%	• Treatment:[a] May require urologic consultation for concomitant indinavir stone if present.
Methotrexate	High-dose IV therapy given for some malignancies	• Crystalluria with amorphous yellow casts • High serum methotrexate level, cytopenias	• Prevention:[a] Urinary alkalinization to pH ≥8 • Treatment:[a] Urinary alkalinization to pH ≥8; leucovorin rescue ± thymidine for extrarenal toxicity until methotrexate level <0.05 μmol/L; for very high methotrexate levels, consider carboxypeptidase G2 versus daily hemodialysis with high-flux membrane.
Sulfonamides	High-dose IV therapy, especially with sulfadiazine.	• Crystalluria with variable shapes from shocks of wheat to spheres • Positive lignin test (orange urine on mixing with 10% hydrochloric acid) • Densities in renal parenchyma and in collection system on imaging are common.	• Treatment:[a] Dose reduction and urine alkalinization to pH >7.1 usually sufficient; may require urologic consultation for concomitant sulfonamide stone if present.
Triamterene	Must distinguish from AIN, which is much more common.	• Crystalluria with birefringent orange casts and spheres • Hyperkalemia out of proportion to renal insufficiency	Treatment: [a] Urine alkalinization to pH >7.5; may require urologic consultation for the more common triamterene stone if obstructed.

[a]Saline loading with concomitant diuretic use when urine output is inadequate is recommended for prevention *and* treatment of all of the crystalline nephropathies when possible.
[b]See text for definition of high-risk features.

AIN, acute interstitial nephritis; AKI, acute kidney injury; ECG, electrocardiogram; EG, ethylene glycol; HGPRT, hypoxanthine–guanine phosphoribosyl transferase; IV, intravenous; LDH, lactate dehydrogenase; TLS, tumor lysis syndrome severe alkalosis. Additionally, early initiation of renal replacement therapy (RRT) can rapidly decrease the concentration of some inciting agents (e.g., phosphate, oxalate, acyclovir, and methotrexate). Again, evidence for improved renal outcome with these maneuvers is lacking. See Table 13-4 for details on specific management strategies for the various causes of crystalline nephropathy. The management of crystalline AKI from TLS and ethylene glycol intoxication is discussed further below.

Management of Tumor Lysis Syndrome

Preventive strategies should be used in patients at high risk for TLS. High-risk patients include patients with high-grade lymphoproliferative malignancies and large tumor burdens about to receive aggressive cytoreductive chemotherapy; those with high pretreatment lactate dehydrogenase, white blood cell count, and serum uric acid values; those with urine uric acid to urine creatinine ratio >1; and/or those with preexisting renal insufficiency or leukemic kidney infiltration. Patients with "laboratory TLS" (modest perturbations in serum electrolytes but no symptoms or evidence of organ dysfunction) should also receive preventive measures. Volume expansion to achieve brisk urine flow and hypouricemic therapy should be initiated 2 days prior to the start of chemotherapy. Urine alkalinization is *not* recommended given the potential risk of calcium phosphate precipitation in alkaline urine. Alkalemia can also worsen hypocalcemia by increasing protein binding of free calcium. Furthermore, data from animal studies revealed no reduction in the occurrence of uric acid nephropathy with urine alkalinization. Two options for hypouricemic therapy exist: allopurinol and rasburicase. **Allopurinol** (400–800 mg total daily dose) competitively inhibits xanthine oxidase thus preventing the *further* production of uric acid. Uric acid levels decrease over the subsequent 2 days. **Rasburicase** is a recombinant uricase enzyme that converts *existing* uric acid to allantoin, which is 5 to 10 times more soluble in urine than uric acid. After intravenous rasburicase administration (0.05–0.20 mg/kg over 30 minutes), uric acid levels decrease by 86% at 4 hours compared with a 12% reduction with allopurinol. However, comparative data between allopurinol and rasburicase regarding meaningful clinical endpoints, such as reductions in AKI, dialysis requirement, or death, do not exist. Therefore, the extremely high cost of rasburicase deters its use in prevention unless an allopurinol allergy is present.

Patients with evidence of organ system dysfunction have "clinical TLS" and require therapeutic rather than preventive interventions. Most patients with AKI will not require dialysis and will recover to their previous renal function, though patient and renal prognosis may be worse with spontaneous TLS. Similar to preventive methods, maintaining adequate urine flow and suppressing further rises in the serum concentration of uric acid and phosphate is essential. In the past, hemodialysis was sometimes initiated early to reduce uric acid levels rapidly, with a 50% reduction occurring after 6 hours of hemodialysis. Rasburicase more promptly reduces the uric acid level and eliminates this indication for RRT. However, when significant hyperphosphatemia is present, early RRT may still be required along with non–calcium-based phosphate binders to prevent further phosphate precipitation and/or hypocalcemia. Indeed, hypocalcemia should not be treated with intravenous calcium without first lowering the phosphorus, unless the patient is symptomatic or there are changes in the electrocardiogram. With intermittent hemodialysis, phosphorus clearance is fairly inefficient and daily or twice-daily treatments may be needed to achieve negative phosphorus balance. Continuous RRT may be more effective at reducing phosphorus levels in this situation.

Management of Ethylene Glycol Intoxication

Management of ethylene glycol intoxication should be focused on decreasing the concentration of toxic metabolites in high-risk ingestions. Patients thought to be at high risk for organ dysfunction are those with serum ethylene glycol levels >20 mg/dL, a known recent ethylene glycol ingestion with an osmolal gap >10 mOsm/L, or strong suspicion of recent ingestion and two of the following: pH <7.3, serum bicarbonate <20 mEq/L, osmolal gap >10 mOsm/L, and/or urinary oxalate crystals. Reductions in the levels of toxic metabolites can be achieved by: (a) limiting *further* organic acid formation through the use of competitive alcohol dehydrogenase inhibitors such as fomepizole or ethanol, (b) increasing metabolite clearance through early initiation of RRT, and (c) conversion to less-toxic metabolites by cofactor supplementation (see Table 13-4 for further details).

MYELOMA CAST NEPHROPATHY

Definition, Pathogenesis, and Epidemiology

Multiple myeloma is a malignancy of plasma cells, most often leading to overproduction of monoclonal immunoglobulin, the so-called M protein. **Myeloma cast nephropathy** (myeloma kidney), refers to the intrinsic AKI that results as the filtered light chain component of the M-protein (the Bence-Jones protein) exerts toxic and obstructive injury to the tubules. The propensity of a particular myeloma light chain to produce cast nephropathy depends somewhat on the amount of Bence-Jones proteinuria but also on its tendency to aggregate together with Tamm-Horsfall protein. Proximal tubular injury from additional insults and decreased effective circulating volume further increase the risk of cast formation, as both may increase the concentration of light chains in the distal tubule. Given these mechanisms at play, many cases of myeloma kidney have an identifiable inciting event:

- Volume depletion, perhaps from hypercalcemia-induced diabetes insipidus
- Infection resulting in ATN or decreased effective circulating volume
- NSAID use, through adverse effects on glomerular filtration
- Iodinated contrast exposure, through its ability to induce afferent arteriolar vasoconstriction

Renal dysfunction is seen in approximately 30% of patients with multiple myeloma at initial diagnosis. Potential etiologies of AKI in patients with myeloma include hypercalcemia-induced volume depletion, hypotension from infection, glomerular diseases such as light chain deposition disease or amyloidosis, and cast nephropathy. In those patients with persistent renal dysfunction despite treatment of hypovolemia and infection, cast nephropathy is the most common cause of AKI. The likelihood of underlying cast nephropathy is increased in cases of more profound AKI.

Clinical Presentation and Diagnosis

Patients with cast nephropathy generally have more advanced myeloma, so other features of the disease are usually present. Patients are often older because myeloma is generally a disease of the elderly. They may have complaints of fatigue, bone pain with pathologic fractures, and recurrent infections. Anemia is often present. Hypercalcemia from myeloma-induced bone resorption is common and may lead to polyuria with signs of volume depletion. The anion gap may be low from both hypercalcemia and the presence of circulating cationic paraprotein. A skeletal survey will usually reveal osteopenia and typical punched-out lesions in bone. The urine sediment is usually bland, with little or no proteinuria noted on urine dipstick because this only measures albuminuria. However, urine protein electrophoresis and/or immunofixation will reveal the presence of a monoclonal light chain in almost all cases. Serum protein electrophoresis with immunofixation will also reveal the paraprotein, though this is less consistent, especially in cases of light chain myeloma where the malignant clone produces only light chains instead of the full immunoglobulin. The serum-free light chain assay is a recently introduced test with greater sensitivity for the detection of paraprotein than protein electrophoresis or immunofixation, and it may further assist in the diagnosis.

The diagnosis of multiple myeloma is typically confirmed by bone marrow biopsy revealing clonal expansion of plasma cells. Definitive diagnosis of myeloma kidney requires kidney biopsy, although kidney-specific therapy may be ineffective. Thus, renal biopsy may only be necessary when considering plasma exchange or other diagnoses. Characteristic eosinophilic casts with "corrugated paper" appearance may be visualized in the lumens of distal tubules on light microscopy. There may be tubular cell toxicity and surrounding interstitial inflammation, occasionally taking the form of a giant cell reaction.

Course and Management

Treatment of cast nephropathy primarily consists of supportive care and treatment of the underlying malignancy. Hypovolemia and hypercalcemia should be corrected, infections should be treated aggressively, and other nephrotoxic insults should be removed. There is no evidence that forced diuresis with loop diuretics improves recovery by washing out obstructing casts. In fact, animal data suggests that there may even be an increase in the tendency to form casts with this strategy. Treatment of the underlying myeloma should be initiated promptly in consultation with an oncologist in order to reduce levels of the paraprotein as rapidly as possible. High-dose corticosteroids are a part of all the available treatment regimens and are the primary noninvasive means to rapidly reduce paraprotein levels. Allopurinol should be started prior to institution of therapy for myeloma to reduce the risk of subsequent TLS.

Plasma exchange has been used for acute treatment of cast nephropathy as a means to more rapidly reduce paraprotein levels. Data regarding its use come from small, usually retrospective studies with conflicting results. The most often-quoted study supporting the use of plasma exchange in myeloma kidney prospectively enrolled 29 patients to either plasma exchange and hemodialysis as needed or daily continuous peritoneal dialysis only, regardless of need. All patients received concomitant corticosteroids and cytotoxic therapy. Renal recovery and survival was better in the hemodialysis and plasma exchange group. A more recent and larger prospective study randomized 104 patients with a clinical diagnosis of myeloma kidney to either plasma exchange or no adjunctive pheresis treatment. All patients received similar chemotherapy and hemodialysis was provided to patients in both groups when indicated. There was no statistically significant difference in outcomes between the two groups. Based on this more recent data, plasma exchange is not recommended for most cases of cast nephropathy, though it may still be considered in those with a rapid decline in renal function, high paraprotein levels, and less chronicity seen on renal biopsy.

The median survival of patients with multiple myeloma is approximately 3 to 4 years. The occurrence of renal insufficiency shortens the median survival to 1.5 to 2 years. There is some potential for renal recovery in cast nephropathy with even severe renal dysfunction, with up to 40% of patients who survive the short-term period being able to regain dialysis independence.

INTERSTITIAL ACUTE KIDNEY INJURY

The causes of intrinsic AKI in which the primary site of pathology is the kidney interstitium include *acute interstitial nephritis* (AIN), *infiltrative malignant processes*, and *acute pyelonephritis* (see Table 13-1). The presence of pyuria and white blood cell casts on urine sediment analysis may allow one to tentatively narrow the differential diagnosis to these interstitial causes of intrinsic renal dysfunction.

ACUTE INTERSTITIAL NEPHRITIS

Definition, Pathogenesis, and Epidemiology

Acute interstitial nephritis is the predominant finding in 10% of biopsies performed in cases of AKI. However, the incidence seems to be increasing, perhaps as a result of more liberal prescribing practices and the availability of new medications. AIN is a hypersensitivity reaction characterized by inflammation in the renal interstitium, sparing the glomeruli. AKI results from immune-mediated tubular injury. The localization of inflammation to the interstitium may occur through several mechanisms, including molecular mimicry with tubular epitopes or deposition of immunogenic portions of the inciting agent at this location in the kidney. Similar to other hypersensitivity reactions, it is not dose dependent, there is recrudescence in disease activity upon re-exposure to compounds with similar biochemical structure, and there is often multiorgan involvement. Both cell-mediated and humoral immunity seem to play a role, though the former seems play a more significant role in pathogenesis.

The **major causes** of AIN are drugs, infections, and systemic diseases (Table 13-5). Prior to the advent of antibiotics, infection was the most common cause of AIN. However, in contemporary medicine, AIN is caused by drugs in 70% of cases. Other less-common etiologies include infections (15%), idiopathic (10%), tubulointerstitial nephritis with uveitis syndrome (TINU) (5%), and sarcoidosis (1%). Among drug-induced AIN, antibiotics and NSAIDS, including salicylates and COX-2 inhibitors, may be responsible for 30% and 40% of cases, respectively.

Clinical Presentation and Diagnosis

The presenting features of AIN can be quite variable, due in part to the multiplicity of agents that can initiate the syndrome. The combination of AKI, urinary symptoms (e.g., flank pain, macroscopic hematuria, or oliguria), and symptoms of hypersensitivity (e.g., rash, fever, or arthralgias) should alert the clinician to the possibility of AIN. However, signs of hypersensitivity may be absent in up to half of AIN cases, especially in those attributable to NSAIDs. The temporal relationship between the initiation of a new drug and the development of renal dysfunction may also aid in the diagnosis. Disease manifestations develop within 3 weeks of initiation of the inciting drug in about 80% of patients, with an average latency of onset of 10 days (range 1 day to >1 year). The duration of onset may be longer with NSAIDs with a mean latent period of 2 to 3 months. In AIN related to infection or systemic diseases, the clinical features of the inciting disease often predominate.

Urinalysis may reveal hematuria and/or sterile pyuria but these are very nonspecific. The presence of white blood cell casts is more specific, although they can also be seen in pyelonephritis and certain proliferative glomerulonephritides. **Eosinophiluria** (urine eosinophils numbering >1% of the urine white blood cell count) can be seen, usually detected more reliably with Hansel stain than with Wright stain. Though the positive predictive value of this test is low, the test's performance characteristics might be improved if other causes of eosinophiluria, such as urinary tract infection and atheroembolic disease, can be excluded. **Mild proteinuria** is common but sometimes it may be in the nephrotic range. Heavy proteinuria is classically associated with NSAIDs, occurring in a third of cases attributable to this drug class and associated with concomitant minimal-change glomerulopathy. Signs of multiorgan dysfunction such as elevated transaminases and hemolysis can occasionally be seen. **Renal imaging** may occasionally reveal normal to large kidneys with increased echogenicity.

Renal biopsy is the gold standard for definitive diagnosis and reveals an edematous interstitium infiltrated mostly by T-cells and macrophages. Neutrophils, eosinophils, and plasma cells can also be found and occasionally there may be granulomatous inflammation. There may be tubulitis or frank tubular necrosis in severe AIN. The glomeruli are usually

TABLE 13-5　CAUSES OF ACUTE INTERSTITIAL NEPHRITIS

Drugs[a]	Infections	Systemic Diseases	Other
Antimicrobial agents	**Bacteria**	Light chain gammopathy	Wasp sting
Penicillins (especially penicillin, ampicillin, and methicillin)	Brucella species	Sarcoidosis	Chinese herbs
	C. jejuni	Sjögren's syndrome	Idiopathic
	C. diphtheriae	Systemic lupus erythematosus	
Cephalosporins	Chlamydia species		
Ciprofloxacin	E. coli	Tubulointerstitial nephritis and uveitis syndrome	
Indinavir	Legionella species		
Rifampin	L. interrogans		
Sulfonamides (including cotrimoxazole)	M. tuberculosis	Wegner's and other vasculitides	
	M. pneumoniae		
NSAIDs, including COX-2 inhibitors and salicylates	Rickettsia species		
	Salmonella species		
Fenoprofen	Staphylococcus species		
Ibuprofen	Streptococcus species		
Indomethacin	Y. pseudotuber-culosis		
Naproxen			
Phenylbutazone	**Viruses**		
Piroxicam	CMV		
Tolmentin	EBV		
Zomepirac	Hantaviruses		
Anticonvulsants	HBV		
Phenytoin	HIV		
Diuretics	HSV		
Furosemide	Measles		
Thiazides	Polyomaviruses		
Gastric antisecretory drugs	**Parasites**		
Cimetidine	L. donovani		
Omeprazole	T. gondii		
Other			
Allopurinol			
Phenindione			

[a]Due to the fact that a very large number of drugs have been associated with acute interstitial nephritis, only drug classes and the most common individual offending medicines are listed here.

COX-2, cyclooxygenase-2; NSAIDs, nonsteroidal anti-inflammatory drugs.

normal, but electron microscopy may reveal foot process effacement in NSAID-associated AIN. A summary of clinical and laboratory features associated with some of the more common causes of AIN is given in Table 13-6.

Course and Management

AIN has a variable clinical course and response to treatment. In the previous prototype for the disease—methicillin-induced AIN—the prognosis was excellent with complete recovery of renal function noted in 90% of patients. In non-methicillin drug-induced AIN, chronic kidney disease persists in 35% to 40% of cases. The prevalence of chronic kidney disease is even higher with NSAID-induced AIN, occurring in 55% of cases. Indeed, the prognosis for AIN may depend on the promptness of elimination of the inciting agent, with those etiologies associated with milder symptoms, and therefore delayed diagnosis (e.g., NSAIDs, chronic infections, or sarcoidosis), having worse prognosis than those with more acute and dramatic presentations (e.g., methicillin, rifampin, or acute bacterial or viral infections). Interestingly, the peak serum creatinine does not seem to correlate with the long-term renal prognosis.

Clearly, the most important therapeutic maneuver in AIN is **prompt removal of the inciting agent**. In those cases associated with infection or other systemic disease, treatment of the underlying cause is necessary. Though it is tempting to combat the hypersensitivity response with **corticosteroids**, the usefulness of this intervention remains uncertain. Retrospective studies, including a series of 100 cases pooled from 7 reports and a recent series of 42 cases, suggest no reduction in the incidence of chronic kidney disease with corticosteroids. However, it might be argued that beneficial effects were not seen because patients with more severe disease were more likely to receive corticosteroids. The best data supporting the use of corticosteroids comes from a small series of 14 patients, all with methicillin-induced AIN. Corticosteroids were associated with complete renal recovery more often than withdrawal of methicillin alone, and the treated group recovered more quickly. Positive observational data with corticosteroids in AIN from other etiologies exist but are limited to small case series. In many reports, the most apparent effect of corticosteroids was a more rapid recovery of renal function. As for the use of other immunosuppressants, the literature is sparse and often describes cases associated with unusual etiologies. Apparently successful treatment has been described using calcineurin inhibitors, cyclophosphamide, azathioprine, and mycophenolate mofetil.

Given these data, a reasonable treatment strategy would be to reserve corticosteroids for patients with idiopathic AIN, systemic diseases for which corticosteroids have a proven role (e.g., sarcoidosis, Sjögren, vasculitides), or cases with poor prognostic features. Predictors of worse prognosis include delayed onset of improvement in renal function after withdrawal of the inciting agent (>1 week), prolonged exposure to the offending agent (>2–3 weeks), preexisting chronic kidney disease, and a renal biopsy characterized by intense and diffuse interstitial infiltrate, granuloma formation, or significant fibrosis and tubular atrophy. A frequently used regimen is oral prednisone, 1 mg/kg, with the duration of therapy guided by the improvement in renal function (usually 3 weeks). The presence of conditions that can be exacerbated by corticosteroid therapy (e.g., slow-healing wounds, brittle diabetes, or *active* infection) should dissuade the clinician from using this therapy. Furthermore, studies have suggested that corticosteroids do not alter the course of NSAID-induced AIN, though if poor prognostic features are present, treatment can still be considered. Other immunosuppressants are occasionally used when corticosteroid therapy has failed.

INFILTRATIVE MALIGNANCIES

Infiltration of the kidneys by malignant cells occurs commonly in lymphoid and myeloid leukemias and lymphomas. In fact, the kidneys are the most common extramedullary

TABLE 13-6 — VARIOUS CAUSES OF ACUTE INTERSTITIAL NEPHRITIS, THEIR CLINICAL AND LABORATORY FEATURES, AND DISEASE COURSES

Inciting Agent	Signs and Symptoms	Laboratory Findings	Course
Drug induced AIN, in general[a]	• Fever, 45%; rash, 42%; arthralgias, 12%; flank pain, 45%; oliguria, 40%; macroscopic hematuria, 17%; new or worsened hypertension, 20%	• Hematuria, 53%; pyuria, 50%; mild proteinuria, 58%; eosinophilia, 40%	• Mean 10-day exposure before presentation • Temporary dialysis required in 32%–50%; CKD persists in 36%–40%
Methicillin	• Hypersensitivity symptoms[b] common; macroscopic hematuria very common	• Hematuria, pyuria, and eosinophiluria in almost all; eosinophilia very common	• CKD persists in only 10%.
NSAIDs	• Hypersensitivity symptoms[b] uncommon	• Nephrotic range proteinuria in 1/3 of cases • Renal biopsy may also show glomerular findings similar to minimal change	• Mean exposure 2–3 mos prior to presentation; CKD persists in 1/2 of cases.
Allopurinol	• Often occurs in setting of renal insufficiency as the causative metabolite accumulates • Hypersensitivity symptoms[b] are very common and robust with signs of vasculitis possible.	• Eosinophilia and hepatitis common • Renal biopsy may sometimes reveal immune complex deposition at tubular basement membrane.	• Death occurs in as many as 1/4 of cases.

Rifampin	• Hypersensitivity symptoms[b] common and robust; oligoanuria in almost all	• Coombs-positive hemolysis, thrombocytopenia, and/or hepatitis occurs. • Almost all have anti-rifampin antibodies.	• Usually occurs with intermittent dosing. • Dialysis is required in almost all cases, though CKD persists only rarely.
Leptospiral nephropathy	• Preceding exposure to animal excrement • Fever, jaundice, hepatomegaly, gingival and or GI bleeding, and purpura very common in 1/2; altered mental status in 1/2; oligoanuria in almost all	• Cholestatic hepatitis, hemolytic anemia, and thrombocytopenia very common; hyponatremia common with hypokalemia from renal potassium wasting in some cases • Positive blood/urine cultures or serology • Renal biopsy reveals inflammation predominating at proximal tubules early on with interstitial hemorrhage possible.	• Leptospiral nephropathy occurs in 1/2 of cases of leptospirosis. • Death in 1/4 of cases; persistent tubular transport defects may remain in 1/3 of cases.
BK nephropathy	• Most often occurs in renal allografts within 1 year after transplant in the setting of aggressive immunosuppression; may occur in other immunosuppressed states as well (e.g., HIV)	• "Decoy cells" (tubular cells with enlarged nucleus and intranuclear inclusions) in urine sediment very common • BK viremia by PCR, 100% sensitive/88% specific • Renal biopsy reveals SV40 stain positive intranuclear inclusion bodies.	• Acute or gradual deterioration in renal function evident • Often resolves with a decrease in immunosuppression

(continued)

TABLE 13-6   VARIOUS CAUSES OF ACUTE INTERSTITIAL NEPHRITIS, THEIR CLINICAL AND LABORATORY FEATURES, AND DISEASE COURSES

Inciting Agent	Signs and Symptoms	Laboratory Findings	Course
Sarcoidosis	• Most often occurs in young adults with higher incidence in blacks • Extrarenal symptoms of sarcoidosis predominate with pulmonary, ocular, and skin symptoms most common	• Hypercalcemia or normocalcemia despite advanced renal failure may be present. • Chest radiography with hilar adenopathy and/or infiltrates very common • Renal biopsy reveals interstitial noncaseating granulomas and giant cells.	• Often a relapsing course responsive to pulse increase in steroids; CKD persists in 90%
TINU	• 3:1 female predominance with median age of onset 15 • Eye pain or redness, fever, and/or weight loss common.	• Elevated serum IgG very common • Renal biopsy may uncommonly reveal granulomas in interstitium.	• Uveitis may precede, follow, or coexist with the renal disease. • Complete renal recovery often occurs spontaneously within 1 year although uveitis recurs in 1/2.

[a]The general characteristics of *drug-induced* interstitial nephritis as a group, together with rates of occurrence, are given in the first row. Features that distinguish between specific causative agents are emphasized in the remaining rows.

[b]Fevers, rash, and/or arthralgias.

ACE, angiotensin-converting enzyme; AIN, acute interstitial nephritis; CKD, chronic kidney disease; GI, gastrointestinal; HIV, human immunodeficiency virus; NSAIDs, nonsteroidal anti-inflammatory drugs; PCR, polymerase chain reaction; SV40, simian virus 40; TINU, tubulointerstitial nephritis with uveitis syndrome.

organs involved by leukemic infiltration, with 63% of autopsies from leukemia patients displaying this finding. In most cases, the phenomenon is clinically silent even though nephromegaly might be evident on imaging. Indeed, kidney enlargement may be seen in 30% of children with acute lymphoblastic leukemia but the incidence of renal dysfunction is much less common. Rarely, leukemic infiltration may be so profound as to cause renal dysfunction. This may be difficult to distinguish from spontaneous TLS, which occurs much more commonly and in similar settings. In both cases, hyperuricemia will be evident since uric acid production is increased in leukemia and renal failure from any cause leads to decreased uric acid excretion. Further complicating this distinction is the fact that leukemic infiltration of the kidneys is a risk factor for TLS.

Examination of the urine sediment is not helpful as it usually reveals nonspecific pyuria and/or hematuria. Definitive diagnosis of AKI from leukemic infiltration requires renal biopsy, which reveals tremendous numbers of malignant cells invading the interstitium, resulting in wide separation and distortion of the tubules. Management involves treatment of the underlying malignancy while employing preventive strategies for TLS (see above). Recovery to near-normal renal function is possible, even in cases of profound renal dysfunction.

ACUTE PYELONEPHRITIS

AKI in the setting of acute pyelonephritis occurs most commonly from prerenal physiology, concomitant obstruction, or ATN from hypotension or nephrotoxic antibiotics. However, the edema and suppurative infiltration of the kidney parenchyma may alone cause AKI in rare cases. Populations at risk for this form of AKI include patients with a single kidney, renal allograft recipients, and malnourished alcoholics. The inflammatory reaction may impinge on the vasa recta which tenuously support the medullary tubules, and frank **papillary necrosis** may occur in vasculopaths such as diabetics. Patients may present with fever, flank pain, or pain over the allograft, though these classic symptoms of pyelonephritis are absent in a significant proportion of patients. The **urinalysis** reveals bacturia and pyuria with or without white blood cell casts. There may be increased renal size on imaging studies. Renal biopsy is indistinguishable from simple pyelonephritis and reveals edema and intense neutrophilic infiltration of the interstitium and tubular lumens with microabscess formation. With concomitant papillary necrosis there may be loss of collecting-duct epithelium. Antibiotic therapy results in slow resolution of the renal dysfunction. Persistent mild to moderate impairment in renal function often occurs as inflammation is replaced by sclerosis.

KEY POINTS TO REMEMBER

- The causes of intrinsic AKI other than ATN can be divided into microvascular, glomerular, tubular, and interstitial etiologies.
- Atheroembolic disease occurs primarily after vascular interventions and may cause progressive, irreversible kidney disease.
- Acute kidney injury following cancer therapy may be due to the effects of the chemotherapy agents, acute uric nephropathy, or acute phosphate nephropathy.
- Acute kidney injury is a common problem in multiple myeloma and may be due to volume depletion, cast nephropathy, or light chain deposition disease.
- Acute interstitial nephritis is usually due to medications. Important clinical findings supporting this diagnosis are sterile pyuria and low-grade proteinuria, sometimes accompanied by eosinophils in the blood or urine.

REFERENCES AND SUGGESTED READINGS

Arellano F, Sacristan JA. Allopurinol hypersensitivity syndrome: a review. *Ann Pharmacother.* 1993;27:337–343.

Baker RJ, Pusey CD. The changing profile of acute tubulointerstitial nephritis. *Nephrol Dial Transplant.* 2004;19:8–11.

Becker K, Jablonowski H, Haussinger D. Sulfadiazine-associated nephrotoxicity in patients with the acquired immunodeficiency syndrome. *Medicine.* 1996;75:185–194.

Boubaker K, Sudre P, Bally F, et al. Changes in renal function associated with indinavir. *AIDS* 1998;12:F249–54.

Brent J, McMartin K, Philips S, et al. Fomepizole for the treatment of ethylene glycol poisoning. *N Engl J Med.* 1999;340:832–838.

Clark WF, Stewart AK, Rock GA, et al. Plasma exchange when myeloma presents as acute renal failure. *Ann Intern Med.* 2005;143:777–784.

Clarkson MR, Giblin L, O'Connell FP, et al. Acute interstitial nephritis: clinical features and response to corticosteroid therapy. *Nephrol Dial Transplant.* 2004;19:2778–2783.

Coomarasamy A, Honest H, Papaioannou S, et al. Aspirin for prevention of preeclampsia in women with historical risk factors: a systematic review. *Obstet Gynecol.* 2003;101:1319–1332.

Covic A, Goldsmith DJ, Gusbeth-Tatomir P, et al. A retrospective 5-year study in Moldova of acute renal failure due to leptospirosis: 58 cases and a review of the literature. *Nephrol Dial Transplant.* 2003;18:1128–1134.

Covic A, Goldsmith DJ, Segall L, et al. Rifampicin-induced acute renal failure: a series of 60 patients. *Nephrol Dial Transplant.* 1998;13:924–929.

Galpin JE, Shinaberger JH, Stanley TM, et al. Acute interstitial nephritis due to methicillin. *Am J Med.* 1978;65:756–764.

Hande KR, Garrow GC. Acute tumor lysis syndrome in patients with high-grade non-Hodgkin's lymphoma. *Am J Med.* 1993;94:133–139.

Hannedouche T, Grateau G, Noel LH. Renal granulomatous sarcoidosis: report of six cases. *Nephrol Dial Transplant.* 1990;5:18–24.

Hirsch HH, Knowles W, Dickenmann M, et al. Prospective study of polyomavirus type BK replication and nephropathy in renal-transplant recipients. *N Engl J Med.* 2002;347:488–496.

Jones SR. Acute renal failure in adults with uncomplicated acute pyelonephritis: case reports and review. *Clin Infect Dis.* 1992;14:243–246.

Keeney RE, Kirk LE, Bridgen D. Acyclovir tolerance in humans. *Am J Med.* 1982;73:176–181.

Knudsen LM, Hjorth M, Hippe E. Renal failure in multiple myeloma: reversibility and impact on the prognosis. Nordic Myeloma Study Group. *Eur J Haematol.* 2000;65:175–181.

Mandeville JT, Levinson RD, Holland GN. The tubulointerstitial nephritis and uveitis syndrome. *Surv Ophthalmol.* 2001;46:195–208.

Markowitz GS, Stokes MB, Rhadhakrishnan J, et al. Acute phosphate nephropathy following oral sodium phosphate bowel purgative: an under-recognized cause of chronic renal failure. *J Am Soc Nephrol.* 2005;16:3389–3396.

Nochy D, Daugas E, Droz D, et al. The intrarenal vascular lesions associated with primary antiphospholipid syndrome. *J Am Soc Nephrol.* 1999;10:507–518.

Perazella MA. Crystal-induced acute renal failure. *Am J Med.* 1999;106:459–465.

Rossert JA, Fischer EA. Acute interstitial nephritis. In Johnson R, Feehally J, eds. *Comprehensive Clinical Nephrology.* 2nd ed. Philadelphia: Mosby; 2003:769–776.

Saftlas AF, Olson DR, Franks AL, et al. Epidemiology of preeclampsia and eclampsia in the United States, 1979–1986. *Am J Obstet Gynecol.* 1990;163:460–465.

Schwarz A, Krause PH, Kunzendorf U, et al. The outcome of acute interstitial nephritis: risk factors for the transition from acute to chronic interstitial nephritis. *Clin Nephrol.* 2000;54:179–190.

Scolari F, Ravani P, Pola P, et al. Predictors of renal and patient outcomes in atheroembolic renal disease: a prospective study. *J Am Soc Nephrol.* 2003;14:1584–1590.

Scolari F, Tardanico R, Zani R, et al. Cholesterol crystal embolism: a recognizable cause of renal disease. *Am J Kidney Dis.* 2000;36:1089–1109.

Solomon A, Weiss D, Kattine AA. Nephrotoxic potential of Bence Jones proteins. *N Engl J Med.* 1991;324:1845–1851.

Steen VD, Costantino JP, Shapiro AP, et al. Outcome of renal crisis in systemic sclerosis: relation to availability of angiotensin converting enzyme (ACE) inhibitors. *Ann Intern Med.* 1990;113:352–357.

Widemann BC, Balis FM, Kempf-Bielack B, et al. High-dose methotrexate-induced nephrotoxicity in patients with osteosarcoma. *Cancer.* 2004;100:2222–2232.

Zucchelli P, Pasquali S, Cagnoli L, et al. Controlled plasma exchange trial in acute renal failure due to multiple myeloma. *Kidney Int.* 1988;33:1175–1180.

Contrast-Induced Nephropathy

14

Ethan Hoerschgen and Anitha Vijayan

INTRODUCTION

Acute decline in renal function can occur shortly after the administration of intravenous iodinated contrast. Currently, contrast-induced nephropathy (CIN) is the third leading cause of hospital-acquired acute kidney injury (AKI). It is essential to understand the risk factors for developing CIN, as well as strategies available to prevent it. The **definition** of CIN varies from study to study, and no consensus has been reached. The most frequent definition of CIN is an elevation of serum creatinine >0.5 mg/dL above baseline, or increase of serum creatinine >25%, within 48 hours after administration of contrast media (CM). Other causes of renal injury must also be excluded.

PATHOGENESIS

The exact pathophysiology of CIN is unclear. However, it appears that there are several mechanisms that have significant roles. Studies have consistently shown that administration of intravenous contrast leads to reduced renal perfusion due to vasoconstriction. Vasoconstriction is most pronounced at the outer medulla, an area highly susceptible to hypoxia and ischemia. The mechanism of vasoconstriction is likely from an increase in regional vasoconstrictors such as endothelin and adenosine, as well as an impaired production of nitric oxide, a potent vasodilator. Research has also demonstrated direct tubular toxicity after CM. CM may also induce renal cellular injury through oxygen-free radicals and decreased antioxidant activity. The ability of antioxidants, such as n-acetyl cysteine, to prevent CIN have been extensively studied for this reason.

RISK FACTORS

It is important to identify those patients at increased risk for CIN prior to exposing them to the potential harm of CM. There are several known risk factors (Table 14-1) for developing CIN. Some of these factors are nonmodifiable, but several can be addressed prior to contrast exposure. The major predictor for those patients at risk for developing CIN is **pre-existing renal impairment**. The risk of developing CIN has been shown to increase as pre-procedure GFR declines or serum creatinine increases. One study showed that renal failure after percutaneous coronary intervention (PCI) was 2.5%, 22.4%, and 30.6% in patients with a serum creatinine of 1.2 to 1.9 mg/dL, 2.0 to 2.9 mg/dL, and >3.0 mg/dL, respectively. **Diabetes mellitus** is likely an independent risk marker, and definitely increases the risk for CIN when diabetic nephropathy is present. The cumulative risk for developing CIN increases as the number of risk factors increases (Table 14-2). **Other**

TABLE 14-1	RISK FACTORS FOR CONTRAST-INDUCED NEPHROPATHY

Nonmodifiable Risk Factors	Modifiable Risk Factors
Advanced age (>75 yrs)	High dose of CM (>100 mL)
Diabetic nephropathy	Osmolarity of CM (high > low > iso)
Chronic kidney disease (SCr >1.5 mg/dL)	Anemia/blood loss (Hct <39% for men, <36% for women)
CHF (New York Heart Classification [NYHC] III–IV, and/or history of pulmonary edema)	Short duration between CM exposures
Acute MI <24 h prior to CM	Hypertension/hypotension
IABP	Hypovolemia
Proteinuria/immunoglobulinopathies	Nephrotoxic agents
Peripheral vascular disease	Aminoglycosides
	NSAIDs
	COX-2 inhibitors
	Amphotericin B
	Cyclosporine
	Tacrolimus
	Diuretics
	Intraarterial injection of CM

NSAIDs, nonsteroidal anti-inflammatory drugs; ACEI, angiotensin-converting enzyme inhibitors; CHF, congestive heart failure; MI, myocardial infarction; CM, contrast media; Hct, hematocrit; SCr, serum creatinine; IABP, intraaortic balloon pump.

modifiable risk factors include high dose of contrast (>100 mL), hypotension, hypertension, hypovolemia, and concomitant administration of nephrotoxic medications

EPIDEMIOLOGY AND CLINICAL COURSE OF CONTRAST-INDUCED NEPHROPATHY

Contrast-induced nephropathy remains a major etiology of AKI, despite the increasing awareness of risk factors, prevention strategies, and safer CM. A rise in serum creatinine is usually seen within 24 to 72 hours after administration of contrast, with a peak around 3 to 5 days. Patients generally remain nonoliguric with decreasing levels of serum creatinine 7 to 10 days after contrast exposure. Return to baseline usually occurs within 2 to 3 weeks. CIN has both immediate and sustained effects. Patients who develop CIN have a higher rate of in-hospital and postdischarge mortality. Patients who develop CIN are also susceptible to other in-hospital events, including myocardial infarction, bleeding diathesis, shock, and respiratory failure. CIN has also been shown to lead to a significant increase in length of hospital stay. The need for hemodialysis from CIN is generally <1%, but increases in high-risk patients, especially those with poor renal function at baseline. CIN must be distinguished from **atheroembolic disease**, which usually presents several days to weeks later with slowly rising creatinine, and may be accompanied by myalgias, intestinal ischemia, lower-extremity rashes and "blue-toe" syndrome.

TABLE 14-2 RISK SCORE PREDICTION

Risk Factor	Points	Risk Score for Risk of CIN
Hypotension	5	0–5; 7.5%
IABP	5	6–10; 14.0%
CHF	5	11–15; 26.1%
SCr >1.5 mg/dL	4	≥16; 57.3%
Age >75	4	
Anemia	3	
Diabetes	3	
Volume of CM	1 point/100 mL	

Modified from Mehran R, Aymong ED, Nikolsky E, et al. A simple risk score for prediction of contrast-induced nephropathy after percutaneous coronary intervention. *J Am Coll Cardiol.* 2004;44: 1393–1399 with permission from Elsevier.

IABP, intraaortic balloon pump; CHF, congestive heart failure; SCr, serum creatinine; CM, contrast media.

Concomitant Medications

There are several medications that can lead to intravascular volume depletion and/or renal vasoconstriction. Inhibitors of prostaglandins, such as nonsteroidal anti-inflammatory medications (NSAIDs) or cyclooxygenase (COX-2) inhibitors, probably should be avoided at least 24 to 48 hours preprocedure, even though there are no randomized controlled studies to support this recommendation. Intravenous diuretics are deleterious if given prior to procedure and should be avoided. There are no recommendations regarding oral diuretics, although they may be continued if patients have been on stable doses at home and are euvolemic. If patients appear to have decreased effective circulating volume, then diuretics should be discontinued. If patients are on stable doses of angiotensin-converting enzyme inhibitors or angiotensin receptor blockers, and are euvolemic, then these may be continued. Titration or initiation of these drugs in the pericontrast period probably should be avoided. Vasoconstrictive, antirejection medications such as tacrolimus or cyclosporine should not be discontinued as this can result in rejection of the transplanted organs. However, the drug levels should be closely monitored and maintained at the recommended levels and hydration protocols should be followed. Ideally, contrast procedures should be avoided when other concomitant nephrotoxins such as aminoglycosides or amphotericin B are being administered, if at all possible. Metformin is not a nephrotoxic agent, but may cause lactic acidosis in the setting of decreased renal function. Even though there is insufficient data to support this approach, the U.S. Food and Drug Administration recommends that metformin be held the day of procedure and 2 to 3 days afterwards, until renal function is checked. Alternative diabetic treatment may be needed.

HMG-CoA Reductase Inhibitors (Statins)

One group of medications that may have a beneficial effect and should be continued are statins. It is believed that statins may prevent CIN by improving endothelial function. Retrospective studies suggest that they may have a prophylactic role in CIN in patients undergoing cardiac catheterization. In one study of more than 29,000 patients, the incidence of CIN was 4.37% in those patients on statins, compared with 5.93% in patients not on the drug prior to procedure. A randomized, controlled trial should be conducted to confirm this finding, but may not be feasible, since statins are recommended for a majority of patients with cardiovascular disorders.

Contrast Media

The osmolarity, type, route of administration, and volume of contrast agent used all can change its nephrotoxic potential. Low-osmolar contrast agents (osmolality ranging from 570–900) have been shown to be superior to high-osmolar (osmolality >2000) agents in preventing CIN. The NEPHRIC study demonstrated that iso-osmolar contrast (osmolality = 270) was superior to low-osmolar contrast in preventing CIN in high-risk patients undergoing coronary or aortofemoral angiography. Studies have suggested an increased risk for CIN with intra-arterial infusion; however this may be complicated by undetected atheroemboli. Although CIN can occur with any volume of contrast, the risk is clearly higher as the dose increases, especially >100 mL. It is recommended that the least amount of CM necessary for the procedure be used. In patients undergoing cardiac catheterization, avoidance of left ventriculogram drastically reduces contrast volume. Repeated contrast exposure, especially <72 hours apart, also increases the risk for CIN. It is preferred to allow 2 weeks between exposures, if possible. If there is a rise in serum creatinine after initial exposure to CM, it is preferable to allow the levels to return to baseline before repeat exposure. One can also consider using noniodinated contrast agents such as gadolinium and carbon dioxide. However, the quality of images may be variable and these agents are not completely free of adverse events. Gadolinium causes pseudo-hypocalcemia due to interference with calcium assay. If the total calcium is low after gadolinium exposure in an asymptomatic patient, ionized calcium needs to be checked before initiating any calcium therapy. A more ominous complication that has been strongly associated with gadolinium is nephrogenic systemic fibrosis and caution must be used when ordering a gadolinium-based imaging study for a patient with renal failure.

PREVENTION OF CONTRAST-INDUCED NEPHROPATHY

Prevention is the fundamental therapy in CIN and intravenous volume expansion is the mainstay of preventive strategies. N-acetylcysteine has also been studied extensively and is administered either orally or intravenously. Other therapies have been studied in very small clinical trials and are not universally recommended.

Volume Expansion

Intravenous volume expansion around the time of contrast exposure is believed to alleviate renal vasoconstriction and improve renal medullary blood flow. Intravenous half-normal saline alone is shown to be superior to half-normal saline plus diuretics (i.e., furosemide and mannitol). **Intravenous normal saline** has been shown to be superior to oral hydration for the prevention of CIN. Normal saline is also superior when compared to half-normal saline. **Intravenous sodium bicarbonate** was compared with normal saline in a randomized study of 141 patients undergoing radiographic procedures. Sodium bicarbonate increases renal tubular pH and the alkaline environment is believed to decrease the release of free radicals. The fluids were given at 3 mL/kg/hour for 1 hour preprocedure and then continued at 1 mL/kg/hour for 6 hours postprocedure. The incidence of CIN was 1.7% in the bicarbonate group, compared with 13.6% in the saline group. This result has been corroborated in two additional trials, which evaluated patients undergoing coronary interventions.

N-Acetylcysteine

N-acetylcysteine (NAC) is thought to prevent CIN by acting as a scavenger of oxygen free radicals. The side-effect profile of NAC is also very favorable, which makes it an attractive prevention strategy. The majority of meta-analyses of NAC and its potential to prevent CIN have shown benefit. However, there is a significant amount of heterogeneity in study analysis. N-acetylcysteine with hydration significantly prevented reduction in renal function in patients with chronic kidney disease after intravenous and intraarterial administration of CM. The standard dose of NAC was 600 mg PO b.i.d. the day before procedure and the day of procedure. One study suggested that the ability of NAC to prevent CIN may be dose dependent. Patients undergoing PCI had significant reduction in CIN with 1200 mg of NAC administered intravenously prior to PCI and 1200 mg twice PO after, when compared with 600-mg doses. It appears than NAC might have some benefit in prevention of CIN and, given its excellent side-effect profile, it is prudent to add NAC to the hydration regimen in patients undergoing high-risk contrast procedures.

Our recommendation is N-acetylcysteine 600 mg PO b.i.d. on the day prior to the procedure and 600 mg PO on the day of the procedure. In high-risk patients undergoing coronary intervention, intravenous NAC can be administered along with volume expansion.

Other Therapies

Several treatments have been successful in preventing CIN in small trials, but are yet to be validated in larger studies. Also, some of the following therapies have a low safety profile. *Ascorbic acid* may prevent CIN through its antioxidant properties, and it has a strong safety profile. Doses of 3 g prior to cardiac angiography, followed by 2 g twice afterwards, showed a significant decrease in CIN. Ascorbic acid is a safe alternative to NAC in prevention of CIN, although further investigation is needed. *Fenoldopam* is a dopamine-1 receptor agonist, which promotes renal and systemic vasodilatation. The CONTRAST trial found no significant reduction in CIN with the use of fenoldopam when compared with placebo. Fenoldopam is not recommended for routine use to prevent CIN. *Theophylline* and *aminophylline* are adenosine antagonists that block the vasoconstrictive properties of adenosine. Studies of these agents for the prevention of CIN have yielded conflicting results. Both have a narrow therapeutic window and dangerous side-effect profile. These agents are not recommended for the prevention of CIN unless patients are at extremely high risk and other alternatives are not available. *Prostaglandin E1* (PGE1) has been studied in the prevention of CIN because of its vasodilator effects. The plasma creatinine increase was lower in patients who received PGE1; however, there were no clinically significant changes in creatinine clearance. The use of PGE1 is limited by significant decline in blood pressure, as hypotension can exacerbate renal injury. Further investigation is needed for PGE1 analog's role in preventing CIN. *Hemofiltration* with CVVH has been investigated in several studies. One group demonstrated that CIN occurred less in high-risk patients receiving hemofiltration when compared with intravenous volume expansion alone. In this study, CIN was defined by a rise in serum creatinine, and hemofiltration alone can alter serum creatinine levels. The hospital and 1-year mortality rates were significantly lower in the hemofiltration group. Hemofiltration is limited by its invasiveness, a need for intensive care support, and cost. Hemodialysis has shown no benefit in preventing CIN. The use of hemofiltration and hemodialysis is not recommended in the prevention of CIN. However, planning for renal replacement therapy and counseling of patients regarding potential need for postprocedure dialysis should be included during renal consultation for those patients at high risk for renal injury.

RECOMMENDATION

Based on the current data, our recommendation for high-risk patients is intravenous sodium bicarbonate 3 mL/kg/hour for 1 hour prior to the procedure, then 1 mL/kg/hour for 6 hours postprocedure. If sodium bicarbonate is not available, then normal saline or half-normal saline can be administered at the same rate. Intravenous fluids must be administered with caution in patients with heart failure and volume status should be monitored closely. The benefit of additional agents (e.g., NAC) combined with this therapy is not known.

KEY POINTS TO REMEMBER

- The presence of renal insufficiency is the most important risk factor for developing CIN.
- Intravascular volume repletion with isotonic fluids before and after CM exposure is the best way to prevent CIN in at-risk patients.
- Intravenous diuretics, NSAIDs, and COX-2 inhibitors should be discontinued prior to administration of CM.
- Intravenous NAC should be considered in those patients at high risk.
- The administration of the lowest volume of iso-osmolar or low-osmolar CM is preferred.
- There is no role for hemofiltration or dialysis in the prevention of CIN.
- In high-risk patients, the discussion should include the risk of CIN and the possible need for dialysis postprocedure.

REFERENCES AND SUGGESTED READINGS

Aspelin P, Aubry P, Sven-Goran F, et al. Nephrotoxic effects in high-risk patients undergoing angiography. *New Engl J Med.* 2003;348:491–499.

Davidson C, Stacul F, McCullough P, et al. Contrast medium use. *Am J Cardiol.* 2006;98[suppl]:42K–58K.

Finn WF. The clinical and renal consequences of contrast-induced nephropathy. *Nephro Dial Transplant.* 2006;[Suppl 1]:i2–i10.

Kay J, Chow WH, Chan TM, et al. Acetylcysteine for prevention of acute deterioration of renal function following elective coronary angiography and intervention. *JAMA.* 2003;289:553–558.

Marenzi G, Assanelli E, Marana I, et al. N-acetylcysteine and contrast-induced nephropathy in primary angioplasty. *New Engl J Med.* 2006;354:2773–2782.

Marenzi G, Lauri G, Campodonico J, et al. Comparison of hemofiltration protocols for prevention of contrast induced nephropathy in high-risk patients. *Am J Med.* 2006;119(2):155–162.

McCullough P, Adam A, Becker C, et al. Epidemiology and prognostic implications of contrast-induced nephropathy. *Am J Cardiol.* 2006;98[suppl]:5K–13K.

McCullough P, Adam A, Becker C, et al. Risk prediction of contrast-induced nephropathy. *Am J Cardiol.* 2006;98[suppl]:27K–36K.

Mehran R, Aymong ED, Nikolsky E, et al. A simple risk score for prediction of contrast-induced nephropathy after percutaneous coronary intervention. *J Am Coll Cardiol.* 2004;44:1393–1399.

Merten GJ, Burgess WP, Gray LV, et al. Prevention of contrast-induced nephropathy with sodium bicarbonate. *JAMA.* 2004;291:2328–2334.

Morcos SK, Contrast-medium induced nephrotoxicity. In Dawson P, Cosgrove DO, Grainger RG, *Textbook of Contrast Media.* San Francisco: Isis Medical Media; 1999:135–148.

Pannu N, Wiebe N, Marcello T. Prophylaxis strategies for contrast-induced nephropathy. *JAMA.* 2006;295:2765–2779.

Rihal CS, Textor SC, Grill DE, et al. Incidence and prognostic importance of acute renal failure after percutaneous coronary intervention. *Circulation.* 2002;105:2259–2264.

Stacul F, Adam A, Becker C, et al. Strategies to reduce the risk of contrast-induced nephropathy. *Am J Cardiol.* 2006;98[suppl]:59K–77K.

Stone G, McCullough P, Tumlin J, et al. Fenoldopam mesylate for the prevention of contrast-induced nephropathy. *JAMA*. 2003;290:2284–2291.

Tepel M, van der Giet M, Schwarzfeld C, et al. Prevention of radiographic-contrast-agent-induced reductions in renal function by acetylcysteine. *New Engl J Med*. 2000;343: 180–184.

Tumlin J, Fulvio S, Adam A, et al. Pathophysiology of contrast-induced nephropathy. *Am J Cardiol*. 2006;98[suppl]:14K–20K.

Renal Replacement Therapy in Acute Kidney Injury

Anitha Vijayan

15

T he mainstay of management of acute kidney injury (AKI) is prevention. The timing of initiation of renal replacement therapy remains controversial. The conventional factors that trigger renal replacement therapy include metabolic acidosis, hyperkalemia, volume overload, and uremia. The exact definition of "uremia" is vague; there is, therefore, extensive variability in the timing of initiation from institution to institution and even among individual nephrologists at the same institution. The important indications for initiation of hemodialysis in AKI are provided in Table 15-1.

MODALITIES OF RENAL REPLACEMENT THERAPY

The available modalities are intermittent hemodialysis (IHD), continuous renal replacement therapy (CRRT), sustained low-efficiency dialysis (SLED), or peritoneal dialysis (PD). The choice depends on the availability of therapies at the institution, physician preference, the patient's hemodynamic status, and the presence of co-morbid conditions. Patients with sepsis or hepatic failure may have potential benefits with continuous therapies. Small studies have shown that intracranial pressure is more stable with CRRT than with IHD in patients with hepatic encephalopathy. High-flow CRRT has been shown to remove inflammatory cytokines in sepsis, but hard endpoints such as mortality, hospital length of stay, and renal recovery are yet to be studied. Intermittent modalities are generally accepted to cause greater fluctuations in blood pressure and produce greater fluid shifts in a short amount of time. Continuous modalities allow for the same solute clearance and fluid removal, but spread out over a 24-hour period, and thus are favored in hemodynamically unstable patients. In the United States, CRRT is performed in approximately 30% of patients with AKI and has almost completely replaced PD in the treatment of AKI. CRRT has not shown improved survival over IHD in critically ill patients. Likewise, randomized trials have not shown a difference in time to renal recovery or length of ICU or hospital stay between groups treated with IHD versus CRRT. Table 15-2 lists the advantages and disadvantages of the different modalities.

The principles of hemodialysis and PD are discussed in other chapters. This section will focus primarily on CRRT, and how this modality compares with IHD in AKI. SLED will also be discussed briefly.

Continuous Renal Replacement Therapy

CRRT utilizes the principles of diffusion, convection, or both, depending on the scheduled technique. *Diffusion* involves the same principles as dialysis and drives solutes such as urea across the dialysis membrane from the blood (higher concentration) to the dialysate (lower concentration), which is running countercurrent to the blood. The dialysate flow rate is about 15 to 40 mL/minute compared with dialysate flow rate in IHD of 300 to

TABLE 15-1	INDICATIONS FOR INITIATION OF DIALYTIC SUPPORT IN AKI

Volume overload refractory to diuretics

Hyperkalemia refractory to medical therapy

Metabolic acidosis refractory to medical therapy

Uremic syndrome

Anorexia, nausea, vomiting

Serositis

Seizures, confusion

Neuropathy

Bleeding

Need to start total parenteral nutrition (volume/solute issues)

Overdoses/intoxications

Refractory hypercalcemia

Refractory hyperuricemia

450 mL/minute. This process is called *continuous venovenous hemodialysis* (CVVHD). During *convection,* solute movement across the membrane is driven by solvent drag. The plasma water is pushed across the membrane by filtrating pressure and takes solutes with it, similar to glomerular ultrafiltration. This large volume loss has to be restored with necessary solutes, and therefore convection requires the addition of replacement fluid solution to the CRRT setup. This is called *continuous venovenous hemofiltration* (CVVH). The *combination* of the two processes utilizes both dialysate and replacement fluid solutions and is termed *continuous venovenous hemodiafiltration* (CVVHDF). Some of the membranes used for CRRT also have adsorptive properties, but it is unclear to what extent this results in significant clearance of substances. Studies have suggested adsorption with polysulfone membranes might result in clearance of cytokines, but, to date, this has not been demonstrated to have clinical benefit. CRRT also can be used without dialysate or replacement fluid to treat volume overload with minimal solute clearance. This process is called *slow continuous ultrafiltration* (SCUF). The nomenclature of CRRT is outlined in Table 15-3.

Fluids in CRRT

Bicarbonate-based solutions have essentially replaced lactate-based solutions in CRRT. Bicarbonate-based solutions are either prepared at individual institutions by the pharmacy or supplied premixed by various manufacturers. Even if they are provided by manufacturers, the final constitution of the fluid is conducted by the local pharmacy as various products have different compositions and mixing instructions. Typically, the bicarbonate concentration is about 35 mEq/L, sodium is 140 mEq/L, chloride is about 106 to109 mEq/L, and magnesium is about 1.0 to 1.5 mEq/L. Potassium concentrations vary and the prescription should reflect the patient's serum levels. Calcium concentration should be zero if citrate anticoagulation is used and calcium should be replaced through a central venous catheter.

Anticoagulation

Slow continuous blood flow through extracorporeal circulation mandates the use of anticoagulation to prevent platelet activation and thrombosis of the circuit. The primary goal of anticoagulation is to prevent clotting of the tubes and filters, thereby preventing the delivery of prescribed therapy. Currently, the two primary methods of anticoagulation

TABLE 15-2	ADVANTAGES AND DISADVANTAGES OF DIFFERENT MODALITIES	
Modality	Advantages	Disadvantages
Intermittent hemodialysis (IHD)	• High-efficiency transport of solutes when rapid clearance of toxins or electrolytes is required • Allows time for off-unit testing	• Hemodynamic intolerance secondary to fluid shifts • "Saw-tooth" pattern of metabolic control between sessions
Continuous renal replacement therapy (CRRT)	• Gentler hemodynamic shifts than IHD • Steady solute control	• Continuous need for specialized nursing • Requires continuous anticoagulation (heparin vs. citrate)
Sustained low-efficiency dialysis (SLED)	• Fewer hemodynamic shifts compared to IHD • Less work for intensive care nursing staff like CRRT • Can be performed at night, avoiding cessation of therapy for procedures • No need for expensive dialysate and replacement fluid and equipment	• Needs to be performed 6 days/week to achieve adequate clearance • Need outcome data, in comparison to IHD and CRRT
Peritoneal dialysis (PD)	• Gentler hemodynamic shifts than IHD	• Requires invasion of peritoneal cavity, which may not be possible in postoperative patients • Less predictable fluid removal rates • Efficiency of urea removal low compared with other therapies

utilized in the United States are (a) intravenous heparin (either provided through the circuit or systemically) to maintain PTT between 60 and 80 milliseconds, and (b) citrate anticoagulation. There are different ways of administering citrate, but the principles remain the same. Citrate administered prefilter chelates the ionized calcium extracorporeal circuit. Calcium is an essential co-factor for the coagulation cascade and its deficiency prevents coagulation in the circuit. To counteract the effect of citrate in the systemic circulation, calcium is given via a central venous catheter to maintain blood-ionized calcium in the normal range. It is of utmost importance to closely monitor ionized calcium levels during citrate anticoagulation. Other methods of anticoagulation used include argatroban and bivalirudin, usually reserved for patients who develop heparin-induced thrombocytopenia.

TABLE 15-3	NOMENCLATURE OF CONTINUOUS RENAL REPLACEMENT THERAPY MODALITIES

Abbreviations

A	Arterio-
V	Venous
C	Continuous
HD	Hemodialysis
H(F)	Hemofiltration
HDF	Hemodiafiltration
UF	Ultrafiltration

Modalities

CVVH	Continuous venovenous hemofiltration
CVVHD	Continuous venovenous hemodialysis
CVVHDF	Continuous venovenous hemodiafiltration
CAVH, CAVHD, and CAVHDF	Continuous arteriovenous hemofiltration, hemodialysis, and hemodiafiltration
SCUF	Slow continuous ultrafiltration
SLED	Slow low-efficiency dialysis

Typical Regimen for CRRT

An example of CRRT orders for a 70-kg patient, assuming 20 mL/kg/hour of replacement fluid and dialysate, serum potassium of 4 mEq/L, is given below:

- Blood flow **180 mL/minute**
- Dialysate flow rate **700 mL/minute**—Replacement fluid flow rate **700 mL/minute**
- Heparin bolus *xx** units loading dose IV, then infusion (1000 units/mL) at *xx* mL/hour
- Dialysate (Prismasate), 0 K, 3.5 Ca—add KCl to make final concentration of K 3 mEq/L
- Replacement fluid (Prismasate), 0 K, 3.5 Ca—add enough KCl to make final concentration of K 3 mEq/L

Note: Heparin is individualized based on patient circumstances.

Drug Dosing in CRRT

Total clearance of any compound depends on its elimination by nonrenal route, residual renal function, and CRRT. Unlike IHD, the clearance of medications is continuous, controlled, and predictable. Patient, drug, and dialysis characteristics determine appropriate dosing schedules to be used. Generally, the nonrenal clearance is taken to be constant, although in critically ill patients with multiorgan system failure, this component may be less than predicted. The CRRT clearance relies on convection, diffusion, and adsorption. *Convective* elimination is determined primarily by the protein-bound fraction of the drug. In *diffusive* elimination, the saturation of the drug in the dialysate (and filtrate) becomes important, and decreases as flow rates increase. By taking these guidelines into consideration, therapeutic doses have been calculated for a variety of drugs used in the ICU. The recommended doses of some of the more commonly prescribed antibiotics are listed in Table 15-4.

Complications

As with any procedure, there are certain complications and adverse events that can be associated with renal replacement therapies. Vigilance for such complications and their immediate rectification are essential to prevent life-threatening situations, especially in the vulnerable population of the ICU. Some are related to the procedure itself, whereas

TABLE 15-4	DOSING OF COMMON ANTIMICROBIAL AGENTS DURING CONTINUOUS RENAL REPLACEMENT THERAPY (ultrafiltration rates of 20–30 mL/minute)
Medication	**Dosing in CRRT**
Vancomycin	500 mg once daily or b.i.d.
Cefepime	2000 mg once daily or b.i.d.
Ceftazidime	500–1000 mg b.i.d.
Cefotaxime	2000 mg b.i.d.
Ceftriaxone	2000 mg once daily
Imipenem	250–500 mg t.i.d. or qid.
Ciprofloxacin	200 mg once daily or b.i.d.
Metronidazole	500 mg t.i.d.
Piperacillin	4000 mg t.i.d.
Amikacin	250 mg once daily or b.i.d.
Tobramycin	100 mg once daily
Fluconazole	100–200 mg once daily
Acyclovir	3.5 mg/kg once daily

others are a result of fluid removal or electrolyte and acid-base disturbances. In addition, the necessity for a central venous catheter places the patient at risk for infection complications.

Hypotension. Hypotension can occur in all clinical settings with all modalities, although it is more commonly seen with IHD and its rapid fluid shifts. Volume-depleted and septic patients are at heightened risk; careful attention to the physical examination and invasive hemodynamic monitoring when indicated can help ensure adequate volume resuscitation prior to initiating the dialysis session. A target central venous pressure of 8 to 12 mm Hg can be used in these settings and may dictate a reduction or stoppage of fluid ultrafiltration. Alternatively, if pulmonary edema or acute lung injury is complicating the picture, then pressor support can be used to maintain blood pressure while continuing ultrafiltration with CRRT. However, this must be done with extreme caution given the risk of peripheral ischemia.

Arrhythmias. Cardiac arrhythmias can occur in the setting of renal replacement therapy and electrolyte shifts. Although generally seen with IHD, arrhythmia can also be seen in CRRT. Potassium, magnesium, and calcium levels must be monitored every 12 to 24 hours during CRRT. If 0 or 1 mEq/L of potassium concentration is being used, then potassium should be monitored every 6 to 8 hours to ensure stable potassium plasma concentration. Patients on digitalis are especially sensitive to hypokalemia. Potassium competes with digitalis for binding at the Na^+/K^+ ATPase pump and reduced serum levels can enhance the medicine's toxicity. Supraventricular arrhythmias can also be triggered during the placement of the dialysis catheter or by a malpositioned dialysis catheter. If the arrhythmia is resulting in hemodynamic compromise, then therapy is discontinued immediately and appropriate measures to treat the arrhythmia should be started.

Central Venous Catheter Problems. Initiation of CRRT, just like IHD, requires the insertion of a nontunneled, large-bore, dual-lumen, central venous catheter into either the internal jugular, subclavian, or femoral veins. Infection risks increase after 3 weeks for internal jugular vein catheters and after 1 week for femoral vein catheters in bed-bound patients. When infection and bacteremia occur, prompt catheter removal is generally recommended unless vascular access is especially difficult. Persistent bacteremia, fever, or an elevated white blood cell count should prompt a search for bacterial endocarditis in this particularly susceptible population. Thrombus or fibrin sheaths can form around or inside the catheters, causing inadequate blood flows for dialysis. Although heparin is usually instilled into the hub of the catheter after each dialysis, this does not necessarily prevent clot formation. An attempt at clot lysis can be made by the local instillation of alteplase 2 mg. Alteplase should not be administered systemically for this purpose. If the catheter malfunctions, then it may be changed over a guidewire or replaced completely, preferably at a different site. In patients with chronic kidney disease, subclavian veins are not used for dialysis catheters as there is a high risk of subclavian venous stenosis, which can prevent the future placement of an arteriovenous fistula for dialysis in that extremity. There are no data to suggest that tunneled catheters are more beneficial regarding infection rates or adequacy of dialysis in intensive care patients with AKI. Tunneled catheters are typically used in patients with multiple malfunctioning temporary catheters, poor chance for early renal recovery, or for those being transferred out of the intensive care to a different facility. For clotted tunneled catheters, interventional radiology consultation is required to perform endoluminal brushing to dislodge thrombi and fibrin sheaths.

Electrolyte Disturbances. Standard CRRT solutions do not contain phosphate, and uninterrupted CRRT can cause dramatic hypophosphatemia. This problem is aggravated by an intracellular shift that occurs during dialysis secondary to alkalemia. Hypokalemia and hypomagnesemia can also result from CRRT and serum electrolytes need to be monitored at least twice a day to avoid such complications. Hypophosphatemia can be corrected by intravenous or oral repletion. Alternatively, phosphorus can be added to the dialysate solution, although this technique is not employed widely at this time. Hypokalemia can be treated by increasing the concentration of potassium in the dialysate and replacement fluid. Hypomagnesemia is usually replaced intravenously or orally. The typical concentration of potassium in the solution is 2 mEq/L. However, potassium can be added by the pharmacist to make the final concentration 3 or 4 mEq/L, depending on serum potassium levels.

Anticoagulation Problems. The use of anticoagulation increases the risk for hemorrhagic episodes. Studies have shown higher incidence with heparin compared with citrate; therefore, citrate should be used preferentially in patients who are at higher risk for bleeding. If a major bleed occurs, then heparin or other systemic anticoagulation should be immediately discontinued. Citrate anticoagulation can be continued, with close attention to bleeding parameters and ionized calcium levels. Heparin can also be associated with heparin-induced thrombocytopenia (HIT). If HIT is suspected, heparin should be discontinued, and alternative agents such as argatroban, bivalirudin, or citrate should be used. The direct thrombin inhibitor, argatroban, can be initiated at 2 μg/kg/minute and adjusted to maintain an activated partial thromboplastin time of 1.5 to 3 times baseline value. Citrate anticoagulation can result in metabolic alkalosis and in the setting of hepatic dysfunction, can lead to life-threatening hypocalcemia. The titration protocol for addressing changes in serum and machine-ionized calcium levels must be closely followed to prevent adverse events. Metabolic alkalosis can be treated by changing the replacement fluid to sodium chloride from a bicarbonate-based product, and hypocalcemia is treated by adjusting the calcium rates.

Hypothermia. Hypothermia is a frequent complication of CRRT, especially at higher flow rates of dialysate and replacement fluid, with an incidence as high as 60% to 70%. Significant amounts of heat are lost from the slow-flowing extracorporeal circuit and can cause decreases in body temperature of 2°C to 5°C. Hypothermia can result in cardiac arrhythmias, hemodynamic compromise, increased risk for infections, and coagulation problems. This can be addressed by warming the replacement fluid being infused or by encasing the venous tubing (blood returning to the patient) with specialized warming devices that can be attached to the machine.

Sustained Low-Efficiency Dialysis (SLED)

Sustained low-efficiency dialysis (slow extended dialysis) combines the benefits of CRRT and IHD. The dialysate flow rates are usually about 100 to 200 mL/minute, similar to the blood flow rates, and the procedure lasts anywhere from 10 to 12 hours. SLED is performed by the dialysis nursing staff and utilizes a modified dialysis machine. It does not require replacement fluids or special filters or machines. Anticoagulation is required in most cases. The therapy is associated with fewer hemodynamic alterations compared with IHD, and because the procedure can be performed at night in the ICU, it leaves the day for various procedures. This is a clear advantage over CRRT, where stopping the therapy for various reasons prevents adequate delivery of dialysis. SLED has been shown to provide adequate urea clearance and has been successfully used in critically ill patients with AKI. More centers are using this option in addition to CRRT and IHD in the treatment of critically ill patients with AKI.

Dose of Dialysis in AKI

The ideal dose of renal replacement therapy in critically ill patients has not yet been conclusively determined. Evidence from end-stage renal disease patients suggests that a thrice-weekly regimen should be performed with a urea reduction of approximately 65% to 68% per session. This correlates to a fractional urea clearance (Kt/V) of 1.2, where K is the dialyzer efficiency, t is the time of treatment, and V is the volume of distribution of urea. Given the acuity of the AKI population, urea clearances are notoriously unreliable, with frequent volume shifts, sepsis, high catabolic state, etc. The current Acute Dialysis Quality Initiative (ADQI) recommendation is to prescribe at least a single-pool Kt/V of 1.3 for each dialysis treatment in AKI. This is based on the assumption that AKI patients should at least receive the dose recommended for end-stage renal disease patients. However, studies have shown that this is rarely achieved in AKI. It has been proposed that benefit may be derived from increasing the renal replacement dose either with higher treatment doses, more frequent treatments, or increasing flow rates in CRRT. A small study published in 2001 suggested that short daily dialysis improved mortality in AKI compared with 3 times/week dialysis (28% vs. 46%). In CRRT, one study demonstrated a survival advantage in critically ill patients who underwent intensive CRRT (35 mL/kg/hour vs. 20 mL/kg/hour). The question of whether intensive renal replacement therapy improves survival will be answered when the results of the Acute Renal Failure Trial Network (ATN) study are published in 2008.

SUMMARY

Renal replacement therapy is initiated after more conservative medical management has failed to control the fluid, electrolyte, and metabolic complications of AKI. Several modalities are available to the clinician and selection between intermittent and continuous forms depends on the availability at the institution, the patient's hemodynamic stability, and co-morbid illnesses. Despite the overall safety of these procedures, complications and adverse events can occur, requiring meticulous attention and, in some cases, frequent laboratory monitoring to anticipate and prevent their occurrence.

KEY POINTS TO REMEMBER

- Renal replacement therapy should be instituted in a timely manner to prevent complications of AKI.
- The decision to use continuous modalities versus intermittent hemodialysis should be based on the patient's condition, as well as physician and nursing knowledge of the modalities.
- Continuous modalities have not shown to have superior outcomes compared with intermittent hemodialysis.

(continued)

KEY POINTS TO REMEMBER (continued)

- The choice of anticoagulation in CRRT depends on the patient's risk for bleeding, his or her co-morbid conditions, and the familiarity of the staff with the therapy.
- Electrolytes must be closely monitored during CRRT.
- Hypocalcemia is a major complication of citrate anticoagulation and ionized calcium levels need to be monitored frequently.
- The dose of dialysis either with IHD or with CRRT remains unknown. The ADOQI guidelines recommend a prescribed Kt/V of 1.3.
- Dose adjustment of medications should be made once patients initiate CRRT.

REFERENCES AND SUGGESTED READINGS

Brause M, Nuemann A, Schumacher T, et al. Effect of filtration volume of continuous venovenous hemofiltration in the treatment of patients with acute renal failure in intensive care units. *Crit Care Mede.* 2003;31:841–846.

Cho KC, Himmelfarb J, Paganini E, et al. Survival by dialysis modality in critically ill patients with acute kidney injury. *J Am Soc Nephrol.* 2006;17:3132–3138.

Dellinger PR, Carlet JM, Masur H, et al. Surviving Sepsis Campaign guidelines for management of severe sepsis and septic shock. *Crit Care Med.* 2004;32:858–873.

Eknoyan G, Levin N. NKF-K/DOQI clinical practice guidelines for hemodialysis adequacy: update 2000. *Am J Kidney Dis.* 2001;37[suppl]:S1–S64.

Kellum J, Angus DC, Johnson JP, et al. Continuous versus intermittent renal replacement therapy: a meta-analysis. *Intensive Care Med.* 2002;28:29–37.

Kroh UF, Holl TJ, Steinhauber W. Management of drug dosing in continuous renal replacement therapy. *Semin Dial.* 1996;9:161–165.

Marshall MR, Golper TA, Shaver MJ, et al. Sustained low-efficiency dialysis for critically ill patients requiring renal replacement therapy. *Kidney Int.* 2001;60:777–785.

O'Reilly P, Tolwani A. Renal replacement therapy III: IHD, CRRT, SLED. *Crit Care Clin.* 2005;21:367–378.

Oliver MJ, Callery SM, Thorpe KE, et al. Risk of bacteremia from temporary hemodialysis catheters by site of insertion and duration of use: a prospective analysis. *Kidney Int.* 2000;58:2543–2545.

Palevsky PM. Renal replacement therapy I: indications and timing. *Crit Care Clin.* 2005; 21:347–356.

Ricci Z, Ronco C. Renal replacement therapy II: dialysis dose. *Crit Care Clin.* 2005;21: 357–366.

Ronco C, Bellomo R, Homel P, et al. Effects of different doses in continuous veno-venous haemofiltration on outcomes of acute renal failure: a prospective randomised trial. *Lancet.* 2000;356:26–30.

Schiffl H, Lang SM, Fischer R. Daily hemodialysis and the outcome of acute renal failure. *New Engl J Med.* 2002;346:305–310.

Venkataraman R. Prevention of acute renal failure. *Crit Care Clin.* 2005;21:281–289.

Vinsonneau C, Camus C, Combes A, et al. Continuous venovenous haemodiafiltration versus intermittent haemodialysis for acute renal failure in patients with multiple-organ dysfunction syndrome: a multicentre randomised trial. *Lancet.* 2006;368:379–385.

Overview and Approach to the Patient with Glomerular Disease

16

Rasa Kedainis

INTRODUCTION

Glomerular diseases are a heterogeneous collection of inflammatory and/or noninflammatory insults to the filtering unit of the kidney. The hallmark of glomerular disease is an alteration in glomerular permeability and selectivity resulting in proteinuria and/or hematuria. Glomerular diseases occurring in the absence of a known systemic process are called *primary. Secondary* glomerular diseases are caused by systemic disease processes. Examples include diabetes mellitus, systemic lupus, certain cancers, or vasculitis. Secondary glomerular diseases often present in a similar fashion to primary glomerular diseases and their pathological and clinical picture may be indistinguishable (primary focal segmental glomerulosclerosis, focal segmental glomerulosclerosis caused by obesity). Sometimes glomerular pathology may be the first manifestation of systemic disease (membranous nephropathy in cancers). Many systemic diseases may be diagnosed on renal biopsy (amyloidosis, drug reactions, sarcoidosis), and in some, the biopsy results indicate disease activity and guide treatment (lupus nephritis). Table 16-1 illustrates the primary pathology and secondary causes of glomerular disease.

CLASSIFICATION OF GLOMERULAR DISEASES

Glomerular diseases are diagnosed by their clinical presentation and histomorphological appearance. Classification of glomerular diseases is based on histological injury patterns with evaluation by light microscopy, immunofluorescence, and electron microscopy. One pattern can have multiple etiological causes (such as membranoproliferative), and one etiology can give different histological patterns (hepatitis B and C, lupus nephritis), so all biopsies must be evaluated with clinical correlations.

Light Microscopy

Light microscopy is useful for determining pattern of disease, cellularity, and assessment of interstitium and vessels. Standard slide preparation includes staining with hematoxylin and eosin (H&E), periodic acid-Schiff (PAS), trichrome, and a silver stain. The glomerulus consists of four regions: Bowman's capsule and space, arterioles, the mesangium, and the glomerular capillary wall. The latter consists of endothelium, basement membrane, epithelium, and podocytes. A normal glomerulus has entire loops patent and approximately two to three mesangial cells per capillary tuft. The basement membrane is about the same thickness as a proximal tubule basement membrane. Bowman's capsule has one layer of cells, and Bowman's space is empty.

- The **lesions** in glomerular diseases can be *diffuse* (affecting the majority of glomeruli) or *focal* (only some of the glomeruli). They also can be *segmental* (only

TABLE 16-1	PRIMARY GLOMERULAR DISEASES AND THEIR SECONDARY CAUSES
Name of Primary Disease	**Secondary Causes**
IgA Nephropathy	Liver disease Henoch-Schönlein purpura Celiac sprue Inflammatory bowel disease Dermatitis herpetiformis
Membranous nephropathy	Malignancy (lung, colon, breast, leukemia, non-Hodgkin lymphoma) Lupus nephritis (Class V) Drugs (NSAIDs, penicillamine, gold, captopril) Infectious diseases (hepatitis B, hepatitis C, syphilis, malaria) Diabetes mellitus
Minimal change disease	Hodgkin disease Heavy metals (lead, mercury) Drugs (NSAIDs, ampicillin/penicillin, trimethadione, lithium) Infections (mononucleosis, HIV)
Focal segmental glomerulosclerosis	HIV Heroin use Morbid obesity Sickle cell disease Drug toxicity (lithium, pamidronate) Genetic (podocin , α–actinin-4, nephrin mutations) Reflux nephropathy
Membranoproliferative glomerulonephritis	Hepatitis C Cryoglobulinemia Lupus nephritis Leukemia and lymphoma Infective endocarditis Malaria

part of a glomerulus involved) or *global* (affecting all regions of any given glomerulus). The best example of a segmental disease would be focal segmental glomerulosclerosis (FSGS). Lesions also can be *hypercellular* or *proliferative* due to mesangial proliferation (IgA nephropathy) or *infiltrative* due to inflammatory cells (leukocytes, monocytes, neutrophils).

- The **mesangium** is composed of cells and matrix. It may expand because of mesangial cell proliferation (hypercellularity) as seen in IgA nephropathy or systemic lupus erythematosus (SLE). Matrix expansion can be seen in diabetic nephropathy or be due to matrix infiltration by abnormal proteins (amyloidosis, fibrillary glomerulonephritis).
- **Crescent** formation refers to cellular or fibrous crescents formed by invasion of cells (proliferating parietal epithelial cells, invading inflammatory cells and fibrous products of those cells) into Bowman's space resulting from severe glomerular injury with capillary leak of cells and proteins.

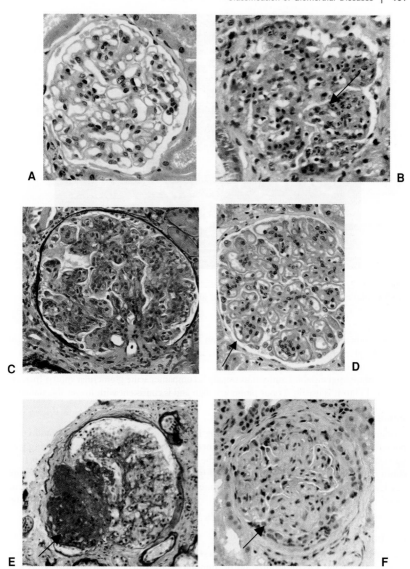

FIGURE 16-1. Pathology of glomerular disease—light microscopy. **(A)** Normal glomerulus in minimal change disease. **(B)** Diffuse hypercellularity, infiltration with neutrophils (*arrow*) in poststreptococcal glomerulonephritis. **(C)** Lobular accentuation due to expansion of mesangial matrix and mesangial hypercellularity in membranoproliferative glomerulonephritis. **(D)** Capillary loop thickening (*arrow*) in membranous nephropathy (Class V lupus nephritis). **(E)** Segmental sclerosis (*arrow*) in focal segmental glomerulosclerosis. **(F)** Crescent formation (*arrow*) in Wegener granulomatosis. (Courtesy of Dr. H. Liapis.)

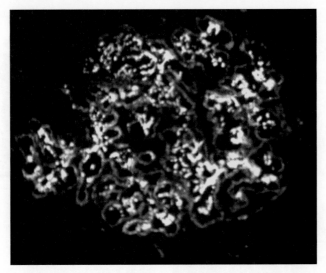

FIGURE 16-2. Pathology of glomerular disease—immunofluorescence microscopy. Postinfectious glomerulonephritis, granular staining. (Courtesy of Dr. H. Liapis.)

- **Basement membrane** proliferation can be assessed by a silver stain. Thickening of the glomerular basement membrane is seen in membranous nephropathy or class V lupus nephritis.
- **Tubulointerstitial** inflammation usually accompanies acute glomerular injury. Interstitial fibrosis is usually a poor prognostic sign and is consistent with irreversible damage.

Immunofluorescence

Immunofluorescence studies include staining for deposition of IgG, IgA, IgM, and components of classic and alternative complement pathways (C3, C4, and C1q). Staining patterns are *linear* (continuous staining along the glomerular capillary wall) or *granular* (discontinuous staining along the capillary wall or in the mesangium). Putative antigens are not known in most cases, but there are some exceptions (e.g., antiglomerular basement membrane [GBM] disease). Several glomerular diseases are diagnosed primarily by immunofluorescent staining. Examples are IgA nephropathy and C1q nephropathy.

Electron Microscopy

Electron microscopy can detect GBM thickness, duplication, infiltration, and podocyte foot process effacement. Precise localization of immune deposits that appear homogeneous and electron dense (subepithelial, subendothelial, mesangial, or within the GBM) is critical for the classification of most primary glomerular renal diseases. Thin basement membrane disease can only be diagnosed by demonstration of abnormally thin areas of basement membrane.

PRESENTATION OF GLOMERULAR DISEASES

History and Physical Exam

- Patients with nephrotic syndrome usually complain of pitting edema (especially periorbital), foamy urine, xanthelasma, Muehrke bands (white bands in fingernails from chronic hypoalbuminemia), elevated blood pressure, infections, or thrombotic complications.

- Patients with nephritic syndrome may complain of oliguria and uremic symptoms. Other findings include elevated blood pressure, gross hematuria, and generalized edema. If the patient has a rapidly progressive glomerulonephritis (RPGN), he may have systemic symptoms of vasculitis—rash, fevers, and pulmonary symptoms (pulmonary-renal syndrome).
- **Timing of recent infections** can be very helpful. In a patient with tea-colored urine, it is important to know about timing of recent infections. IgA nephropathy patients will have hematuria within 1 to 3 days after onset of respiratory infection. In contrast, hematuria from postinfectious glomerulonephritis will develop 1 to 2 weeks after the streptococcal upper respiratory infection or up to 6 weeks after a skin infection.
- **Family history** of renal failure and deafness may suggest Alport syndrome. Family history of thin basement membrane disease, IgA nephropathy, FSGS, and hemolytic-uremic syndrome (HUS) is important because those diseases may be inherited.
- **Medications** should be evaluated. Prescriptions, over-the-counter medications, and herbal preparations should be reviewed. Particular attention should be paid to the use of NSAIDs and antibiotics.
- **Malignancies** (Hodgkin disease; graft-versus-host disease after bone marrow transplant; solid tumors of lung, breast, and colon) are also associated with glomerular disease and renal disease may be the initial presentation.

Clinical Presentations

Patients with glomerular diseases generally present with one of the following clinical syndromes.

Asymptomatic Hematuria

This **syndrome** is defined as >2 to 3 red blood cells (RBCs) per high-power field in spun urine (microscopic), or painless brown/red macroscopic hematuria without clots in patients who have normal renal function and no evidence of systemic diseases known to affect kidneys. The differential diagnosis is broad and urological problems (bladder, prostate, urethra, stones, and renal tumors) account for up to 80% of all cases of hematuria. The presence of RBC casts and/or dysmorphic RBCs indicates a glomerular cause for the hematuria. The most common diseases presenting as asymptomatic hematuria are thin basement membrane disease, IgA nephropathy, hereditary nephritis, and sickle cell disease. Kidney biopsy is usually not done to evaluate asymptomatic hematuria.

Asymptomatic Proteinuria

Proteinuria in the range of 150 mg to 3 g/day (in 24-hour urine collection) or as measured as spot protein-to-creatinine ratio ranging from 0.2 to 3 g protein per gram creatinine is usually asymptomatic. It is sometimes referred to as *nonnephrotic proteinuria*. It may occur with glomerular or nonglomerular diseases such as tubulointerstitial diseases or orthostatic proteinuria (usually <1 g/day). Any type of glomerular disease can cause proteinuria in this range with FSGS, membranous nephropathy, and diabetic nephropathy being common examples.

Nephrotic Syndrome

This **syndrome** is a clinical pentad of proteinuria >3 g/day, hypoalbuminemia <3.5 g/dL, edema, hypercholesterolemia, and lipiduria (most specific finding is presence of oval fat bodies in urinalysis). Complications of nephrotic syndrome include:

- *Hypercoagulability* due to loss of hemostasis control proteins such as antithrombin III, and increased hepatic synthesis of protein C, fibrinogen, and von Willebrand factor. Venous thrombosis is more common than arterial thrombosis.

- *Infection* due to loss of immunoglobulins and immunosuppressive drugs
- *Hyperlipidemia* and *atherosclerosis*

The most common glomerular diseases presenting as nephrotic syndrome are primary diseases such as minimal change disease, membranous nephropathy, and FSGS, as well as secondary forms such as diabetic nephropathy, amyloidosis, and light chain deposition disease.

Nephritic Syndrome

This **syndrome** presents as proteinuria, usually <3 g/day, hematuria with dysmorphic RBCs and/or RBC casts, edema, hypertension, and reduction in glomerular filtration rate (GFR) with or without oliguria. Distinction between nephrotic and nephritic syndromes is usually based on clinical and laboratory evaluation. The most common diseases presenting as nephritic syndrome are poststreptococcal glomerulonephritis, other postinfectious diseases (endocarditis, abscess), IgA nephropathy, vasculitis, and lupus nephritis.

Rapidly Progressive Glomerulonephritis (RPGN)

This **presentation** is the most severe form of the nephritic syndromes. In this case, glomerular injury is so acute that renal failure develops over the course of a few days to weeks. RPGN usually presents as proteinuria <3 g/day, hematuria with dysmorphic RBCs and/or red cell casts, with or without signs of systemic vasculitis. A specific finding on kidney biopsy is crescent formation. The most common diseases presenting as RPGN are Goodpasture disease, Wegener granulomatosis, microscopic polyangiitis, pauci-immune crescentic glomerulonephritis, lupus nephritis, and essential mixed cryoglobulinemia.

Chronic Glomerulonephritis

This **terminology** is sometimes used to describe patients thought to have some form of previous glomerular disease presenting with hypertension, chronic kidney disease (CKD), proteinuria >3 g/day and small, atrophic, smooth kidneys on ultrasound. Any glomerulonephritis can slowly progress to kidney failure, so chronic glomerulonephritis may be the presumptive diagnosis when patients present with shrunken kidneys and biopsy is not appropriate.

Routine Laboratory Evaluation

The routine initial evaluation of patients with suspected glomerular disease should include the following tests:

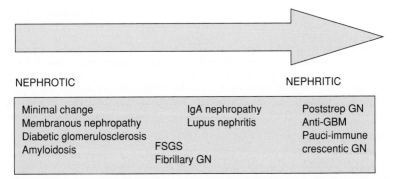

NEPHROTIC   NEPHRITIC

Minimal change	IgA nephropathy	Poststrep GN
Membranous nephropathy	Lupus nephritis	Anti-GBM
Diabetic glomerulosclerosis		Pauci-immune
Amyloidosis	FSGS	crescentic GN
	Fibrillary GN	

FIGURE 16-3. Spectrum of glomerular diseases with nephrotic and nephritic features. FSGS, focal segmental glomerulosclerosis; GBM, glomerular basement membrane; GN, glomerulonephritis; MPGN, membranoproliferative glomerulonephritis; strep, streptococcal.

- *Urinalysis.* The presence of protein and/or RBCs on microscopic exam of the urine sediment is helpful. RBC casts or dysmorphic RBCs are specific for glomerular disease and always warrant further testing. The presence of other formed elements in urine (e.g., granular casts, WBCs, WBC casts) is less specific. Oval fat bodies, fatty casts, and hyaline casts may be seen in the urine sediment of patients with nephrotic syndrome.
- *Serum creatinine* (Cr) and *BUN* should be measured. Prior values may be important to determine the duration of disease.
- *Urine protein quantification.* Spot protein-to-Cr (mg/dL) ratio provides a rough estimation of 24-hour urine protein excretion in g/day. A 24-hour urine collection for protein and Cr can provide more precise quantification of both protein excretion and estimation of Cr clearance. See Chapter 4.
- *Urine culture.* Patients with hematuria should have a urine culture to rule out cystitis or prostatitis.
- *Renal ultrasound.* Patients with hematuria should undergo kidney ultrasound to evaluate for anatomical abnormalities such as polycystic kidney disease (PKD), cysts, renal masses, stones, and kidney size. The presence of atrophic smooth kidneys (<9 cm) suggests CKD, which is usually irreversible. This finding should limit use of aggressive diagnostic workup (including renal biopsy, which carries greater risk with small, scarred kidneys) and aggressive immunosuppressive therapies. Large kidneys (>14 cm) can be associated with nephrotic syndrome from diabetes mellitus, amyloid infiltration, or HIV-associated nephropathy.

Specialized Laboratory Evaluation

Several serologic studies should be considered in all nephritic presentations, nephrotic syndrome, and in selected patients with proteinuria and/or hematuria. The decision as to which of these tests to order in a particular patient depend on the age, gender, and features of the presentation.

- **Antinuclear antibody (ANA)** and **anti–double-stranded-DNA antibody** tests evaluate the presence of SLE.
- **Cryoglobulins and rheumatoid factor** should be measured to support a diagnosis of cryoglobulinemia.
- **Anti-GBM antibodies** support a diagnosis of Goodpasture's disease.
- **Anti-neutrophil cytoplasmic antibodies (ANCAs):** C-ANCA/PR3 are typically positive in Wegener granulomatosis and P-ANCA/MPO are often present in microscopic polyangiitis and Churg-Strauss syndrome.
- **Antistreptolysin-O antibody (ASO), Anti-DNAse B** in poststreptococcal glomerulonephritis. Other streptococcal antibodies are also available.
- **Hepatitis B and C serologies:** Infections with these viruses have been associated with membranoproliferative glomerulonephritis, membranous nephropathy, vasculitis, and cryoglobulinemia.
- **HIV antibodies** for HIV-associated nephropathy should also be measured.
- **SPEP /UPEP** can detect light chain or heavy chain paraproteins that are commonly seen in amyloidosis, multiple myeloma, or light chain deposition disease.
- **Complement levels (C3, C4, and CH50)** are decreased in a limited spectrum of diseases and can be useful in limiting the differential diagnosis (Fig. 16-4). **Renal biopsy** is usually required to establish diagnosis and treatment of most glomerular diseases. Biopsy is usually **not required** in the following special patient groups:
  - Children who present with features typical of minimal change disease and who respond appropriately to steroid trial.

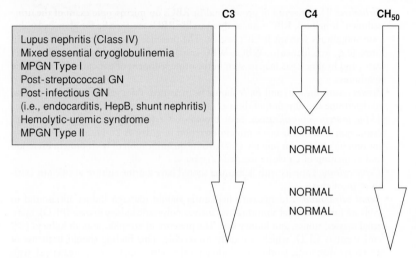

FIGURE 16-4. Complement levels in various glomerular diseases. GN, glomerulonephritis; HepB, hepatitis B; MPGN, membranoproliferative glomerulonephritis.

- Longstanding diabetes with evidence of microvascular complications of diabetes (e.g., retinopathy, peripheral neuropathy) and other features typical of diabetic nephropathy.
- History of preceding streptococcal infection with features typical of poststreptococcal glomerulonephritis
- Mild, asymptomatic urine abnormalities (microscopic hematuria, nonnephrotic proteinuria) with preserved renal function. These patients have excellent prognosis and biopsy results would be unlikely to alter management.

GENERAL PRINCIPLES OF TREATMENT OF GLOMERULAR DISEASES

Treatment of glomerular diseases consist of disease-specific treatment and symptomatic treatment of proteinuria, hypertension, hyperlipidemia, and control of edema. Patients with **proteinuria** should be treated with ACE inhibitors and/or angiotensin receptor blockers (ARBs) to reduce proteinuria to <1 g/day. Use caution with these agents in patients with accelerating renal failure or a tendency toward hyperkalemia. Serum chemistries, including potassium and Cr, should be monitored within 1 to 2 weeks of initiation of therapy. Creatinine increases of up to 30% from baseline are acceptable. Control of **blood pressure** is essential in order to preserve kidney function. Blood pressure should be controlled, with a goal of <135/80 mm Hg. In patients with proteinuria, ACE inhibitors or ARBs should be the first-line therapy.

Control of **edema** or **volume overload** requires the use of dietary salt and water restriction in conjunction with diuretics. Loop diuretics are the most effective agents.

Treatment of **hyperlipidemia** usually consists of hydroxymethylglutaryl coenzyme-A reductase inhibitors (statins). Most patients with nephrotic syndrome should be on statin therapy to prevent coronary and other atherosclerotic long-term complications.

Clinical/laboratory features suggestive of glomerular disease:
- Proteinuria
- Microscopic/macrocopic hematuria in absence of urologic cause
- Dysmorphic RBCs and RBC casts
- Nephrotic syndrome: edema, proteinuria >3g/day, hypoalbuminemia, hypercholesterolemia
- Hypertension
- Acute oliguria

↓

Laboratory evaluation in all patients:
- Urinalysis, microscopic evaluation of urine sediment
- Serum Cr, BUN, eGFR calculation
- Spot protein to spot creatinine ratio for proteinuria calculation
- Renal ultrasound

↓

Etiology of glomerular disease is readily identifiable (biopsy may not be needed):
- Children with features typical for MCD who respond to steroids
- Longstanding DM with retinopathy with typical diabetic nephropathy features
- Precedings streptococcal infection with typical poststreptococcal GN presentation
- Mild asymptomatic urine abnormalities in setting of normal renal function

Additional laboratory evaluation required (biopsy usually indicated):
- ANA, anti-dsDNA: SLE
- Cryoglobulins, RF: cryoglobulinemia
- Anti-GBMAb: anti GBM disease
- ANCA:
  c-ANCA: Wegener's granulomatosis
  p-ANCA: PAN
- ASO, anti-DNAse-B: poststrep GN
- Hep B Ag, HCV ab: MPGN
- HIV ab: HIVAN
- SPEP/UPEP: amyloid, LCDD

↓

Appropriate treatment

**Renal biopsy
Appropriate treatment**

FIGURE 16-5. Algorithm for initial evaluation of the patient with suspected glomerular renal disease. Ab, antibody; Ag, antigen; ANA, antinuclear antibody; ANCA, anti-neutrophil cytoplasmic antibodies; ASO, antistreptolysin-O; Cr, creatinine; DM, diabetes mellitus; ds, double-stranded; GBM, glomerular basement membrane; GFR, glomerular filtration rate; GN, glomerulonephritis; HCV, hepatitis C virus; Hep, hepatitis; HIVAN, HIV-associated nephropathy; HUS, hemolytic-uremic syndrome; LCDD, light chain deposition disease; MCD, minimal change disease; MPGN, membranoproliferative glomerulonephritis; PAN, polyarteritis nodosum; RF, rheumatoid factor; RPGN, rapidly progressive glomerulonephritis; SPEP, serum protein electrophoresis; UPEP, urine protein electrophoresis.

Disease-specific therapy is most often guided by results of renal biopsy and by supplemental lab evaluation. A final decision regarding the initiation and intensity of immunosuppressive therapy and use of other potentially toxic agents must include consideration of the patient's age and other medical conditions, the likelihood of reversibility of the kidney disease, and compliance with the medical regimen. These therapies will be discussed in the next several chapters on primary and secondary glomerular diseases.

PREVENTION OF COMPLICATIONS OF IMMUNOSUPPRESSIVE REGIMENS

Infection

It is thought that the risk of infections is increased with immunosuppressive therapies. Much of the data for prevention of infection during immunosuppression is derived from the solid organ transplant literature. The following options should be considered when treating glomerular diseases. The intensity of immunosuppression and other patient risk factors should also be factored into the decision.

- Trimethoprim/sulfamethoxazole, 80 mg/400 mg, one tablet daily for prophylaxis against *Pneumocystis jiroveci*
- Low-dose acyclovir, 200 mg daily for prevention of herpes zoster
- Vaccination for *Pneumococci* and influenza is advised to prevent fatal infections
- Monitoring for the development of oropharyngeal thrush, which is usually treatable with nystatin oral suspension

Other Medical Complications

- Histamine-2 blockers to prevent steroid-induced gastritis
- Oral bisphosphonates and calcium supplementation for the prevention of osteoporosis in patients requiring prolonged courses of corticosteroids
- Gonadotropin-releasing hormone agonists (leuprolide) to suppress gonadal function (to protect against gonadal failure before treatment with cytotoxic agents) where indicated
- Although patients with hypoalbuminemia due to nephrotic syndrome are at much higher risk to develop thrombotic events, prophylactic anticoagulation is controversial. If there is documented thrombosis, the patient should receive long-term anticoagulation while still nephrotic.

Adverse effects of disease-specific therapy should be considered in all patients receiving aggressive immunosuppressive regimens for the treatment of glomerular diseases. Some adverse effects of **high-dose corticosteroids** include:

- Steroid-induced osteoporosis
- Glucose intolerance
- Worsening diabetic control
- Opportunistic infections
- Change in body fat distribution, striae, and cushingoid facies

Cyclosporin A carries the following adverse effects:

- Nephrotoxicity requires monitoring of serum Cr. Trough levels of cyclosporine A between 70 and 120 ng/mL may reduce the chances of nephrotoxicity.
- Glucose intolerance, hypertension, and dyslipidemia
- Multiple drug interactions

Use of **cyclophosphamide** may cause the following effects:

- Leukopenia is common with some therapies and the WBC count should be monitored every 1 to 2 weeks. During therapy with cyclophosphamide, the dose should be held if the absolute neutrophil count falls to $<2000/\mu L$ and restarted at a lower dose when leukocyte counts recover.
- Hemorrhagic cystitis incidence can be reduced by aggressive hydration with a daily urine output of >2000 mL/day and with 2-mercaptoethane sulfonate sodium (MESNA) given concomitantly with cyclophosphamide. This agent binds toxic metabolites in the bladder and may be used to reduce cystitis risk.
- Irreversible gonadal failure incidence may be reduced with pretreatment with leuprolide to suppress gonadal function.
- Hair thinning
- Increased risk of bladder cancer
- Nausea and vomiting

Mycophenolate mofetil use places the patient at risk for the following:

- Increased risk of lymphoma or other malignancies
- Neutropenia
- GI upset, diarrhea

Azathioprine use carries the following risks:

- Leukopenia
- Developing certain types of cancer, especially skin cancer and lymphoma

Rituximab is associated with the following adverse effects:

- Severe infusion reactions within the first 24 hours after start of the infusion including angioedema and bronchospasm
- Lymphopenia
- Neutropenia
- Prolonged pancytopenia

KEY POINTS TO REMEMBER

- The presence of dysmorphic RBCs, RBC casts, or nephrotic-range proteinuria can identify glomerular renal diseases, although nonnephrotic proteinuria is nonspecific for glomerular pathology.
- The classification of glomerular diseases is largely based on pathology at the time of renal biopsy with specific features on light microscopy, immunofluorescence, and electron microscopy suggesting the diagnosis.
- Serologic evaluation is supportive of a particular diagnosis in the evaluation of patients with nephritic presentations, nephrotic syndrome, and in selected patients with hematuria or nonnephrotic proteinuria.
- Nonspecific therapies to reduce proteinuria include strict blood pressure control using ACE inhibitors and/or angiotensin receptor blockers, diuretics to control edema, and statins to control hyperlipidemia are warranted.
- Disease-specific therapy is guided by findings on renal biopsy.
- Prophylaxis against complications of steroid or cytotoxic therapy and infections should be considered in all patients.

REFERENCES AND SUGGESTED READINGS

Clarkson M, Brenner B. *Pocket Companion to Brenner & Rector's The Kidney*. 7th ed. London: WB Saunders; 2005.

Couser WG. Glomerulonephritis. *Lancet*. 1999;353:1509.

Dinits-Pensy M. The use of vaccines in adult patients with renal disease. *Am J Kidney Dis*. 46;2005:997–1011.

Greenberg A, ed. *Primer on Kidney Diseases*. 4th ed. London: WB Saunders; 2005.

Hricik DE, Chung-Park M, Sedor JR. Medical progress: glomerulonephritis. *N Engl J Med*. 1998;339:888–899.

Johnson RJ, Feehally JF, eds. *Comprehensive Clinical Nephrology*. 2nd ed. London: Harcourt; 2003.

Orth SR, Ritz E. Medical progress: the nephrotic syndrome. *N Engl J Med*. 1998;338:1202–1211.

Sarasin FP, Schifferli JA. Prophylactic oral anticoagulation in nephrotic patients with idiopathic membranous nephropathy. *Kidney Int*. 1994;45:578–585.

Primary Glomerulopathies

17

David Windus

INTRODUCTION

Primary glomerular diseases are a group of disorders in which the main mainfestations of disease are directly related to kidney involvement rather than as part of a systemic disease process. Systemic diseases associated with glomerular disease are discussed in the following chapter. Primary glomerular diseases can present with nephrotic syndrome, asymptomatic proteinuria, isolated hematuria, or a nephritic picture. In many cases, they are described as being idiopathic without known association or cause. For each of the primary glomerulopathies, secondary causes are also discussed. For instance, medications, infections, and malignancies are all associated with glomerular pathology that is otherwise indistinguishable from the idiopathic forms. Proper diagnosis and management of the primary glomerulopathies requires an understanding of patient characteristics, risk of progressive kidney disease, and safe use of immunosuppressive agents. These cases should be managed in conjunction with physicians experienced in evaluation and treatment of kidney diseases.

FOCAL SEGMENTAL GLOMERULOSCLEROSIS

Focal segmental glomerulosclerosis (FSGS) has become the most important form of primary glomerular disease, both because of increasing incidence and because of its contribution to the growth of end-stage renal disease (ESRD) in the United States. FSGS is a group of disorders that shares several histologic features. Renal biopsy shows some glomeruli (focal) with sclerosis in part of the glomerular tuft (segmental). Patients with these abnormalities often present with nephrotic syndrome but may also have asymptomatic proteinuria. Several means of categorizing FSGS are in use. First, one can discuss FSGS as a *primary* or *secondary* disorder associated with a range of causes and potential differences in treatment. For instance, primary FSGS is usually treated with corticosteroids or immunosuppressive regimens, while secondary disease is not. Second, histologic variants have been described that take into account subglomerular localization of the sclerotic lesion, presence of proliferation, and presence of glomerular capillary collapse. The value of the latter system is thought to arise from better prediction of causation and outcomes. The collapsing FSGS variant is associated with HIV and some drug-associated diseases. The idiopathic form of the collapsing variant is notable for a poor renal prognosis. Table 17-1 summarizes the histologic variants and some of their associations. In addition, a variant of FSGS has been termed *C1q nephropathy*.

TABLE 17-1	HISTOLOGIC VARIANTS OF FOCAL SEGMENTAL GLOMERULOSCLEROSIS	
Name	Histology	Comments
FSGS (NOS)	Segmental increase in matrix, obliterating capillary loop	Most common form
Perihilar variant	Perihilar hyalinosis in >50% of affected glomeruli	Seen in primary and secondary FSGS
Glomerular tip lesion	Segmental sclerosis adjacent to proximal tubular pole of Bowman's capsule, with accumulation of foamy protein droplets in adjacent glomerular capillary loops and podocytes	May correlate with better prognosis and increased responsiveness to steroids
Mesangial hypercellular variant	Localized areas of proliferation and sclerotic lesions	Associated with poor prognosis
Collapsing FSGS	Segmental sclerotic lesions associated with global collapse of the glomerular tuft, visceral epithelial cell hyperplasia, and tubulointerstitial injury	More aggressive with rapid progression to ESRD Associated with secondary FSGS

NOS, not otherwise specified.

PRIMARY IDIOPATHIC FOCAL SEGMENTAL GLOMERULOSCLEROSIS

Clinical Features

FSGS is responsible for approximately 25% of kidney disease in a series of adults with ≥2 g of protein per 24 hours, and up to 35% if nephrotic syndrome is present. The disease is markedly more common in blacks and the mean age of onset in adults is 40 years. In children, FSGS is responsible for about 10% of cases of nephrotic syndrome. However, children with nephrotic syndrome are usually treated empirically with corticosteroids without definitive biopsy diagnosis. In addition to proteinuria, common features on presentation are hypertension (30%–50%), microscopic hematuria (25%–75%), and renal insufficiency (30%–60%). Serologic testing and complement levels should be normal.

Outcomes of Primary FSGS

Spontaneous remission of primary FSGS is unusual (<5% of cases). Poor prognostic indicators are high-grade persistent proteinuria (>10 g/day), higher plasma creatinine (>2.5 mg/dL) at time of diagnosis, greater degree of glomerulosclerosis or tubulointerstitial fibrosis, presence of collapsing lesions or cellular variant, black race, and initial poor response to corticosteroids. FSGS has a significant risk of progression to ESRD with 5- and 10- year renal survival rates of 76% and 57% in those initially presenting with nephrotic syndrome. Nonnephrotic proteinuria is associated with greater than 90% 10-year kidney survival.

Treatment of Primary FSGS

The poor renal outcomes in FSGS have led clinicians to develop aggressive therapies. Traditionally, standard therapy is initiated with high-dose daily *corticosteroids* (prednisone, 1 mg/kg of ideal body weight/day to maximum dose of 80 mg/day or 2 mg/kg alternate-day treatment). Treatment with high-dose daily or alternate-day steroids should be continued for at least 8 weeks. With this regimen, remission is achieved in approximately 40% of patients. Treatment duration for up to 6 months or more will increase remission rates further. However, potential morbidities associated with steroid-related side effects need to be considered if this approach is planned. If remission occurs, the steroids may be tapered slowly. Longer courses may be used in patients who achieve only partial remission or who relapse with steroid tapering. *Cyclosporine* (5 mg/kg ideal body weight/day in divided doses) for steroid-resistant FSGS has been studied by the North American Collaborative Study of Cyclosporine in Nephrotic Syndrome. The remission rate in this trial was >70% (complete or partial) in steroid-resistant patients. In addition to reduction in proteinuria, slower progression of kidney disease was found. However, relapse is common after cyclosporine is discontinued. Cyclophosphamide or chlorambucil plus steroid-based regimens have not been tested in randomized controlled trials. Only 15% to 20% of steroid-resistant patients have historically responded to these regimens. Recurrence of FSGS after renal transplantation is common (up to 30%) and is associated with decreased graft survival. Plasmapheresis has been used with limited success in the management of posttransplant FSGS recurrence.

SECONDARY FOCAL SEGMENTAL GLOMERULOSCLEROSIS

Genetic Causes of FSGS

Familial variants of FSGS secondary to mutations in podocyte proteins, including alpha-actinin-4 and podocin, have been described. These conditions are more often detected in children and tend to be resistant to corticosteroid treatment.

Viral Infection

HIV-associated nephropathy may occur at any time during the course of HIV infection, although it is usually diagnosed when CD4 count falls below 200. The glomerular disease appears to result from direct infection of podocytes leading to podocyte proliferation and de-differentiation. Up to 95% of HIV-associated nephropathy cases occur in young black men with HIV infection contracted by any route (mean age, 33 years; male-to-female ratio, 10:1). The clinical presentation includes nephrotic or nonnephrotic proteinuria, elevated plasma creatinine, and microscopic hematuria. Laboratory evaluation reveals HIV seropositivity, normal C3, normal C4, and CD4 count usually <200. Renal ultrasound shows enlarged kidneys with increased echogenicity. The pathology of HIV-associated nephropathy includes collapsing FSGS, mesangial proliferation, hypertrophied podocytes with protein resorption droplets, microcystic dilated tubules filled with hyaline casts, and edematous interstitium. *Parvovirus B19* infection has also been associated with collapsing FSGS.

Drugs

Drugs associated with FSGS include pamidronate, heroin, lithium, and alpha-interferon. Pamidronate has been associated with the collapsing form. Secondary FSGS was attributed to heroin use in older studies. These cases presented with nephrotic syndrome and with rapid progression to ESRD. More recent studies have shown that the incidence of heroin-associated disease has declined markedly.

Sickle Cell Nephropathy

Kidney disease can occur in persons with sickle cell disease. The prevalence of proteinuria was 26% in one series. Chronic kidney disease has been seen in 7% to 30% of patients with long-term follow-up. Hyperfiltration and increased glomerular pressure are thought to be the mechanism for injury. The most common lesion on kidney biopsy is FSGS, although other histology can sometimes be found (e.g., membranoproliferative glomerulonephritis [MPGN]).

Other

Other causes of secondary FSGS include reduced renal mass (unilateral renal agenesis, renal ablation, and renal allograft), chronic vesicoureteral reflux, morbid obesity, congenital cyanotic heart disease, malignancy, and sarcoidosis.

Treatment of Secondary FSGS

Therapy for the underlying disorder is first-line management. Lesions of FSGS may regress with management of the underlying condition. Nonspecific therapy to reduce edema and proteinuria with diuretics, dietary sodium restriction, and ACE inhibitor/angiotensin receptor blocker therapy should be aggressively pursued. Steroid treatment as for idiopathic FSGS can be considered in refractory cases, but limited data do not support the use of aggressive immunosuppressive or cytotoxic agents.

OTHER FSGS VARIANT: C1Q NEPHROPATHY

Distinctive features of C1q nephropathy are a predominance of C1q staining in the glomerulus and mesangial electron-dense deposits. Persons with this diagnosis are predominantly African American women. Proteinuria is usually in the nephrotic range and hematuria is present in around 20%. The best treatment for this lesion is unclear but should include antiproteinuric strategies, such as ACE inhibitors.

MINIMAL CHANGE DISEASE

Clinical Presentation

Minimal change disease is the most common cause of nephrotic syndrome in children (~ 65%) and up to 10% to 15% of cases in adults. The peak incidence of minimal change disease is in children 2 to 7 years old, but the disease may occur at any age. Children presenting with typical features of nephrotic syndrome usually undergo empiric steroid therapy without a definitive diagnosis by renal biopsy. Steroid responsiveness in this group is equated with a diagnosis of minimal change disease. The typical presentation of minimal change disease is nephrotic syndrome (proteinuria >3 g/day, hyperlipidemia, edema). Clinical presentation is usually characterized by rapid onset of edema, often with periorbital edema, marked weight gain, pleural effusions, and ascites. Acute kidney injury can occur in up to 18% of adults. Major risk factors for this presentation are older age and a prior history of hypertension. Other complications of minimal change disease include sepsis, peritonitis in ascitic fluid, and thromboembolism. The *pathophysiology* remains unknown but may be related to a specific T-cell defect with release of a glomerular permeability factor. The majority of cases are idiopathic. *Laboratory evaluation* reveals low plasma albumin and elevated cholesterol. In children, the urine sediment is usually normal other than Maltese-cross oval fat bodies under polarized light. In adults, microscopic hematuria is present in about 30%. Complement levels and other serologic markers are normal. A urine protein electrophoresis will show that the negatively charged protein albumin predominates. This has been termed *selective proteinuria*. Renal biopsy is required for diagnosis, especially in adults.

Secondary Causes of Minimal Change Disease

Minimal change disease can be induced by exposure to drugs (most commonly NSAIDs or interferon-alpha), heavy metals (mercury, lead), or systemic allergic reactions to environmental allergens or vaccines. Minimal change disease is also associated with hematologic malignancies, most notably Hodgkin disease.

Pathology

Light microscopy is typically normal, although mild mesangial hypercellularity may be found. Tubular and interstitial structures are normal. Immunofluorescence may reveal IgM and C3 trapped in damaged capillary loops and mesangium. Heavy mesangial deposits of IgM are associated with worse prognosis and poor response to treatment (so-called IgM nephropathy). Electron microscopy reveals diffuse glomerular epithelial foot process fusion; this is indistinguishable from foot process fusion seen in podocyte injury from other causes.

Treatment and Outcomes

The initial treatment of *adults* with minimal change disease is corticosteroids. Typical regimens are daily dosing with prednisone 1 mg/kg or alternate-day dosing with 2 mg/kg every other day. These approaches appear to have similar initial response rates. If response has occurred by 8 weeks, the dose is tapered over the ensuing 2 to 3 months. Studies find that approximately 60% of adults will achieve a complete remission by 8 weeks and 90% will ultimately respond if corticosteroids are continued for up to 18 to 20 weeks. Adults who initially respond to corticosteroids will experience at least one relapse around 70% of the time. Relapses are usually treated with a second course of corticosteroids. In *children*, nephrotic syndrome is often treated with empiric treatment. As in adults, the mainstay of therapy is corticosteroids (prednisone, 1 mg/kg of ideal body weight/day, not to exceed 80 mg/day). This regimen is usually continued for 4 weeks after resolution of proteinuria and then tapered by 10 mg on an alternate day regimen every 2 weeks (total course of 3–4 months in steroid responders). The typical course is remitting and relapsing, with approximately 75% of patients who initially achieve remission on steroids relapsing within 5 years. Shorter courses of prednisone (6–10 weeks) can generally be used to treat relapses. Steroid resistance can also be encountered and is characterized by failure to reach remission within 4 months of steroid treatment. These subsets of patients are most susceptible to complications of steroid therapy (osteoporosis, avascular necrosis, abnormal fat deposition) and are often maintained on low-dose daily or every-other-day prednisone. Alternative therapy in these patients should be considered. Alkylating agents may be as effective in preventing relapses. Options for management are oral cyclophosphamide (1.5 mg/kg of ideal body weight/day) or chlorambucil (0.1–0.2 mg/kg of ideal body weight/day) for 8 to 12 weeks after steroid induction. Alternate regimens, including cyclosporine have also been used with some success in those patients with frequent relapses. A small percentage of adults initially thought to have minimal change disease will progress to ESRD. Repeat biopsies show FSGS in these patients.

Minimal Change Disease Variant: IgM Nephropathy

The term *IgM nephropathy* is used by some to describe patients presenting with nephrotic syndrome and with the findings of mesangial proliferation on renal biopsy. Controversy exists regarding whether to include this constellation of findings as a variant of minimal disease or FSGS or as part of a continuum related to both entities. The majority of patients will have some response initially to corticosteroid therapy. In one series, 23% progressed to ESRD over 15-year follow-up.

MEMBRANOUS NEPHROPATHY

Epidemiology

Membranous nephropathy is a common cause of nephrotic syndrome due to primary glomerular disease in adults with an incidence that roughly equals that of FSGS (~35%). In addition, it is the most common cause of nephrotic syndrome in persons >60 years of age and has a male predominance (~2–3:1). It is distinctly uncommon in children and adolescents. Most cases (90%) are idiopathic.

Secondary Causes of Membranous Nephropathy

A diagnosis of membranous nephropathy should prompt a thorough evaluation for other related diseases. It is associated with a variety of autoimmune, infectious, and malignant diseases, as well as with toxic or drug exposures. Autoimmune diseases associated with membranous nephropathy include systemic lupus erythematosus (SLE—WHO class V), type 1 diabetes mellitus, rheumatoid arthritis, mixed connective tissue disease, Sjögren syndrome, Hashimoto thyroiditis, and myasthenia gravis. Associated infectious diseases are hepatitis B, hepatitis C (HCV), syphilis, malaria, and HIV. Malignancies associated with membranous nephropathy include lung, stomach, breast, colon, or prostate adenocarcinoma, non-Hodgkin lymphoma, and leukemia. Nephrotic syndrome may precede clinical evidence of malignancy by up to 1 year. NSAIDs, gold, penicillamine, hydrocarbons, mercury, formaldehyde, captopril, and certain antiepileptics have been reported in association with membranous nephropathy.

Clinical Features

Membranous nephropathy presents as nephrotic syndrome in 80% of patients. Microscopic hematuria may be found in 50% of cases, but RBC casts are unusual. As with the other causes of nephrotic syndrome, a renal biopsy is necessary to make the diagnosis. Plasma complement levels are normal in the idiopathic form. Decreased C3 or C4 should prompt further evaluation for SLE or other systemic disorders associated with hypocomplementemia. There is an increased incidence of thromboembolism, especially renal vein thrombosis. Membranous nephropathy is characterized by slow progression of renal insufficiency (<20% of patients have renal insufficiency at time of presentation). Hypertension develops only with advancing renal insufficiency and is usually not characteristic of membranous nephropathy at earlier stages.

Pathogenesis

The pathogenesis of membranous nephropathy is thought to be due to autoimmunity via specific nephritogenic autoantibodies, although the putative antigens have not been identified in humans. Heymann nephritis is a rat model of this disease that is induced by inoculation with *megalin*, a large (516-kDa) glycoprotein extracted from rat cortical nephrons. Formation of antigen-antibody complexes are seen at the podocyte level, with complement activation and formation of the membrane attack complex (C5b–9). This leads to destruction of the glomerular base membrane (GBM) and shedding of the immune complexes to form the characteristic subepithelial deposits.

Pathology

Light microscopy is normal at early stages and later progresses to thickened glomerular capillary wall with epithelial "spikes" seen by methenamine silver staining. There is a notable absence of leukocyte infiltration with no evidence of hypercellularity or proliferative lesions. Immunofluorescence demonstrates characteristic IgG granular subepithelial staining in all portions of the glomerular capillary loop. In idiopathic membranous nephropathy, staining is exclusively IgG. Presence of IgM or IgA staining suggests class V lupus nephritis. Complement C3 and light chains also present with similar localization to IgG in approximately 50% of cases. Electron microscopy demonstrates the diagnostic subepithelial electron-dense deposits in stages:

- **Stage I:** subepithelial dense deposits without adjacent projections of GBM; normal light microscopy
- **Stage II:** adjacent GBM projections forming spikes around immune deposits
- **Stage III:** GBM projections surrounding deposits completely
- **Stage IV:** markedly thickened GBM with electron-lucent zones replacing the dense deposits

These stages reflect the duration of disease but do not correlate well with prognosis. The finding of extensive mesangial electron-dense deposits should prompt consideration of membranous nephropathy secondary to SLE.

Treatment and Outcomes

Factors associated with poor prognosis include male gender, age >50 years, presence of hypertension, decreased GFR (plasma creatinine >1.2 mg/dL in women, >1.4 mg/dL in men), nephrotic syndrome of >6 months' duration, and >20% interstitial fibrosis on renal biopsy specimen. Spontaneous, partial or complete remission is seen in up to 50% of patients with membranous nephropathy within 3 to 5 years of diagnosis. Those with partial remission continue to experience non–nephrotic-range proteinuria and stable GFR. In these cases, management is targeted at continued aggressive blood pressure control, ACE inhibition, and lipid-lowering therapy. Up to one-fourth of patients who remit may experience a relapse of nephrotic-range proteinuria that may require disease-specific therapy.

All patients with membranous nephropathy should be managed with blood pressure control (goal, <130/85 mm Hg), dietary sodium restriction, ACE inhibition or angiotensin receptor blockade, and lipid-lowering therapy. Patients with documented renal vein or other venous thrombosis should be anticoagulated with warfarin. Disease-specific therapy is indicated in a subset of patients with membranous nephropathy at the discretion of the treating physician. Aggressive cytotoxic therapy is reserved for patients considered to be at higher risk for kidney disease progression, as the natural history can be relatively benign in up to one-half of affected patients. The higher risk group has decreased kidney function or has persistent nephrotic range proteinuria after achieving blood pressure control with ACE inhibitors, angiotensin receptor blockers, and other agents.

Disease-specific therapy for membranous nephropathy includes the *Ponticelli protocol* for the treatment of membranous nephropathy (10-year follow-up study by Italian group):

- **Months 1, 3, and 5:** Methylprednisolone, 1 g IV for 3 days followed by prednisone, 0.5 mg/kg of ideal body weight PO daily for the remainder of the 4 weeks.
- **Months 2, 4, and 6:** Chlorambucil, 0.1 to 0.15 mg/kg of ideal body weight PO daily for 4 weeks.

At 10-year follow-up, 88% of patients treated with this protocol had partial or complete remission compared with 47% of controls. The original study reported using chlorambucil 0.2 mg/kg. However, these doses are limited by bone marrow toxicity of chlorambucil and lower doses may be a more prudent course. *Cyclophosphamide* and *corticosteroids* have been used as an alternative therapy. Cyclophosphamide, 1.5 to 2 mg/kg of ideal body weight/day PO daily plus prednisone, 0.5 mg/kg of ideal body weight/day PO daily can be given for 3 to 6 months. This regimen has been found to be comparable to the original Ponticelli protocol in smaller studies. In both regimens, WBC counts should be carefully monitored. Typically, the WBCs are monitored weekly with both chlorambucil and cyclophosphamide use. Alternative regimens include cyclosporine, 3.5 to 5 mg/kg of ideal body weight/day, which usually requires a more prolonged course (1–2 years) to sustain remission.

MEMBRANOPROLIFERATIVE GLOMERULONEPHRITIS

MPGN is a pathologic diagnosis based on the finding of diffuse mesangial proliferation, thickening of the capillary wall, subendothelial immune deposits, and hypercellularity. Most cases are associated with circulating immune complexes and hypocomplementemia.

Clinical Presentation of MPGN

Clinical presentation of patients with MPGN types 1 and 2 can range from nephrotic syndrome and microscopic or gross hematuria to acute nephritic syndrome with rapid decline of kidney function. Onset of nephritis may be preceded by upper respiratory infection. Idiopathic MPGN type 1 is most common in adolecents and young adults. Hypertension is present in a majority of cases. MPGN type 1 associated with cryoglobulins is the most common form found in adults. MPGN type 2 is most often seen in children. Diagnosis of MPGN should prompt investigation for underlying causes, including blood cultures to rule out infective endocarditis; serologies for hepatitis B, HCV, and HIV; evaluation for malignancy; chronic liver disease; or SLE.

Laboratory findings include decreased complement levels:

- **Type I and cryoglobulinemic MPGN:** low C3, low or normal C4, low CH_{50}
- **Type II:** low C3, normal C4, low CH_{50}, C3 nephritic factor present in approximately 60% of cases
- **Type III:** low C3, low C5–C9

Classification

Type I MPGN

Pathology. Type I MPGN is defined by subendothelial and mesangial immune deposits seen on electron microscopy at renal biopsy. Light microscopy reveals expanded mesangium with increased matrix and cellularity with a classic lobular appearance to the glomeruli. Immunofluorescence reveals heavy C3 deposition. Type I MPGN is frequently idiopathic but is also often associated with cryoglobulinemia, chronic HCV infection, chronic hepatitis B viral infection, endocarditis, or malarial infection.

Pathogenesis. The pathogenesis includes glomerular deposition of immune complexes that preferentially localize to the mesangium and subendothelial space, with subsequent complement activation via classic pathway with resultant inflammation, leukocyte infiltration, and cellular proliferation. Type I MPGN can also be associated with hereditary complement deficiencies (C2, C3, C6, C7, C8) or with defective clearance of immune complexes. C3 and CH_{50} are reduced in most cases; C4 is reduced in some cases.

Type II MPGN (Dense Deposit Disease)

Pathology. Type II MPGN is defined by the presence of mesangial electron-dense deposits on electron microscopy. Immunofluorescence reveals C3 staining on either side of the GBM, creating the classic "railroad track" appearance.

Pathogenesis. Type II MPGN is associated with C3 nephritic factor (a circulating autoantibody that binds to C3 convertase and prevents its inactivation), which leads to constitutive activation of the alternate pathway of complement and damage to the GBM. The condition is associated with partial lipodystrophy in up to 25% of pediatric patients, leading to marked reduction in subcutaneous fat tissues, especially in the face and upper body. C3 and CH_{50} are reduced in most cases; C4 is usually normal.

Type III MPGN

Type III MPGN is defined by diffuse subendothelial deposits and electron-dense deposits within the GBM and in the subepithelial spaces. The pathogenesis includes activation of the classic or terminal pathway of complement activation.

Mixed Cryoglobulinemia

Cryoglobulins are monoclonal (IgM) and polyclonal (IgG and IgM) Ig-containing proteins that precipitate in the cold. The presence of cryoglobulins is strongly associated with chronic HCV infection in up to 90% of patients. Associations have also been noted with hepatitis B and Epstein-Barr virus. Type II (monoclonal, usually IgM-kappa, and polyclonal components) and type III (polyclonal) cryoglobulinemia are associated with MPGN.

Natural History and Treatment of MPGN

Untreated MPGN progresses to death or ESRD in 50% of adults within 5 years and up to 90% in 20 years. The presence of prolonged nephrotic syndrome carries with it a poor prognosis. The disease can recur after renal transplantation, especially type II and MPGN associated with HCV. When MPGN is diagnosed in a patient who already has chronic kidney disease, only general supportive measures to reduce proteinuria and control blood pressure are appropriate, as treatment is aimed at preserving renal function. The role of alternate-day, high-dose steroids and cytotoxic agents in MPGN remains controversial, with the majority of longer trials performed in children demonstrating equivocal or no effect. Cyclosporine has also been administered to some patients with MPGN and is of unclear benefit.

Other Therapies

Antiplatelet therapies, such as aspirin or dipyridamole, have been studied in several trials. Although proteinuria was reduced in the treatment group, no differences in renal function were observed. Systemic anticoagulation with warfarin has also been studied in the MPGN population and is of unclear benefit with substantial bleeding risks. HCV-associated cryoglobulinemia has been successfully treated with interferon-alpha (3 million units SC 3 times/week for 6–12 months) plus ribavirin in the setting of stable renal function. If renal function is rapidly deteriorating (commonly termed *fulminant cryoglobulinemia*), high-dose steroid therapy is indicated, with or without cytotoxic therapy and plasma exchange.

IGA NEPHROPATHY AND HENOCH-SCHÖNLEIN PURPURA

Epidemiology

IgA nephropathy (also known as *Berger's disease*) is the most common form of glomerular disease diagnosed worldwide. The incidence in the United States and Canada is substantially lower than that in Europe, Asia, and Japan. This discrepancy may be due to rates of routine urinalysis in the United States compared with Asian countries and due to attitudes toward doing kidney biopsies in patients with asymptomatic hematuria. The male-to-female ratio is 2.5:1. Henoch-Schönlein purpura is a syndrome associated with IgA deposition in the kidney with other systemic features. This disorder is seen predominantly children and adolescents.

Clinical Presentation

Microscopic or gross hematuria is almost always part of the initial presentation of IgA nephropathy. Asymptomatic microscopic hematuria with variable degrees of proteinuria is found in 30% to 40% of cases. Acute macroscopic hematuria concurrent with upper respiratory tract infection is seen in roughly in 50% of patients. The timing of the hematuria after the infection is usually within 1 to 2 days. This is in contrast to poststreptococcal glomerulonephritis, in which the hematuria (often associated with nephritic syndrome) occurs 10 to 14 days after pharyngitis. Occasionally, patients will present with nephrotic syndrome or acute kidney injury syndromes. Progressive renal insufficiency and hypertension are seen in a minority of patients, occasionally with rapid course and glomerular epithelial crescents on biopsy (<10%). Laboratory evaluation demonstrates normal complement levels and increased plasma IgA levels in approximately 50% of patients. Diagnosis is made by renal biopsy.

Henoch-Schönlein purpura is a syndrome with IgA nephropathy associated with systemic vasculitis caused by IgA deposition. It usually presents with arthralgias, purpuric skin rash, abdominal pain, ileus, or GI bleeding. Renal involvement may be transient.

Secondary Causes of IgA Nephropathy

IgA deposition associated with mesangial cell proliferation can appear secondary to systemic diseases associated with decreased IgA clearance or increased IgA production (e.g., cirrhosis, celiac sprue, inflammatory bowel disease, GI tract cancer).

Pathology and Diagnosis

Light microscopy reveals global or segmental mesangial hypercellularity with some sclerosis and tubulointerstitial fibrosis. Immunofluorescence demonstrates mesangial IgA deposition, co-deposition of C3, and, less commonly, IgG and IgM co-deposition. Electron microscopy shows mesangial electron-dense deposits and focal thinning of GBM.

Natural History of IgA Nephroathy

The majority of patients with IgA nephropathy do not progress to ESRD and experience a benign disease course. Several markers predicting a better outcome are minimal proteinuria, normal blood pressure, and normal renal function on presentation. In addition, lack of fibrosis of glomeruli and tubulointerstitium are good prognostic signs. Approximately 30% of patients with IgA nephropathy will experience progressive disease. These patients often have poor prognostic features including poorly controlled hypertension, older age at diagnosis, persistent proteinuria, reduced renal function at diagnosis, and tubulointerstitial fibrosis or more advanced glomerular lesions on renal biopsy.

Treatment of IgA Nephropathy

Little controversy exists in the general management of patients with IgA nephropathy. Blood pressure control with ACE inhibition is indicated in all hypertensive patients with IgA nephropathy and may be of some benefit despite normal blood pressure at presentation. Beyond these general recommendations, there are a wide range of study outcomes and opinions regarding the use of other nonimmunosuppressive and immunosuppressive therapies. The effect of *fish oil containing omega-3 fatty acids* has been studied by several groups. One group found that the patients receiving fish oil (12 g daily) had a significantly lower rate of progression of renal insufficiency and lower rate of progression to ESRD compared with placebo. Other studies have shown no benefit. It remains unclear if certain subgroups would benefit from this therapy. *Corticosteroid* therapy has been shown to reduce proteinuria in several studies of IgA nephropathy. However, progressive GFR decline does not appear to be prevented. Patients presenting with nephrotic syndrome may have a better response to steroid therapy. Corticosteroid therapy is also likely to be of benefit when crescentic changes are present on biopsy. Studies of other immunosuppressive drugs suggest that patients with severe or progressive disease may benefit from combination therapy with cyclophosphamide and corticosteroids. In sum, the use of immunosuppressive regimens needs to be tailored to the severity (and thus prognosis) of disease.

Children in whom recurrent bouts of tonsillitis appear to correlate with episodes of IgA nephropathy may benefit from *tonsillectomy*. Of all the glomerular diseases, IgA nephropathy recurs with greatest frequency after renal transplantation, but the majority of recurrences do not worsen graft outcome and have a benign course.

KEY POINTS TO REMEMBER

- Minimal change disease is the most common cause of nephrotic syndrome in children. Most cases are responsive to steroids.
- Spontaneous resolution in FSGS is quite uncommon. Response to steroid therapy is often not as complete or sustained as response in minimal change disease.
- Membranous nephropathy is a heterogeneous disease with variable progression and complication rates; careful determination of each patient's risk for disease progression should be made before instituting therapy.
- MPGN is associated with circulating immune complexes and hypocomplementemia. There is a strong association between mixed cryoglobulinemia and chronic HCV infection.
- IgA nephropathy has a variable disease course with proteinuria and hypertension being the major risk factors for progressive kidney disease.

REFERENCES AND SUGGESTED READINGS

Banfi G, Moriggi M, Sabadini E, et al. The impact of prolonged immunosuppression on the outcome of idiopathic focal-segmental glomerulosclerosis with nephrotic syndrome in adults. *Clin Nephrol.* 1991;36:53.

Cattran DC, Appel GB, Hebert L, et al. A multicenter trial of cyclosporine in patients with steroid resistant focal and segmental glomerulosclerosis. *Kidney Int.* 1999;56:2220.

D'Amico G. Natural history of IgA nephropathy: role of clinical and histological prognostic factors. *Am J Kidney Dis.* 2000;36:227.

Donadio JV Jr, Grande JP, Bergstrahl EJ, et al. The long term outcome of patients with IgA nephropathy treated with fish oil in a controlled trial. The Mayo Clinic Collaborative Group. *J Am Soc Nephrol.* 1999;10:1772.

Donadio JV, Grande JP. Medical progress: IgA nephropathy. *N Engl J Med.* 2002;347: 738–748.

Fujimoto S, Yamamoto Y, Hisanaga S, et al. Minimal change nephrotic syndrome in adults: response to corticosteroids therapy and frequency of relapse. *Am J Kidney Dis.* 1991;150:380.

Gulati S, Pokhariyal S, Sharma RK, et al. Pulse cyclophosphamide therapy in frequently relapsing nephrotic syndrome. *Nephrol Dial Transplant.* 2001;16:2013.

Kamar, N. Rostoing, L, Alric, L. Treatment of hepatitis C-virus-related glomerulonephritis. *Kidney Int.* 2006; 69:436.

Korbet SM. Clinical picture and outcome of primary focal segmental glomerulosclerosis. *Nephrol Dial Transplant.* 1999;14[Suppl 3]:68.

Lai, KN. Membranous nephropathy: when and how to treat. *Kidney Int.* 2007;71:841.

Lefaucheur, C, Stengel, B, Nochy, D, et al. Membranous nephropathy and cancer: epidemiologic evidence and determinants of high-risk cancer association. *Kidney Int.* 2006;70:1510.

Levin A. Management of membranoproliferative glomerulonephritis: evidence-based recommendations. *Kidney Int.* 1999;70[suppl]:S41.

Mak SK, Short CD, Mallick NP. Long-term outcome of adult-onset minimal-change nephropathy. *Nephrol Dial Transplant.* 1996;11:2192.

Markowitz, GS, Schwimmer, JA, Stokes, MB. C1q nephropathy: a variant of focal segmental glomerulosclerosis. *Kidney Int.* 2003;64:1232.

Matalon A, Markowitz GS, Joseph RE, et al. Plasmapheresis treatment of recurrent FSGS in adult transplant recipients. *Clin Nephrol.* 2001;56:271.

Matalon A, Valeri A, Appel GB. The treatment of focal segmental glomerulosclerosis. *Semin Nephrol.* 2000;20:309.

Nolin L, Courteau M. Management of IgA nephropathy: evidence-based recommendations. *Kidney Int.* 1999;70[suppl]:S56.

Ponticelli C, Altieri P, Scolari F, et al. A randomized study comparing methylprednisolone plus chlorambucil versus methylprednisolone plus cyclophosphamide in idiopathic membranous nephropathy. *J Am Soc Nephrol.* 1998;9:444.

Ponticelli C, Zucchelli P, Passerini P, et al. A 10-year follow-up of a randomized study with methylprednisolone and chlorambucil in membranous nephropathy. *Kidney Int.* 1995;48:1600.

Ponticelli C, Zucchelli P, Passerini P, et al. Methylprednisolone plus chlorambucil as compared with methylprednisolone alone for the treatment of idiopathic membranous nephropathy. *N Engl J Med.* 1992;327:599.

Rydel JJ, Korbet SM, Borok RZ, et al. Focal segmental glomerular sclerosis in adults: presentation, course, and response to treatment. *Am J Kidney Dis.* 1995;25:534.

Schwimmer JA, Markowitz GS, Valeri A, et al. Collapsing glomerulopathy. *Semin Nephrol.* 2003;23:209.

Thomas, DB, Franceschini, N, Hogan, SL, et al. Clinical and pathologic characteristics of focal segmental glomerulosclerosis pathologic variants. *Kidney Int.* 2006;69:920.

Waldman M, Crew RJ, Valeri A, et al. Adult minimal-change disease: clinical characteristics, treatment, and outcomes. *Clin J Am Soc Nephrol.* 2007;2:445.

Weiner NJ, Goodman JW, Kimmel PL. The HIV-associated renal diseases: current insight into pathogenesis and treatment. *Kidney Int.* 2003;63:1618.

Glomerulonephritis in Multisystem Disorders

18

Nadine D. Tanenbaum

RENAL DISEASE IN SYSTEMIC LUPUS ERYTHEMATOSIS

Epidemiology and Clinical Presentation

Systemic lupus erythematosus (SLE) is an autoimmune disease characterized by multi-organ involvement and the production of antinuclear antibodies (ANAs), particularly antibodies directed against **double-stranded DNA (dsDNA)** and the **Smith antigen (Sm)**, the latter which consists of nonhistone nuclear proteins. In many patients, titers of anti-dsDNA antibodies correlate with disease activity, whereas titers of anti-Sm antibodies tend to be more constant, regardless of disease activity. Most patients with untreated active disease have low complement levels. Clinical criteria for distinguishing SLE from other rheumatologic disorders were revised in 1982 by the American College of Rheumatology and are listed in Table 18-1. The presence of ≥4 of these criteria have a specificity and sensitivity of 96% for the diagnosis of SLE.

Although SLE can occur at any age, it is most common in women between ages 15 and 40. It is 3 to 4 times more common in African Americans than in whites. Precipitating factors for flares in susceptible individuals include sunlight, infections, surgery, stress, and pregnancy. Renal abnormalities occur in up to 60% of adults and 80% of children with SLE, usually within 3 years of diagnosis. Almost all patients with renal involvement in SLG, also called lupus nephritis (LN), have some degree of proteinuria; 45% to 65% have nephrotic syndrome. Other observed findings include microscopic hematuria, granular or RBC casts, renal insufficiency, hypertension, and distal renal tubular acidosis associated with either hypo- or hyperkalemia. With current treatment, about 10% to 15% of patients with SLE develop end-stage renal disease (ESRD). Some patients have a decrease in systemic disease activity once on dialysis but others do not. Kidney transplantation in patients with SLE remains an excellent option for those who have progressed to ESRD, with <4% incidence of allograft loss secondary to SLE.

Renal Pathology

Most patients with LN have **immune-complex mediated glomerulonephritis** (GN) characterized by positive glomerular immunofluorescence (IF) for IgG and usually IgM, IgA, C3, and C1q. The ISN 2003 classification of the pathological categories of LN has replaced the prior WHO classification and is presented in Table 18-2. Additionally, other **nonglomerular lesions** can be seen in LN, including tubulointerstitial nephritis and vascular lesions such as immunoglobulin vascular deposits, arteriosclerosis, vasculitis, arteriolar thrombi, or overt thrombotic microangiopathy. Arteriolar thrombi and overt microangiopathy often occur in the presence of antiphospholipid antibodies.

Renal biopsy in patients with suspected active LN is essential for confirming the diagnosis and for guiding management, as prognosis and treatment options depend on the pathological class of GN. Furthermore, biopsy results cannot be reliably predicted based

TABLE 18-1	AMERICAN COLLEGE OF RHEUMATOLOGY CRITERIA FOR THE DIAGNOSIS OF SLE

Malar rash
Discoid rash
Photosensitivity
Oral ulceration
Nonerosive arthritis
Serositis (pleuritis, pericarditis)
Renal involvement (proteinuria, hematuria, or the presence of casts)
Neuropsychiatric involvement
Leukopenia, hemolytic anemia, and/or thrombocytopenia
Positive antiphospholipid antibody, anti–double-stranded DNA antibody, anti-Smith antibody, or false-positive antitreponemal test
Positive ANA

From Tan EM, Cohen AS, Fries JF, et al. The 1982 revised criteria for the classification of systemic lupus erythematosus. *Arthritis Rheum.* 1982:25:1271.

on clinical features (e.g., degree of proteinuria, renal insufficiency). Recurrence of LN, even after years of remission, occurs in 50% of patients. Patients can transition between the various classes of LN at any time in their course. Commonly, class III progresses to class IV nephritis, and class IV nephritis transitions into class V nephritis.

Treatment of Lupus Nephritis

Class I and II
Patients with mesangial lupus have an excellent prognosis and do not require specific treatment for their renal disease.

Class III and IV
Patients with mild class III disease are generally treated like those with class I and II LN. Patients with severe class III and class IV disease have traditionally received **induction therapy** with monthly IV cyclophosphamide ($0.5–1.0$ g/m^2) for 6 months. Pulse methyl-prednisolone (500—1000 mg IV daily for 3 days) is followed by prednisone (0.5–1.0 mg/kg PO daily), which is tapered over a period of months as directed by extrarenal symptoms. Others have used oral cyclophosphamide (1.5–2.0 mg/kg/day PO) for 8 to 12

TABLE 18-2	ISN CLASSIFICATION OF LUPUS NEPHRITIS (LN)

Class Definition

I	Minimal mesangial LN
II	Mesangial proliferative LN
III	Focal proliferative LN
IV	Diffuse proliferative LN
V	Membranous LN
VI	Advanced sclerosis LN

weeks, in addition to prednisone, as induction therapy. More recently, mycophenolate mofetil (MMF) (2–3 g PO per day) with oral prednisone has been shown to be equally efficacious as induction therapy in relatively short-term follow-up. This has been studied in patients with baseline normal creatinine.

After achieving remission, **maintenance therapy** with MMF (1–2 g/day PO) or aza-thioprine (2 mg/kg PO daily) with low-dose prednisone is generally continued for at least 24 months with a subsequent slow taper. This maintenance approach appears to be associated with fewer complications and improved renal and patient survival than using maintenance IV cyclophosphamide every 3 months. In patients unresponsive to stan-dard therapies, less well-studied treatments such as rituximab and IV immunoglobulin have been used.

Class V

The treatment for membranous class V lupus is controversial. The natural history is not well defined, but some patients go into spontaneous remissions or have long-term stable renal function. Patients with declining renal function and/or severe nephrotic syndrome are generally treated like class IV patients. Cyclosporine (3–5 mg/kg PO daily) with low-dose prednisone for 4 to 6 months has been used in patients with less severe nephrotic syndrome.

POSTSTREPTOCOCCAL GLOMERULONEPHRITIS

Epidemiology and Clinical Presentation

Poststreptococcal GN (PSGN) is an immune-complex mediated GN that is caused by certain nephritogenic strains of group A streptococci. Typically, there is a sudden onset of hematuria or tea-colored urine, hypertension, and edema that occurs about 1 to 6 weeks after pharyngitis or a skin infection. Oliguria and, less commonly, anuria may occur. Although the peak incidence of PSGN is in the first decade, in some series 30% to 40% of people with PSGN are over the age of 40. Subclinical forms of PSGN man-ifested by microscopic urinary abnormalities and/or transient low complement levels may occur. The nature of the nephritogenic antigen and the mechanisms that lead to renal immune complex deposition are not clearly established and are an area of much study.

Laboratory Features

Patients with PSGN typically have hematuria with RBC casts, dysmorphic RBCs, granu-lar casts and sometimes WBC casts. Proteinuria is common, but only 5% to 20% have nephrotic syndrome. Many patients have elevated titers of antistreptococcal antibodies. The most commonly tested antistreptococcal antibodies are antistreptolysin O (ASO) and antideoxyribonuclease-B (anti-DNase-B). Titers of the latter are more commonly elevated in skin infections than are ASO titers. Serum complement levels, especially C3 and CH50 levels, are almost always depressed during an acute episode and generally normalize by 6 weeks after diagnosis. Other findings include a low urine FeNa and a high urine specific gravity.

Renal Pathology

Renal biopsy is not required if the clinical and laboratory features are consistent with PSGN, particularly in children in which PSGN is most common. Biopsy should be per-formed if the diagnosis is in question or if there is failure to improve spontaneously.

Kidneys are enlarged in PSGN, with enlarged diffusely involved hypercellular glomeruli on light microscopy. Typically, there is an abundance of polymorphonuclear neutrophils (PMNs) in the endocapillary space. Rarely, crescents can be seen. On IF, glomerular capillary walls stain positive for IgG and C3, and occasionally IgM, in a granular pattern. On electron microscopy (EM), glomerular subepithelial electron-dense deposits ("subepithelial humps") are characteristic; smaller mesangial and subendothelial deposits are also seen.

Natural History and Treatment

In general, the prognosis of PSGN is excellent, especially in children. Resolution of acute symptoms occurs within 4 to 6 weeks and progression to ESRD is extremely rare. Microscopic proteinuria and hematuria may persist for up to 6 months after the acute event while mild proteinuria can be seen for years. Treatment is generally supportive and includes salt restriction, diuretics for edema, and blood pressure control. If there is evidence of a remaining infection, antibiotics should be given. Family members and close contacts with an acute infection should receive antibiotics. There are anecdotal reports of pulse glucocorticoids being used for crescentic PSGN, but the benefits of this are not well studied.

PAUCI-IMMUNE GLOMERULONEPHRITIS: WEGENER'S GRANULOMATOSIS, CHURG-SRAUSS SYNDROME, AND MICROSCOPIC POLYANGIITIS

Pauci-immune GN is characterized by crescentic, necrotizing GN with minimal immune deposits by IF. Pauci-immune GN is a common feature of Wegener's granulomatosis (WG), Churg-Strauss syndrome (CSS), and microscopic polyangiitis (MPA). These three diseases are all systemic small-vessel vasculitides that are associated with antineutrophilic cytoplasmic antibodies (ANCAs).

Wegener's Granulomatosis

Epidemiology and Clinical Features
WG is characterized by necrotizing, granulomatous inflammation that typically involves the upper and lower respiratory tracts and the kidneys. Almost any other organ can be involved. The mean age of diagnosis is 55, but WG can occur at any age. Clinical features may include fever, malaise, weight loss, purpura, proptosis, facial nerve paralysis, hearing loss, septal perforation (saddle nose deformity), sinusitis, pulmonary hemorrhage, and rapidly progressing GN (RPGN). At least 80% of patients eventually have renal involvement, which typically presents with a nephritic urine sediment, variable degrees of proteinuria, and often a rapid decline in renal function. Plasma ANCA titers in some, but not all patients, may reflect disease activity.

Renal Pathology
Although ANCAs (typically c-ANCA directed against proteinase-3) are positive in up to 90% of WG patients with generalized disease, tissue biopsy of the suspected organ involved is considered mandatory to confirm the diagnosis, given the potential toxicity of treatment. On renal biopsy, a crescentic GN with fibrinoid necrosis and a lack of immunoglobulin staining by IF is seen. Only rarely are granulomas or actual vasculitis seen on renal biopsy.

Disease Course, Treatment, and Transplantation
Without treatment, the 1-year mortality rate of WG is 80%. The relapse rate is about 50% and typically occurs in the first year after immunosuppression is discontinued, but can occur later. Therefore, lifelong monitoring is critical.

    Induction treatment for most patients consists of cyclophosphamide, 1.5 to 2.0 mg/kg/day PO (adjusted for renal function), with prednisone 1 mg/kg/day (pulse methylprednisolone 250–1000 mg IV daily × 3 days prior to starting prednisone can be given in severe disease). Remission can be induced in about 90% of patients. Prednisone can be tapered after a couple months and discontinued after 6 to 9 months. Most clinicians treat with cyclophosphamide until remission is induced (usually between 3 and 6 months) before changing to maintenance therapy. Some patients with mild disease and normal or near-normal renal function can be considered for induction therapy with methotrexate (20–25 mg/kg/week maximum dose) and prednisone. For patients with life-threatening disease who are dialysis dependent at presentation, have pulmonary hemorrhage, or concomitant anti-GBM antibodies, plasma exchange should be considered.

Maintenance therapy consists of azathioprine (2 mg/kg PO daily) or methotrexate (20–25 mg/week maximum) if serum creatinine is <2.0 mg/dL. Some clinicians continue low-dose prednisone. The optimal duration of maintenance therapy is not known but is generally continued for 12 to 18 months. A longer course of oral cyclophosphamide (1.5 mg/kg/day PO) can be considered as maintenance therapy in some patients. The use of other treatments such as rituximab and MMF is being investigated but has not been studied in large numbers of patients to date.

Between 11% and 40% of WG patients develop ESRD. Poor prognostic indicators are an elevated creatinine or dialysis dependence at diagnosis. However, 20% to 70% who require dialysis at diagnosis may recover enough renal function to come off dialysis. If there is no improvement in renal function after 2 to 3 months of cytotoxic therapy, treatment should be guided by extrarenal involvement. Renal transplantation remains a good option in WG patients who have quiescent disease for at least 6 months prior to transplant. Disease occurs in the allograft in about 16% with a roughly 5% graft loss from WG.

Churg-Strauss Syndrome (CSS) and Microscopic Polyangiitis (MPA)

CSS is a small-vessel vasculitis like WG that is characterized by necrotizing granulomatous inflammation. In addition, patients with CSS have asthma and peripheral blood eosinophilia. About 40% have p-ANCA (against myeloperoxidase); 40% to 50% may not have detectable ANCAs. MPA is clinically similar to WG and is characterized by a positive p-ANCA in 50%–70% of patients. **MPA** is generally a diagnosis of exclusion in the presence of pauci-immune GN and systemic vasculitis and the absence of granulomas, eosinophilia, and asthma. Renal biopsy when the kidney is involved cannot distinguish between these diseases, except to exclude MPA if a granuloma is seen. MPA may have a less-relapsing course than WG. The treatment regimens for CSS and MPA are the same as for WG.

ANTIGLOMERULAR BASEMENT MEMBRANE ANTIBODY DISEASE

Epidemiology and Clinical Features

Antiglomerular basement membrane (anti-GBM) antibody disease is characterized by necrotizing crescentic GN in association with antibodies against the noncollagenous 1 domain of the $\alpha 3$ chain of type IV collagen. Type IV collagen is also found in the alveoli, and about 70% of patients have pulmonary hemorrhage (Goodpasture disease). Incidence of disease peaks in both the third and sixth decades. Renal disease typically presents as RPGN with rapid decline in renal function, hematuria, and oliguria. Pulmonary disease presents with hemoptysis, cough, and dyspnea with alveolar infiltrates on chest x-ray. Lung involvement is more common in young men and is often seen in cigarette smokers. Other types of lung injury, such as cocaine use, may trigger the disease. Up to 30% of anti-GBM patients have a positive ANCA, typically p-ANCA and may have other features of a systemic vasculitis such as fever, malaise, or weight loss. Patients with a negative ANCA typically do not have systemic features. In X-linked Alport syndrome, the Goodpasture antigen is often not expressed or exposed, and after renal transplantation these individuals can develop de novo anti-GBM antibody disease.

Renal Pathology and Diagnosis

Renal biopsy is important for prognosis and to confirm the presumptive diagnosis obtained from serology testing. On light microscopy, diffuse crescentic GN with segmental glomerular necrosis, rare evidence of vasculitis, and interstitial infiltrates are seen. IF reveals the classic pattern of linear IgG and C3 staining (sometimes with IgA or IgM staining) along the GBM.

Natural History and Treatment

Untreated, anti-GBM antibody disease has a fulminant course, thus emphasizing the need for a high level of suspicion for this disease and early diagnosis and treatment. In those who require dialysis within 72 hours of presentation, renal survival is only 8% at 1 year. Conversely, the 1-year renal survival rate in those not requiring dialysis at presentation is 95% in those with a creatinine <5.7 mg/dL and 82% in those with a creatinine >5.7 mg/dL. Treatment includes daily plasma exchange for 14 days or until anti-GBM antibody titers have decreased (typically 4L exchange for 5% albumin, or fresh frozen plasma (FFP) if recent biopsy or pulmonary hemorrhage is present). Adverse effects of plasma exchange, including hypocalcemia, coagulopathy, metabolic alkalosis, and thrombocytopenia, must be closely monitored. Cyclophosphamide (2 mg/kg/day PO for 3 months) and prednisone (1 mg/kg/day PO, with taper to 20 mg/day by 6 weeks and slow taper to off by 6 months) are recommended. Patients who do not have pulmonary disease and are dialysis dependent at diagnosis, particularly those with crescents in all glomeruli, have a very poor renal prognosis and may not benefit from aggressive immunosuppression.

THROMBOTIC MICROANGIOPATHIES: THROMBOTIC THROMBOCYTOPENIA PURPURA–HEMOLYTIC UREMIC SYNDROME

Thrombotic microangiopathies (TMAs) are pathologic processes of systemic platelet consumption and formation of intraluminal platelet thrombi, resulting in thrombocytopenia, microangiopathic hemolytic anemia, renal involvement, and other systemic manifestations. Causes of TMAs that can present with changes on renal biopsy identical to thrombotic thrombocytopenia purpura–hemolytic uremic syndrome (TTP-HUS) that are not discussed here include malignant hypertension, scleroderma, and the antiphospholipid antibody syndrome. Thus, differentiating the different types of TMAs is dependent on the clinical history.

Epidemiology and Clinical Features

Classic childhood Shiga toxin-mediated HUS, or diarrhea positive (D+) HUS, occurs most commonly in children in the summer and is preceded by an acute hemorrhagic diarrheal illness caused by certain *E. coli* strains (usually O157:H7) or other enteric infections (Shigella, Salmonella, Campylobacter, Yersinia). Transmission is from contaminated food (e.g., undercooked meat) or secondary person-to-person contact. The Shiga toxin triggers the microangiopathic process by entering the circulation via inflamed colonic tissue and causing endothelial damage and platelet activation. Clinical features of HUS include oligoanuric renal failure, pallor, and mental status changes (lethargy, confusion, coma, seizures) preceded by 1 week of diarrheal illness. Hypertension, purpuric rash, jaundice, and pancreatitis can be seen in some patients. Laboratory features include schistocytes on peripheral blood smear, elevated LDH, thrombocytopenia, elevated BUN and SCr, and normal PT and PTT.

Diarrhea negative (D–) HUS is less well understood and accounts for 5% to 12% of HUS cases. In some cases, D– HUS is familial and relapsing. Abnormalities in regulatory proteins of the alternative complement pathway (such as factor H, membrane cofactor protein, and Factor I) are seen in some cases.

The classic pentad of **TTP** (fever, CNS dysfunction, thrombocytopenia, microangiopathic anemia, and renal failure) is seen in only 40% of patients; and in the right clinical setting, thrombocytopenia with microangiopathic hemolytic anemia is sufficient to diagnose TTP. Unlike classic D+ HUS, TTP is not preceded by a diarrheal illness and is a disease generally of adults, disproportionately affecting African American women. In general, the renal involvement is less severe in TTP than in HUS and neurological manifestations often predominate. However, the distinction between D– HUS and TTP is often murky. In many cases, the pathogenesis of TTP is linked to inherited or acquired deficiencies of von Willebrand factor (vWF)–cleaving protease. Mutations in the ADAMTS13 gene, which encodes the vWF-cleaving protease, or inhibitory autoantibodies to vWF-cleaving protease result in abnormally large vWF, which promotes platelet activation and aggregation.

Oftentimes, TTP is idiopathic but it may be familial or related to pregnancy, collagen vascular diseases such as SLE, malignancy, infections (HIV, parvovirus), bone marrow transplantation, or medications. Oral contraceptives, ticlopidine (and less commonly clopidogrel), mitomycin C, gemcitabine and multiple other chemotherapeutics, calcineurin inhibitors, interferon-alpha, and quinine have all been associated with TTP.

Renal Pathology

Renal biopsy in TTP-HUS reveals fibrin and platelet thrombi in glomerular capillaries, arterioles, and arteries. Arterioles and arteries demonstrate muscular hypertrophy and intimal thickening causing luminal narrowing. Capillary wall double contours may be seen. Ischemic glomeruli may have wrinkled, partially collapsed capillaries. IF demonstrates diffuse fibrin staining in vascular walls, without immune complexes. On EM, widened subendothelial zones containing altered fibrin are seen.

Course and Treatment

In classic D+ HUS, treatment is supportive only and includes attention to fluid-electrolyte imbalances, bowel rest, and dialysis and RBC transfusions if needed. Plasma exchange is not beneficial. Antibiotics are not recommended if *E. coli* O157:H7 is the causative agent. Antimotility agents should be avoided. Up to 90% have a partial recovery, although up to 40% may have reduced GFR and residual proteinuria.

In adults with nondiarrheal-associated HUS-TTP, **plasma exchange** is life saving and should be initiated promptly, with seven consecutive daily treatments exchanging 1 to 1.5 times the patient's predicted plasma volume with FFP followed by alternate-day treatments as the condition improves. Twice-daily exchanges may be required initially. Plasma exchange likely acts both to deplete acquired protease inhibitors as well as to replace the deficient vWF-cleaving protease. However, the use of monitoring ADAMTS13 activity to guide plasma exchange remains unclear, and patients with normal ADAMTS13 activity who clinically have TTP appear to benefit from plasma exchange as much as those with low ADAMTS13 activity. Other therapies such as glucocorticoids, IV Ig infusions, and splenectomy have been used with variable efficacy.

Platelet transfusions are contraindicated except in cases of life-threatening bleeding as they may worsen symptoms.

AMYLOIDOSIS AND LIGHT CHAIN DEPOSITION DISEASE

Amyloidosis

Amyloidosis occurs when amyloid proteins deposit in various tissues where they assemble into characteristic fibrils. Amyloid fibrils are 7.5 to 10 nm wide and are randomly oriented and nonbranching. The filaments that make up the fibril each have a regular antiparallel beta-pleated sheet configuration. Amyloid deposits are tightly associated with glycosaminoglycans and the serum amyloid-P component. All amyloid fibrils stain with Congo red and demonstrate apple-green birefringence under polarized light.

There are multiple types of amyloid proteins. The most common kind of amyloidosis is **primary amyloid** (AL-amyloidosis), in which the deposits are from immunoglobulin light chains (or, rarely, heavy chains). Multiple myeloma or another lymphoproliferative disorder will be found in 20% of patients with AL-amyloidosis.

Clinical features include proteinuria, renal insufficiency, and monoclonal light chains detected by serum (SPEP) or urine protein electrophoresis (UPEP) (in up to 90%). Deposits in other organs can cause restrictive cardiomyopathy, hepatosplenomegaly, orthostatic hypotension, macroglossia, and GI motility, hemorrhage, or absorption problems.

Renal pathology in AL-amyloidosis demonstrates progressive nodular mesangial deposits that lack hypercellularity. IF may demonstrate light chains in the deposits but is sometimes negative. Characteristic fibrils as described above are seen on EM. Performance of Congo red staining should be requested if amyloidosis is suspected.

Treatment regimens for AL-amyloidosis, with or without myeloma, consists of melphalan and glucocorticoids. Selected patients may be candidates for high-dose melphalan and autologous stem cell transplantation.

In **secondary amyloidosis** (AA-amyloidosis), the deposits are from serum amyloid A (SAA) protein. This condition is associated with inflammatory conditions such as granulomatous or pyogenic infections (10%–20%), autoimmune diseases (70%), and inflammatory bowel disease (5%–10%). Eprodisate, which interferes with the interaction between amyloid fibrils and glycosaminoglycans, may have some benefit in slowing renal progression in AA-amyloidosis. Familial Mediterranean Fever, which is prevalent in Sephardic Jews, is an autosomal recessive cause of AA-amyloidosis. Colchicine (1 mg/day PO) is beneficial in treating this disease.

Light Chain Deposition Disease

Light chain deposition disease (LCDD) typically manifests as proteinuria with renal insufficiency and is not associated with Congo red staining on biopsy. In 50% to 60% of cases, LCDD is associated with a lymphoproliferative disorder, most commonly multiple myeloma. Unlike AL-amyloidosis, the light chain in LCDD is usually of the kappa subtype. Up to 30% of patients may have a negative UPEP and SPEP. Like amyloidosis, light chain infiltration of the heart and liver can occur. On renal pathology, nodular mesangial matrix expansion with hypercellularity is seen. By IF, monoclonal light chain staining is seen in the GBM, the mesangium, and along tubular basement membranes. No fibrillar structures are seen on EM. Treatment regimens have been based on melphalan and prednisone. Prognosis is better in patients with LCDD than in those with AL-amyloidosis. Four-year patient and renal survival rates are 52% and 40%, respectively. LCDD recurs in renal allografts in at least 80% of patients.

KEY POINTS TO REMEMBER

- Lupus nephritis may have diverse histopathologic features, but class IV disease (diffuse proliferative) as well as severe class III disease (severe focal proliferative nephritis) require immunosuppressive agents to induce and maintain remission, as these classes of nephritis have an aggressive course with rapid progression to ESRD.
- Poststreptococcal GN typically occurs 7 to 28 days after a pharyngeal or skin streptococcal infection. The disease is generally self-limiting and requires only supportive care.
- The pauci-immune GNs are characterized by an aggressive necrotizing crescentic GN with no immune deposits, and are associated with positive serum ANCAs. For severe renal disease, treatment consists of glucocorticoids and 3 to 6 months of induction cyclophosphamide followed by maintenance azathioprine or methotrexate for another 12 to 18 months.
- Early diagnosis and treatment are critical in anti-GBM antibody disease, as renal prognosis is poor in patients who present with dialysis dependence.
- Patients with HUS and TTP present with microangiopathic hemolytic anemia, thrombocytopenia, and variable degrees of neurologic and renal compromise. Plasma exchange is beneficial in TTP and should be initiated promptly.
- Renal amyloidosis and LCDD result from the accumulation of fibrils or monoclonal Ig components within the glomerulus. They are associated with plasma cell dyscrasias or other inflammatory conditions in a high percentage of cases.

REFERENCES AND SUGGESTED READINGS

Cameron JS. Lupus nephritis. In: Johnson RJ, Feehally J, eds. *Comprehensive Clinical Nephrology.* Edinburgh: Elsevier; 2003:357–372.

Contreras G, Pardo V, Leclercq B, et al. Sequential therapies for proliferative lupus nephritis. *N Engl J Med.* 2004;350(10):971–980.

de Lind van Wijngaarden RA, Hauer HA, Wolterbeek R, et al. Clinical and histologic determinants of renal outcome in ANCA-associated vasculitis: a prospective analysis of 100 patients with severe renal involvement. *J Am Soc Nephrol.* 2006;17:2264–2274.

Dember LM, Hawkins PN, Hazenberg BP, et al. Eprodisate for the treatment of renal disease in AA amyloidosis. *N Engl J Med.* 2007;356(23):2349–2360.

Dooley MA, Nachman PH. Kidney manifestations of systemic lupus erythematosus and rheumatoid arthritis. In: Greenberg A, ed. *Primer on Kidney Diseases.* Philadelphia: National Kidney Foundation; 2005:235–240.

George JN. Clinical practice. Thrombotic thrombocytopenic purpura. *N Engl J Med.* 2006;354(18):1927–1935.

Gertz MA, Lacy MQ, Dispenzieri A, et al. Transplantation for amyloidosis. *Curr Opin Oncol.* 2007;19(2):136–141.

Ginzler EM, Dooley MA, Aranow C, et al. Mycophenolate mofetil or intravenous cyclophosphamide for lupus nephritis. *N Engl J Med.* 2005;353(21):2219–2228.

Jayne D, Rasmussen N, Andrassy K, et al. A randomized trial of maintenance therapy for vasculitis associated with antineutrophil cytoplasmic autoantibodies. *N Engl J Med.* 2003; 349:36–44.

Laszik ZG, Silva G. Hemolytic uremic syndrome, thrombotic thrombocytopenic purpura, and other thrombotic microangiopathies. In: Jennette JC, Olson JL, Schwarz MM, et al., eds. *Heptinstall's Pathology of the Kidney.* Philadelphia: Lippincott Williams & Wilkins; 2007:701–764.

Levy JB, Turner AN, Rees AJ, et al. Long-term outcome of anti-glomerular basement membrane antibody disease treated with plasma exchange and immunosupression. *Ann Intern Med.* 2001;134:1033–1042.

Nadasdy T, Silva FG. Acute postinfectious glomerulonephritis and glomerulonephritis caused by persistent bacterial infection. In: Jennette JC, Olson JL, Schwarz MM, et al., eds. *Heptinstall's Pathology of the Kidney.* Philadelphia: Lippincott Williams & Wilkins; 2007:321–365.

Pozzi C, D'Amico M, Fogazzi GB, et al. Light chain deposition disease with renal involvement: clinical characteristics and prognostic factors. *Am J Kidney Dis.* 2003;42: 1154–1163.

Raff A, Hebert T, Pullman J, et al. Crescentic post-streptococcal glomerulonephritis with nephrotic syndrome in the adult: is aggressive therapy warranted? *Clin Nephrol.* 2005;63(5):375–380.

Rodriguez-Iturbe B, Batsford S. Pathogenesis of poststreptococcal glomerulonephritis a century after Clemens von Pirquet. *Kidney Int.* 2007;71(11):1094–1104.

Skinner M, Sanchorawala V, Seldin DC, et al. High-dose melphalan and autologous stem-cell transplantation in patients with AL amyloidosis: an 8-year study. *Ann Intern Med.* 2004;140:85–93.

Tan EM, Cohen AS, Fries JF, et al. The 1982 revised criteria for the classification of systemic lupus erythematosus. *Arthritis Rheum.* 1982:25:1271.

Weening JJ, D'Agati VD, Schwartz MM, et al. The classification of glomerulonephritis in systemic lupus erythematosus revisited. *J Am Soc Nephrol.* 2004;15(2):241–250.

Wegener's Granulomatosis Etanercept Trial (WGET) Research Group. Etanercept plus standard therapy for Wegener's granulomatosis. *N Engl J Med.* 2005;352:351–361.

White ES, Lynch JP. Pharmacological therapy for Wegener's granulomatosis. *Drugs.* 2006;66(9):1209–1228.

Diabetic Nephropathy

19

Steven Cheng

EPIDEMIOLOGY

Diabetic nephropathy is the most common cause of chronic kidney disease in the United States. According to data from the United States Renal Data System (USRDS), diabetic nephropathy accounted for 49% of patients reaching end-stage renal disease (ESRD) between the years 2000 to 2004. Although both type 1 and type 2 diabetes can result in progressive kidney disease, the majority of diabetic patients with ESRD have type 2 diabetes, likely reflecting the greater prevalence of this form of the disease. Diabetic nephropathy (DN) imparts a significant increase in both morbidity and mortality, and the diabetic dialysis patient has a mortality rate that is 50% higher than that of nondiabetic patients. Early detection and aggressive intervention is crucial for the optimal management of this population.

DEFINITION

DN is a clinical syndrome characterized by a progressive loss of kidney function resulting from diabetes. The development of *albuminuria* is a hallmark of this condition and is used to screen patients for DN. Although definitive evidence of diabetic kidney disease requires a kidney biopsy, clinical characteristics are usually sufficient to make the diagnosis.

CAUSES

Pathophysiology

Hyperglycemia plays a central role in the development of DN by mediating hemodynamic and structural changes in the kidney. The direct exposure to sustained high blood glucose concentrations results in glycosylation of mesangial proteins, leading to mesangial expansion and injury. Furthermore, the hyperglycemic milieu induces several overlapping biochemical pathways that are injurious to renal architecture. These include the generation of advanced-glycosylation end products (AGEs) and reactive oxygen species, the stimulation of transforming growth factor β (TGF β) and proinflammatory cytokines, and the decrease in mesangial PPAR γ. Hemodynamic changes also likely contribute to the progression of renal disease. Hyperfiltration at the glomerulus can be seen preceding the onset of microalbuminuria, reflecting impaired autoregulation and increasing glomerular pressures.

Histopathology

Many of these structural changes can be appreciated on renal biopsy. Glomerular hypertrophy can be seen early in DN, coinciding with mesangial expansion and thickening of the glomerular basement membrane. This typically progresses to a nodular pattern of glomerulosclerosis, known as *Kimmelstiel-Wilson nodules*. Although this is often considered the most pathognomonic lesion in DN, nodular glomerular lesions can also be seen in other conditions, such as light-chain nephropathy and amyloidosis.

Structural lesions outside of the glomerulus include changes in renal vasculature, tubular architecture, and the interstitium. Hyalinosis of both afferent and efferent arterioles can be seen, and may be particularly noticeable in patients with concurrent hypertension. Tubular changes include thickening of the tubular basement membrane and the Armanni-Ebstein lesion, a specific, albeit rarely appreciated, manifestation of tubular glycogen deposition and subsequent tubular vacuolization. Tubulointerstitial fibrosis can be featured prominently in patients with longstanding DN and is suggestive of irreversible chronicity of the disease process.

PRESENTATION

Natural History

The natural history and progression of kidney disease is likely similar in both types of diabetes. However, the early course of diabetic kidney disease is better studied in type 1 diabetes due to a more accurate correlation between the onset of disease and the time of diagnosis.

In type 1 diabetes, the first 5 years are typically characterized by normal laboratory values for serum creatinine, electrolytes, and urine protein levels. However, high glucose levels lead to glomerular hyperfiltration and the initiation of subtle histopathological changes. Microalbuminuria typically develops between 5 and 10 years from diagnosis. This is one of the earliest markers for diabetic kidney involvement and forms the cornerstone of the screening process for diabetic nephropathy. Fifteen to 20 years from the time of diagnosis of diabetes, albuminuria and hypertension develop, with a fairly steep decline to ESRD occurring after 20 years.

SCREENING

Screening for DN consists of regular evaluations for microalbuminuria. **Microalbuminuria** refers to a small quantity of albumin that can be detected in the urine during early DN. Normal individuals excrete <30 mg of albumin in the urine over a 24-hour period. Microalbuminuria is the excretion of between 30 and 300 mg of albumin in a 24-hour period, and albuminuria (sometimes called *macroalbuminuria*) is the excretion of >300 mg of albumin in a 24-hour period. Twenty-four hour collections can be cumbersome and are often difficult to interpret due to improper sampling and the logistical difficulties of saving urine through 24 hours. A ratio of albumin to creatinine excretion has sufficient correlation to 24-hour protein excretion and can be used instead. This study is often called a *spot microalbumin test* or a *microalbumin/creatinine ratio*. The ratio of albumin excreted per gram of creatinine correlates to the amount of albumin excreted in a 24-hour period (Table 19-1). As a result, microalbuminuria is defined as 30 to 300 mg of albumin per gram of creatinine, and albuminuria is defined as >300 mg of albumin per gram of creatinine.

Screening is conducted yearly in patients with type 2 diabetes, but can be deferred for the first 5 years in those with type 1 diabetes. Because screening for microalbuminuria requires the detection of minute elevations in urine albumin, a routine urinalysis should not be used for screening of DN. If a routine urine dipstick is negative for protein, a spot microalbumin screening test should still be checked, as microalbuminuria may not be detected by dipstick alone. If a routine urine dipstick is positive for protein, a spot microalbumin screening test remains necessary to quantify the extent of albumin excretion.

TABLE 19-1	CLASSIFICATION OF ALBUMINURIA	
	24-hour Collection (mg/24 hours)	Adjusted for U Cr (mg/g creatinine)
Normal	<30	<30
Microalbuminuria	30–300	30–300
Albuminuria	>300	>300

RISK FACTORS

Among modifiable risk factors, control of blood glucose levels is perhaps the most obvious and most important. A number of large studies, including the UKPDS trial and the Diabetes Control and Complications Trial, have shown that poor glycemic control is associated with an increased risk of developing microalbuminuria and other microvascular complications of diabetes, such as retinopathy and neuropathy. The risk is increased for all hemoglobin A1C levels above the nondiabetic range and greatest at levels >12%. Hypertension is also clearly associated with the development of nephropathy. A number of factors may contribute to the development of hypertension in these patients, including hyperinsulinemia, fluid retention, increased arterial stiffness, and the development of nephropathy. Blood pressure measurements consistently higher than the current goal of 130/80 mm Hg expose diabetic patients to an increased risk for the development or progression of DN. Obesity further increases this risk, although it is uncertain whether this effect is independent of diabetic and glycemic control.

Nonmodifiable risk factors are also well documented. Some have suggested that certain variations of the gene encoding the angiotensin-converting enzyme (ACE) are associated with the aggravation of proteinuria and overt nephropathy. A genetic predisposition is also supported by the fact that certain ethnicities are at greater risk for DN; particularly those of Mexican American, African American, and Pima Indian descent. Age, in conjunction with duration of diabetes, was associated with an increased risk of albuminuria in a study of type 2 diabetes from Australia. The correlation of age with renal disease progression is still unclear in type 1 diabetes, though those diagnosed prior to the age of 5 are typically at low risk for progression to ESRD.

EVALUATION

Diabetic patients are frequently referred to the nephrology clinic with albuminuria or elevations in serum creatinine levels. A complete evaluation of such patients requires a detailed evaluation for the presence of DN risk factors, manifestations of extrarenal microvascular disease, and a thorough review of long-term patterns in biochemical markers such as hemoglobin A1C, serum creatinine, and urine albumin levels. The goal of this detailed investigation is twofold. First, it is necessary to establish whether the underlying renal condition is consistent with the pattern and progression of DN. Second, it is crucial to identify the presence of modifiable risk factors and to establish appropriate goals of therapy.

History

A detailed history should elicit the duration of diabetes, the level of glycemic control, and the presence of diagnoses suggesting other end-organ microvascular disease associated with diabetes. As mentioned previously, patients typically develop microalbuminuria 5 to

10 years after the onset of disease. The risk of DN is further increased in those with poor glycemic control. During each visit, patients should be asked about adherence to the diabetic diet and their current level of glycemic control. A written log of recorded blood sugars is often helpful in tracking overall trends and daily variations in glucose levels. A concurrent history of retinopathy or neuropathy often supports the diagnosis of DN. Persons with type 1 diabetes and nephropathy almost always manifest evidence of retinopathy and/or neuropathy. However, the association is less established in type 2 diabetes. Although the absence of retinopathy should not exclude consideration of DN in these patients, physicians should consider alternative diagnoses as well.

Physical Exam

Blood pressure recordings should be checked routinely at each office visit. Hypertension is a common co-morbidity among diabetic patients and plays an important role in both the development and progression of DN. The patient's volume status should also be carefully assessed, since an expansion of the body's interstitial fluid compartment, manifesting as edema, may reflect avid sodium retention in hypertension or a loss in oncotic pressure due to nephrotic-range urinary albumin excretion. Evidence of retinopathy and neuropathy may reflect concurrent microvascular disease and should be evaluated with a fundoscopic and neurologic exam.

Laboratory Analysis

Recent laboratory data should always be interpreted in the context of long-term trends and current clinical contexts. A single elevation in serum creatinine or urine albumin should be confirmed with repeat testing, especially if there are clues to suggest a transient rise in such markers (dehydration, febrile illnesses, urinary tract infections, and new medications). Diabetic nephropathy is confirmed by the persistence of albuminuria in two separate samples separated by 3 to 6 months. Because the changes in renal function with DN typically follow a gradual but progressive course over time, serum creatinine would initially be expected to rise slowly, and small subtle increments are often noted when lab trends over the preceding months and years are scrutinized. Sudden fluctuations in laboratory data warrant confirmation with repeat values and consideration of alternative diagnoses (see below).

DIFFERENTIAL DIAGNOSES

While the term *diabetic nephropathy* specifically refers to the glomerular disease caused by the mechanisms discussed above, there are other forms of kidney injury that can occur in the diabetic patient. Of the other glomerular diseases, membranous nephropathy is associated with diabetes, and can occur in long-standing diabetic patients between the ages of 40 and 60 years. Diabetic patients are also susceptible to the development of renal vascular disease, which may be unmasked with the initiation of an angiotensin antagonist, and obstructive nephropathy, which is a particular concern among the 40% of diabetic patients who develop autonomic neuropathy of the bladder. Diabetic patients are more prone to developing certain infectious sequelae as well, such as renal papillary necrosis or renal tuberculosis (TB). The former may present in individuals with frequent urinary tract infections (UTIs) who develop hematuria, pyuria, and mild kidney disease. A small degree of proteinuria is also common. Renal TB may also present with sterile pyuria, hematuria, and azotemia; the diagnosis is based on clinical suspicion and the growth of mycobacterial species in the urine.

In a diabetic patient who develops proteinuria or renal insufficiency, the following should raise suspicion of a diagnosis other than DN:

- Development of albuminuria <5 years from diabetic disease onset
- Acute kidney injury
- Active urine sediment
- Thrombosis associated with nephrotic syndrome
- Absence of retinopathy or neuropathy, particularly in type 1 diabetes

MANAGEMENT

Treatment

Modifiable risk factors of hyperglycemia and hypertension are the primary target of both preventive and treatment strategies. Weight loss and smoking cessation are also thought to mediate some protective benefit from DN. Optimal care includes the reduction of hemoglobin A1C to levels <7% and the reduction of blood pressure to levels <130/80.

Glycemic Control

Glycemic control remains the most important modifiable risk factor and should be pursued to a goal Hemoglobin A1C of <7%. Some guidelines now propose a stricter goal of Hgb A1C <6.5%. Studies have demonstrated that treatment with early and aggressive glycemic control results in a decreased incidence of microalbuminuria, as well as a decrease in the prevalence of hypertension. In type 1 diabetic patients, intensive insulin therapy has also been shown to reduce the rate of progression from microalbuminuria to overt albuminuria by 54%. However, once patients develop overt nephropathy and marked albuminuria, the evidence that strict glycemic control slows progressive renal dysfunction is controversial. Some suggest that a lack of apparent benefit may be due to the significant contribution of concurrent hypertensive disease. This clearly emphasizes the importance of preventive interventions and early, comprehensive treatment in the diabetic population.

Hypertension

The current K/DOQI and JNC VII treatment guidelines support a blood pressure target of ≤130/80 in patients with diabetes and patients with chronic kidney disease. In hypertensive diabetic patients without proteinuria, angiotensin inhibitors and thiazide diuretics are often prescribed as first-line agents. Many clinicians favor the initiation of a thiazide diuretic based on lower cost and the results of the ALLHAT trial, which showed that cardiovascular outcomes were better in hypertensive diabetic patients treated with a thiazide diuretic. On the other hand, inhibitors of the angiotensin system are known to decrease proteinuria and are the only agents associated with a significant reduction in the risk of developing microalbuminuria. Some speculate that further benefit is conferred through anti-inflammatory effects of angiotensin inhibition, and not merely through blood pressure control and the reduction of intraglomerular pressure by efferent vasodilation. In practice, the argument of which agent is to be preferred is somewhat attenuated by the fact that almost all such patients require two agents to reduce blood pressure to target goal, and that the combination of a diuretic with an ACE inhibitor or angiotensin receptor blocker (ARB) is usually necessary as well as optimally protective.

Once patients develop microalbuminuria, the control of hypertension becomes a crucial intervention to prevent progression of nephropathy and the incidence of additional diabetic complications. Data suggests that each 10-mm Hg reduction in systolic blood pressure is correlated with a 12% reduction in diabetic complications. Additionally, a more aggressive goal of 125/75 may be more beneficial in slowing the progression of renal disease in patients with >1 gram of proteinuria per day. In the context of increased urinary albumin excretion, angiotensin-inhibiting agents become a clear first choice among antihypertensive drugs based on their ability to reduce both blood pressure and albuminuria.

Albuminuria

Albuminuria is often used as a surrogate marker for the extent of renal involvement, but there is expanding evidence to suggest that it is an independent risk factor associated with further disease progression. Furthermore, the reduction of albuminuria with ACE inhibitors and ARBs has become an important target of therapy. Studies suggest that a reduction in albuminuria may confer improvements in both renal and cardiovascular outcomes. In trials using ACE inhibitors and ARBs in diabetic patients with proteinuria, the reduction of proteinuria was associated with a decreased risk of progression to ESRD as well as improved outcomes in DN. This beneficial effect is independent of blood pressure reduction, and has been demonstrated in trials comparing angiotensin-inhibiting agents to other antihypertensive medications titrated to equivalent blood pressure control.

The question of whether ACE inhibitors and ARBs are equivalent has not yet been fully answered, though in clinical practice they are frequently used interchangeably. One comparison of ACE inhibitors and ARBs in type 2 diabetic patients showed no significant differences in the primary endpoint (decline in glomerular filtration rate) or secondary endpoints (blood pressure control, albuminuria, serum creatinine, ESRD, cardiovascular endpoints, and death). Another area of controversy involves the combination of ACE inhibitors and ARBs for maximal reduction of proteinuria. This combination has been shown to be beneficial in proteinuric nondiabetic patients, and while this data is commonly extended to the diabetic population, long-term data to confirm the additional benefit specifically in the diabetic population is pending.

FOLLOW-UP

Patients with overt nephropathy should be followed regularly in the nephrology clinic. Achievement of glycemic goals, attainment of adequate blood pressure control, and maximal reduction of albuminuria should be checked at each visit. In those with progressive nephropathy, management of common complications of chronic kidney disease, including anemia and renal osteodystrophy, should be addressed as discussed elsewhere in this book.

COMPLICATIONS

Clinical complications that may result from DN or the treatment of DN include hypoglycemia, acute renal failure, hyperkalemia, and metabolic acidosis.

Hypoglycemia

Pharmacological agents should be dosed with careful consideration of diminished renal clearances in patients who develop DN. While glycemic control should be pursued by any means possible, the degree of renal insufficiency must be considered in the selection and titration of pharmacological agents. The clearance of the biguanide metformin is notably decreased in the setting of impaired renal function, predisposing patients with renal disease to lactic acidosis. Metformin is thus not recommended for patients with a creatinine clearance of <60 to 70 mL/minute. Sulfonylureas are also not recommended in patients with a clearance of <50 mL/minute due to the increased risk of severe hypoglycemia. Routine calculations of a patient's estimated renal function can be done using formulas described elsewhere in this book and may serve as a reminder to dose drugs appropriately in the clinical setting.

Acute Renal Failure

Acute renal failure is manifested by a sudden increase in creatinine which exceeds the predicted gradual decline of function seen with DN. Both pre- and postrenal etiologies should be kept in mind as diabetic patients are prone to both intravascular depletion and obstruction due to autonomic neuropathies. An elevation in creatinine is often encountered in patients initiating on an angiotensin-inhibiting agent. This usually reflects an expected physiological response to the change in glomerular filtration with efferent arterial vasodilation. However, a rise in creatinine of >30% should prompt the cessation of the ACE inhibitor or ARB until renal function returns to baseline. A slow retitration with gradual dose increments is warranted for most patients, given the known benefits of angiotensin inhibition in this population. An evaluation for unmasked renal artery stenosis may be appropriate as well.

Hyperkalemia

Hyperkalemia is another complication often associated with the institution of angiotensin-inhibiting agents in diabetic patients. Serum potassium levels <5.5 mEq/L can be managed medically. Dietary potassium restriction and the titration of diuretics, particularly loop diuretics, are usually sufficient to lower potassium levels and promote kaliuresis. For more severe cases of hyperkalemia, a decrease or cessation of dose may be necessary. After normalization of potassium levels and dietary education, a gradual retitration can be attempted.

Diabetic patients with chronic kidney disease may also develop a type 4 renal tubular acidosis which may manifest as hyperkalemia with a nonanion gap metabolic acidosis. The hyperkalemia, which results from hyporeninemic hypoaldosteronism, impairs the generation of ammonia necessary for sufficient acid excretion, resulting in a metabolic acidosis. Although type 4 renal tubular acidosis can be managed with mineralcorticoid replacement, the potential for exacerbation of fluid retention or hypertension often limits clinical application. The institution of dietary potassium restriction and the stimulation of potassium excretion with diuretics can be used to control the hyperkalemia and restore normal ammoniagenesis.

KEY POINTS TO REMEMBER

- Patients with diabetes should be screened for DN regularly at yearly intervals.
- The prevention of microalbuminuria by treatment of modifiable risk factors should be pursued aggressively.
- Progression to diabetic nephropathy is associated with an increase in morbidity and mortality.
- Hemoglobin A1C levels of <7% should be targeted. Agents used to lower blood sugars should be dosed with consideration of renal function.
- Blood pressure should be kept to a target of ≤130/80 mm Hg.
- The institution of an ACE inhibitor or ARB is desirable for both blood pressure control and reduction of Albuminuria.

REFERENCES AND SUGGESTED READINGS

Adler AI, Stevens RJ, Manley SE, et al. Development and progression of nephropathy in type 2 diabetes: the United Kingdom Prospective Diabetes Study (UKPDS). *Kidney Int.* 2003;63(1):225–232.

ALLHAT Officers and Coordinators for the ALLHAT Collaborative Research Group. The Antihypertensive and Lipid-Lowering Treatment to Prevent Heart Attack Trial. Major outcomes in high-risk hypertensive patients randomized to angiotensin-converting enzyme inhibitor or calcium channel blocker vs diuretic: ALLHAT. *JAMA.* 2002;288:2981.

Barnett AH, Bain SC, Bouter P, et al. Angiotensin-receptor blockade versus converting-enzyme inhibition in type 2 diabetes and nephropathy. *N Engl J Med.* 2004;351: 1952–1961.

Brenner BM, Cooper ME, de Zeeuw D, et al. Effects of Losartan on renal and cardiovascular outcomes in patients with type 2 diabetes and nephropathy. *N Engl J Med.* 2001;345:861.

Chavers BM, Mauer SM, Ramsay RC, et al. Relationship between retinal and glomerular lesions in IDDM patients. *Diabetes.* 1994;43:441.

Chobanian AV, Bakris GL, Black HR, et al. The seventh report of the joint national committee on prevention, detection, evaluation, and treatment of high blood pressure: the JNC 7 report. *JAMA.* 2003;289:2560.

Dahl-Jorgensen K, Bjoro T, Kierulf P, et al. Long-term glycemic control and kidney function in insulin-dependent diabetes mellitus. *Kidney Int.* 1992;41(4):920–923.

De Zeeuw D, Remuzzi G, Parving HH, et al. Proteinuria, a target for renoprotection in patients with type 2 diabetic nephropathy: lessons from RENAAL. *Kidney Int.* 2004;65(6):2309–2320.

Fioretto P, Steffes MW, Brown DM, et al. An overview of renal pathology in insulin-dependent diabetes mellitus in relationship to altered glomerular hemodynamics. *Am J Kidney Dis.* 1992;20(6):549–558.

Fliser D, Wagner K, Loos A, et al. Chronic angiotensin II receptor blockade reduces intrarenal vascular resistance in patients with type 2 diabetes. *J Am Soc Nephrol.* 2005; 16(4):1135–1140.

Jeffers BW, Estacio RO, Raynolds MV, et al. Angiotensin-converting enzyme gene polymorphism in non-insulin dependent diabetes mellitus and its relationship with diabetic nephropathy. *Kidney Int.* 1997;52:473.

Klahr S, Levey AS, Beck GJ, et al. The effects of dietary protein restriction and blood-pressure control on the progression of chronic renal disease. *N Engl J Med.* 1994; 330(13):877–884.

Lewis EJ, Hunsicker LG, Bain RP, et al. The effect of angiotensin-converting-enzyme inhibition on diabetic nephropathy. The Collaborative Study Group. *N Engl J Med.* 1993;329:1456.

Lewis EJ, Hunsicker LG, Clarke WR, et al. Renoprotective effect of the angiotensin-receptor antagonist irbesartan in patients with nephropathy due to type 2 diabetes. *N Engl J Med.* 2001;345:851.

Makita Z, Radoff S, Rayfield EJ, et al. Advanced glycosylation end products in patients with diabetic nephropathy. *N Engl J Med.* 1991;325:836.

Nakao N, Yoshimura A, Morita H, et al. Combination treatment of angiotensin-II receptor blocker and angiotensin-converting enzyme inhibitor in non-diabetic renal disease (COOPERATE): a randomized controlled trial. *Lancet.* 2003;361(9364): 1230.

Nelson RG, Knowler WC, Pettitt DJ, et al. Diabetic kidney disease in Pima Indians. *Diabetes Care.* 1993;16(1):335–341.

Parving HH, Lehnert H, Brocher-Mortensen J, et al. The effect of irbesartan on the development of diabetic nephropathy in patients with type 2 diabetes. *N Engl J Med.* 2001;345:870.

Ritz E, Orth SR. Nephropathy in patients with type 2 diabetes mellitus. *N Engl J Med.* 1999;341(15):1127–1133.

Sharma K, Eltayeb B, McGowan TA, et al. Captopril-induced reduction of serum levels of transforming growth factor-beta 1 correlates with long-term renoprotection in insulin-dependent diabetic patients. *Am J Kidney Dis.* 1999;34:818.

Strippoli G, Craig M, Schena FP, et al. Antihypertensive agents for primary prevention of diabetic nephropathy. *J Am Soc Nephrol.* 2005;16:3081–3091.

The Diabetes Control and Complications Trial Research Group. The effect of intensive treatment of diabetes on the development and progression of long-term complications in insulin-dependent diabetes mellitus. *N Engl J Med.* 1993;329:977–986.

U.S. Renal Data System. *USRDS 2006 Annual Data Report.* Bethesda, MD: National Institutes of Health, National Institute of Diabetes and Digestive and Kidney Diseases; 2006.

Wolf G, Ziyadeh FN. Molecular mechanisms of diabetic renal hypertrophy. *Kidney Int.* 1999;56:393.

Renal Artery Stenosis and Renovascular Hypertension

20

Matthew C. Lambert

INTRODUCTION

Renovascular hypertension (RVHTN) is a common cause of secondary hypertension in adults. The structural finding of a narrowed renal artery alone defines renal artery stenosis (RAS). RVHTN is the resultant increase in blood pressure produced from decreased renal perfusion because of a stenotic lesion in the renal artery(s). Injury to the renal parenchyma can occur from decreased renal perfusion as well, resulting in a decrease in kidney function known as *ischemic nephropathy*. It is often thought that hypertension in a patient with RAS is caused by the stenotic lesion and the physiologic response of the kidney. However, it is likely to be a more complex process. RAS can be found incidentally in patients without hypertension and with normal renal function. Moreover, fixing the lesion may or may not improve blood pressure control or improve renal function. Thus, the diagnosis and management of renal artery disease and hypertension requires experience, use of clinical and prognostic factors, and a good understanding of interventions and outcomes.

CAUSES OF RENAL ARTERY STENOSIS

Atherosclerotic renal vascular disease (ASRVD) is the most common cause of renal artery stenosis (80% of cases). **Fibromuscular dysplasia** (FMD) is the second most common cause of renal artery stenosis (~20%). **Other causes of renal artery stenosis** include vasculitis (i.e., polyarteritis nodosa, Takayasu arteritis), aortic or arterial aneurysm (including dissection), embolic disease, trauma, radiation, or mass effect.

Epidemiology

Atherosclerosis

The prevalence of RAS in the general population is unclear as most data is from autopsy series or patients undergoing angiography for evaluation of other atherosclerotic disease (e.g., cardiac catheterization or lower extremity angiography). In addition, methods and criteria for defining a significant stenosis vary. Furthermore, the prevalence of RAS does not equal the prevalence of RVHTN because a causal relationship is not always clear. A large autopsy study found RAS in 4.3% of examinations. If a history of type 2 diabetes was found, 8.3% had RAS. A combined history of type 2 diabetes and hypertension was associated with a 10% risk of RAS. Population-based studies using Doppler techniques in persons older than 65 years found RAS in 6.8% (males, 9.1%; females, 5.5%). RAS was unilateral in 88% of cases and bilateral in 12%. Medicare claims from 1999 to 2001 showed an incidence of newly diagnosed ASRVD of 3.7 per 1000 patient years. Follow-up of this group for another 2 years showed that cardiovascular events from atherosclerotic heart disease in the incident ASRVD patients were higher than in the general population (304 vs.

73 per 1000 patient years). It stands to reason that patients with atherosclerotic disease of other vascular beds would be more likely to have ASRVD. For instance, RAS of >50% can be found incidentally in up to 20% of patients undergoing coronary angiography. A finding of RAS of >75% in this setting is an independent predictor of all-cause mortality. In patients undergoing angiography for atherosclerotic disease in the aorta or legs, RAS of >50% can be found up to 50% of the time. **Ischemic nephropathy** is defined as the diminution of renal function due to low blood flow caused by an obstructive lesion in the renal artery. According to the U.S. Renal Data System (USRDS) report from 2000 to 2004, the incidence of ESRD from RAS was 1.8%. Other studies suggest that ischemic nephropathy may be the cause of ESRD in up to 11% to 15% of cases. As the elderly population in the United States is steadily increasing, it is also expected that the incidence of RAS will rise.

Fibromuscular Dysplasia
Fibromuscular dysplasia (FMD) is most common in women with onset of hypertension who are younger than 30 years of age or in women under 50 with refractory or suddenly worsening hypertension. The most common form of FMD is medial fibroplasias and presence with the classic "string of beads" appearance on angiogram. Other arteries may also be affected in this disease.

Pathophysiology
In 1934, Goldblatt experimentally produced hypertension in dogs by clamping their renal arteries demonstrating that decreasing perfusion to the kidney(s) could cause systemic hypertension. For a lesion to cause significant hemodynamic impairment of blood flow through the renal artery, it must occlude the luminal diameter of the artery by 75% to 80%. When this critical level of stenosis is reached, numerous mechanisms are activated in an attempt to restore renal perfusion. Fundamental to this process is the production of renin in the juxtaglomerular apparatus, which then activates the renin angiotensin aldosterone system (RAAS). Subsequently, systemic arterial pressure increases until renal perfusion is restored or improved. By experimentally blocking the RAAS, medically or by genetic knockout animal models for the angiotensin II 1A receptor, this rise in systemic arterial pressure can be prevented. Other mechanisms may play a larger role in the long-term elevation of blood pressure such as chronic activation of the sympathetic nervous system, activation of oxidative stress pathways, impaired nitric oxide production, endothelin production, and hypertensive nephrosclerosis.

Maintenance of Hypertension
Mechanisms of continued RVHTN depend on whether the RAS affects one or both kidneys. The terminology that has evolved from experimental animal models illustrate pathophysiologic concepts in human disease. The 1-clip 2-kidney (1C2K) model represents unilateral RAS in a patient with two functioning kidneys. Central to this concept is that the kidney contralateral to the stenosis is normal and experiences increased perfusion pressure. This kidney adapts to the increased arterial pressure with local suppression of the RAAS and excretion of excess sodium and water. Because of normalization of volume status, poor perfusion to the stenotic kidney is maintained and persistent activation of the RAAS in this kidney occurs. This model is known as *angiotensin II–dependent* RVHTN. The 1-clip 1-kidney (1C1K) model means that the entire renal mass is distal to a hemodynamically significant stenosis, whether this is bilateral RAS in a patient with two functioning kidneys or unilateral RAS in a patient with a single functioning kidney. In the 1C1K model, the entire renal mass is underperfused, leading to RAAS activation with sodium retention and volume expansion leading to increased renal perfusion pressure. Once this occurs, the RAAS is then suppressed and hypertension is thought to be more related to

TABLE 20-1 CLINICAL CHARACTERISTICS SUGGESTIVE OF RVHTN

Incident HTN <30 (FMD) or >50 years of age (ASRVD)
Negative family history for HTN
Worsening of previously controlled HTN
HTN refractory to multiple medications
Recurrent flash pulmonary edema
Unexplained heart failure
Evidence of end organ damage from malignant HTN
Abdominal bruit
Hypokalemia and metabolic alkalosis with HTN
Increase in serum creatinine after initiation of ACE inhibitor or angiotensin II
  receptor blocker
Renal asymmetry of >1.5 cm

persistent volume expansion. This scenario is known as *angiotensin-independent* or *volume-dependent* RVHTN.

CLINICAL MANIFESTATIONS

There are no clinical characteristics that absolutely differentiate RVHTN from other causes of hypertension. Features that may be of use include onset of moderate to severe hypertension early or late in life, short duration, and hypertension refractory to standard therapy. A list of characteristics that raise clinical suspicion are given in Table 20-1. In addition, improved and more aggressive medical treatments for hypertension make refractory hypertension less common. Early recognition of RVHTN is thought to be important, as success of revascularization appears to be inversely related to the duration of hypertension. Episodes of recurrent flash pulmonary edema with accelerated hypertension should raise the suspicion of RVHTN and are more commonly found in patients with bilateral disease. This is related to the pathophysiology of the 1C1K model and the resultant tendency toward volume overload and to left ventricular hypertrophy with diastolic dysfunction. One series showed that RVHTN was present in 30% of patients reporting to the emergency department with accelerated hypertension and severe hypertensive retinopathy (grade III/grade IV Keith-Wagner changes). A significant rise (at least 30%–40%) in serum creatinine after initiation of an ACE inhibitor or angiotensin II receptor blocker (ARB) suggests the presence of bilateral RAS or RAS in a patient with a single functioning kidney. Other characteristics associated with RVHTN include smoking, elevated cholesterol, increased body mass index, and progressive renal failure. Reports suggest that RVHTN may rarely be associated with nephrotic-range proteinuria. Patients may have polydipsia with hyponatremia secondary to the dipsogenic properties of angiotensin II and may have hypokalemia related to increased aldosterone activity.

DIAGNOSTIC TESTING

Before embarking on a diagnostic evaluation for renal artery disease, the clinician should consider whether further intervention will occur if disease is found. Renal artery disease is a relatively common unsuspected finding in certain high-risk groups as discussed above. Most experts only advocate looking for RAS if it is deemed that the patient would benefit

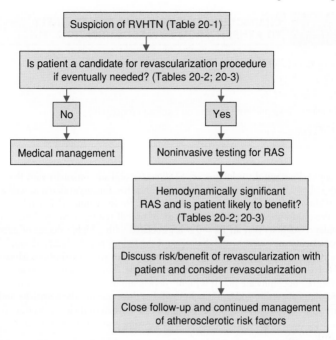

FIGURE 20-1. Approach to treatment.

from revascularization therapy. Factors such as co-morbid conditions, age, and risk of intervention should be considered in the decision process. Given that functional tests measuring renin activity in the blood lack statistical power for diagnosis, radiographic imaging of the renal vasculature has become the primary approach to RAS diagnosis. The test chosen depends on institutional expertise but less-invasive tests are generally preferred initially.

Renal Ultrasound with Doppler

Blood flow velocities in the renal arteries and aorta are measured using ultrasound with Doppler examination for RAS. Higher velocities indicate a narrowed luminal diameter. Doppler ultrasound is widely available, relatively inexpensive, and extends little if any risk

TABLE 20-2	CHARACTERISTICS OF PATIENTS LIKELY TO BENEFIT FROM REVASCULARIZATION

Recent onset or accelerated HTN
Recent onset or progressive renal failure
Bilateral disease or stenosis in a single functioning kidney
Recurrent flash pulmonary edema

Possibly

Resistive index <0.8
Physiologically significant stenosis on captopril renogram

TABLE 20-3	CHARACTERISTICS OF PATIENTS NOT LIKELY TO BENEFIT FROM REVASCULARIZATION

Pre-existing longstanding HTN (>3 yr)

Kidney size <8 cm

Resistive index >0.8

Physiologically insignificant stenosis on captopril renogram

Advanced age

to the patient. Peak systolic velocities of >180 cm/second are consistent with RAS. Ultrasound also allows for assessment of kidney size, and therefore asymmetry, as well as other structural abnormalities such as cysts or obstruction. Resistive index (RI) can be measured by Doppler ultrasonography and is a measure of overall resistance to renal arterial blood flow. Evidence suggests that an RI >0.8 is associated with a higher degree of irreversible intrarenal vascular or parenchymal disease, and the kidney may be less functional. Therefore, the RI may be helpful in predicting the response to revascularization. More studies are needed to further determine its predictive value, however. *Disadvantages* of renal Doppler ultrasonography are that it is highly dependant on patient body habitus, operator skill, interpreter expertise, and equipment used. For these reasons, the sensitivity and specificity vary in the literature, but can be as high as 98% when proficiency is great. Technology and expertise with Doppler ultrasound is growing and it is now often utilized as an initial test for RAS.

Spiral CT Scan and CT Angiography

CT scanning with CT angiography is a highly sensitive and specific, noninvasive tool for the diagnosis of RAS. However, this requires that iodinated contrast be given to a patient who is likely at increased risk for contrast-induced nephropathy.

Magnetic Resonance Angiography (MRA)

MRA is being increasingly used as the initial test for RAS. It is also highly sensitive and specific and is noninvasive. It is less operator dependent compared with Doppler ultrasound. Iodinated contrast is not required, as in CT angiography. On the other hand, gadolinium has been associated with nephrogenic systemic fibrosis (NSF) and should be avoided with more-advanced degrees of renal insufficiency. Because of issues related to maximum spatial resolution, MRA tends to slightly overestimate the severity of a stenotic lesion when compared with angiography. MRA is contraindicated in patients with pacemakers, cochlear implants, intracranial aneurysm clips, or other metallic implants.

Renal Angiography

The gold standard for the diagnosis of RAS is still angiography. Problems with this procedure include its invasiveness and risk of catheter-induced injury, such as cholesterol crystal embolization and arterial dissection. Patients are also at risk for contrast nephropathy, although digital imaging procedures and CO_2 contrast can minimize this complication. Angiography is now usually performed only at the time of a percutaneous intervention after another less-invasive test has made the diagnosis of RAS very likely. If noninvasive testing is inconclusive, angiography should be performed.

FUNCTIONAL TESTING

Knowledge of the pathophysiology of RVHTN can be used to help determine the physiologic significance of a stenotic lesion and possibly whether or not it is contributing to or causing RVHTN. These tests are most helpful in patients with unilateral disease and with normal renal function.

Captopril Plasma Renin Activity

Although increased renin production, measured as plasma renin activity (PRA), is fundamental to the initial rise in blood pressure, the chronic elevation of blood pressure in RVHTN is thought to be from other mechanisms (see Pathophysiology, above) and renin levels can fall within a few weeks. Renin levels are also highly dependent on other factors such as sodium intake, posture, age, race, gender, and medications. Consequently, the usefulness of PRA alone in the evaluation of RVHTN is extremely limited. On the other hand, the predictive value of PRA measurement can be increased by measuring it 1 hour after administration of 25 to 50 mg of captopril, a rapid-acting ACE inhibitor. This is called the *captopril PRA* or the *captopril stimulation test*. If RVHTN is being maintained by high angiotensin II levels, renin will be suppressed by normal negative feedback mechanisms. ACE inhibition will remove this suppression and renin production from the stenotic kidney should increase. A major limitation of this test is that antihypertensive medications including ACE inhibitors, ARBs, diuretics, and beta blockers must be held for up to 2 weeks prior to the test and this should not be done in patients with congestive heart failure, edema, cardiovascular instability, or significant renal dysfunction. Sensitivities and specificities in the literature, when done properly, have ranged from 75% to 100% and 60% to 95%, respectively.

Captopril Radionuclide Renogram

Radionuclide imaging of the kidneys can be helpful in evaluating the individual contribution of each kidney to the glomerular filtration rate (GFR). However, its use in diagnosing RAS has a false positive rate of up to 25%. When combined with the administration of captopril, similar to the captopril PRA, the predictive value can be improved. A rapid-acting intravenous ACE inhibitor, such as enalaprilat, is used at some institutions. In the kidney distal to a stenosis, GFR is maintained by the efferent arteriolar constrictive effects of angiotensin II. When angiotensin II is blocked by captopril, efferent arteriolar dilatation occurs and GFR in the stenotic kidney often decreases, usually with a corresponding increase in GFR in the nonstenotic kidney. When a radioactive isotope such as DTPA is given in this setting to measure GFR, the stenotic kidney will exhibit decreased uptake with a delayed peak time and a slower washout time compared with the nonstenotic kidney. ACE inhibitors or ARBs must be held prior to this test, but other antihypertensive agents can be continued and loop diuretics may even enhance the sensitivity. A positive captopril renogram indicates the presence of a physiologically significant stenosis that is likely causing RVHTN. Furthermore, there is evidence to suggest that it can predict a good blood pressure response after percutaneous transluminal renal angioplasty (PTRA) with a sensitivity of 90%. This test has a lower sensitivity in chronic kidney disease and is generally not used in this setting.

MANAGEMENT

Natural History

As with any disease, the approach to management must take into account the natural history of the disease. Recent prospective studies using Doppler ultrasound show that progression of ASRVD may not occur as frequently and rapidly as was once thought. Progression can occur in as many as 30% of higher-risk patients at 3 years, or as little as 4% in lower-risk patients followed out to 8 years. Progression of disease is related to the initial degree of stenosis. Progression to complete occlusion may develop in up to 3% to 7% of patients. Risk factors for progression are still poorly understood but appear to be similar to risk factors for general atherosclerotic disease. Complicating matters further, progression of a stenotic lesion may not translate clinically into worsening hypertension or renal function. In a group of patients with high-grade RAS (>70%) followed for just over 3 years, only 8% eventually required revascularization for refractory hypertension. In the entire group, antihypertensive medication requirement increased but blood pressure remained relatively unchanged and creatinine rose from 1.4 to 2 mg/dL. This increase in serum creatinine was more pronounced in patients with bilateral RAS. Mortality in this group was 30% and was primarily due to cardiovascular disease. As described above, the finding of a high-grade stenosis has been shown to be an independent predictor for all-cause mortality and patients with ASRVD have been shown to have a higher incidence of atherothrombotic cardiovascular events than the general population. It is possible that the long-term neuroendocrine defects caused by ASRVD could contribute to worsening cardiovascular disease. Therefore, endpoints of therapy should not only be targeted at blood pressure control and preservation of renal function, but should include reduction in cardiovascular events overall.

Indications for Intervention

Patients with newly diagnosed, accelerated hypertension and rapidly progressive kidney disease found to have RAS will most likely benefit from revascularization. Other indications for revascularization include recurrent episodes of congestive heart failure or flash pulmonary edema. The most common dilemma regarding intervention is the patient with ASRVD who has stable hypertension and stable renal function. Even though the presence of ASRVD portends a higher likelihood of a future cardiovascular event, intervening may or may not change that risk. This issue is currently under study, but evidence to date suggests that there is no advantage to revascularization over medical management alone. Present therapy available for RVHTN and ischemic nephropathy includes medical management, PTRA with or without stent placement, and surgical revascularization.

Medical Management

Aggressive medical therapy targeted at reducing atherosclerotic disease is recommended in all patients with ASRVD. This includes smoking cessation, control of dyslipidemia (usually with statins and LDL goal of <70 mg/dL), glycemic control, aspirin, and blood pressure control according to JNC 7 goals. Given the pathophysiology of RVHTN and their proven benefits on cardiovascular disease in general, ACE inhibitors and ARBs are the preferred first-line agents. It is rare for patients to experience a clinically significant drop in their GFR after initiation of these agents, but close monitoring of serum creatinine and optimization of volume status after initiation of these drugs is recommended. If GFR does decline, it is usually in a patient with bilateral disease or RAS in a single functioning kidney and revascularization should be considered. Refractory hypertension is generally defined as inadequate control with three medications, and in this case revascularization may be beneficial. Even after successful revascularization is performed, medical management is usually necessary and the ability to discontinue all antihypertensive drugs is rare.

Angioplasty and Stent Placement

PTRA is the preferred revascularization procedure in most institutions. Due to high rates of restenosis with balloon angioplasty alone, especially with ostial lesions, stent deployment has been increasingly utilized. This has improved technical success and is now the most widely used procedure for revascularization of RAS. Unfortunately, technical success does not guarantee "cure" of hypertension. In fact, three recent prospective randomized controlled trials comparing PTRA with medical therapy alone failed to show a blood pressure difference between the groups. Reported flaws in study design have questioned the validity of these conclusions. In other analyses, the literature has concluded that there is evidence to support trends toward improvement (not cure) in blood pressure control and renal function with angioplasty compared with medical therapy alone. Another problem is that prospective randomized controlled trials to date have only evaluated PTRA without stent placement. A prospective randomized controlled trial is underway that will evaluate PTRA with stent placement compared with medical therapy alone.

Risks of PTRA

Restenosis is estimated to occur in 15% to 20% of cases. Contrast nephropathy complicates the procedure up to 13% of the time but is self-limited. Conversely, acute and progressive deterioration in renal function has been reported to have an incidence of up to 20% in some series. Atheroembolic disease is thought to be responsible for a majority of these cases. Studies using distal filter devices after stent placement show that atheroembolic debris can be recovered almost all of the time and that by using these devices postprocedure renal function deterioration is less frequent. Other complications are renal artery dissection, renal artery thrombosis, and segmental renal infarction. Periprocedural death or cardiovascular events each occur with a reported incidence of up to 3%.

Surgery

Before the era of interventional radiology, surgery was the definitive treatment for RAS. Now, it is reserved for situations in which revascularization is necessary but cannot be achieved by the percutaneous route.

Treatment of Fibromuscular Dysplasia

The decision to perform revascularization with PTRA or surgery is less controversial with FMD than with atherosclerotic disease and is usually recommended. Intervention results in a cure or improvement of hypertension in 70% to 90% of patients.

KEY POINTS TO REMEMBER

- RAS does not equate to RVHTN because the stenosis may not be physiologically significant.
- Significant RAS appears to be an independent predictor for overall cardiovascular disease.
- Clinical presentation of RVHTN can be indistinguishable from other causes of hypertension and knowledge of clinical clues is important in suspecting the diagnosis.
- Evaluation for RAS should be based not only on clinical suspicion, but also on whether or not the patient is likely to tolerate and benefit from revascularization.
- Know your center's proficiency in the various methods for evaluating RAS and RVHTN.
- All patients require medical therapy. Some patients may benefit from revascularization, although this is not without risk and this decision must be made on an individualized basis.
- There is no conclusive data to suggest that revascularization of RAS has an advantage over medical therapy alone in stable patients.

REFERENCES AND SUGGESTED READINGS

Balk E, Raman G, Chung M, et al. Effectiveness of management strategies for renal artery stenosis: a systematic review. *Ann Intern Med.* 2006;145:901.

Caps MT, Perissinotto C, Zierler RE, et al. Prospective study of atherosclerotic disease progression in the renal artery. *Circulation.* 1998;98:2866.

Chabova V, Schirger A, Stanson AW, et al. Outcomes of atherosclerotic renal artery stenosis managed without revascularization. *Mayo Clin Proc.* 2000;75:437.

Chen, R, Novick, AC, Pohl, M. Reversible renin mediated massive proteinuria successfully treated by nephrectomy. *J Urology.* 1995;153:133–134.

Conlon PJ, Little MA, Pieper K, et al. Severity of renal vascular disease predicts mortality in patients undergoing coronary angiography. *Kidney Int.* 2001;60:1490–1497.

Cooper CJ, Murphy TP, Malsumoto A, et al. Stent revascularization for the prevention of cardiovascular and renal events among patients with renal artery stenosis and systolic hypertension: rationale and design of the CORAL trial. *Am Heart J.* 2006;152:59–66.

Davis BA, Crook JE, Vestal RE, et al. Prevalence of renovascular hypertension in patients with grade III or IV retinopathy. *N Engl J Med.* 1979;301:1273.

Erbsloh-Moller B, Dumas A, Roth D, et al. Furosemide-131I-hippuran renography after angiotensin-converting enzyme inhibition for the diagnosis of renovascular hypertension. *Am J Med.* 1991;90:23.

Hansen KJ, Edwards MS, Craven TE, et al. Prevalence of renovascular disease in the elderly: a population based study. *J Vasc Surg.* 2002;36:443–451.

Kalra PA, Guo H, Kausz AT, et al. Atherosclerotic renovascular disease in United States patients aged 67 years or older: risk factors, revascularization, and prognosis. *Kidney Int.* 2005;68:293–301.

Krijnen P, van Jaarsveld BC, Steyerberg EW, et al. A clinical prediction rule for renal artery stenosis. *Ann Intern Med.* 1998;129:705–711.

Mailloux LM, Mossey RT. Renal vascular disease causing end-stage renal disease, incidence, clinical correlates, and outcomes: a 20-year clinical experience. *Am J Kidney Dis.* 1994;24:622–629.

Mann SJ, Pickering TG. Detection of renovascular hypertension. State of the art: 1992. *Ann Intern Med.* 1992;117:845.

Maxwell MH. Cooperative study of renovascular hypertension: current status. *Kidney Int.* 1975;8[suppl]:S153.

Olin JW, Melia M, Young JR, et al. Prevalence of atherosclerotic RAS in patients with atherosclerosis elsewhere. *Am J Med.* 1990;88(1N):46N–51N.

Olin JW, Piedmonte MR, Young JR, et al. The utility of duplex ultrasound scanning of the renal arteries for diagnosing significant renal artery stenosis. *Ann Intern Med.* 1995;122:833.

Pearce JD, Craven BL, Craven TE, et al. Progression of atherosclerotic renovascular disease: a prospective population-based study. *J Vasc Surg.* 2006;44:955.

Pickering, TG, Devereux, RB, James, GD, et al. Recurrent pulmonary edema in hypertension due to bilateral renal artery stenosis: treatment by angioplasty or surgical revascularization. *Lancet.* 1988;2:551.

Plouin P-F, Chatellier G, Darne B, et al., for the Essai Multicentrique Medicaments vs. Angioplastie (EMMA) Study Group. Blood pressure outcome of angioplasty in atherosclerotic renal artery stenosis: a randomized trial. *Hypertension.* 1998;31:823.

Plouin P-F. Controversies in nephrology: stable patients with atherosclerotic renal artery stenosis should be treated first with medical management—pro. *Am J Kidney Dis.* 2003;42(5):851.

Radermacher J, Chavan A, Bleck J, et al. Use of Doppler ultrasonography to predict the outcome of therapy for renal-artery stenosis. *N Engl J Med.* 2001;344:410.

Rihal CS, Textor SC, Breen JF, et al. Incidental renal artery stenosis among a prospective cohort of hypertensive patients undergoing coronary angiography. *Mayo Clin Proc.* 2002;77:309–316.

Safian RD, Textor SC. Renal-artery stenosis. *N Engl J Med.* 2001;344:431–442.

Sawicki PT, Kaiser S, Heinemann L. Prevalence of renal artery stenosis in diabetes mellitus—an autopsy study. *J Intern Med.* 1991;229:489–492.

Slovut DP, Olin JW. Fibromuscular dysplasia. *N Engl J Med.* 2004;350:1862.

Textor SC. Controversies in nephrology: stable patients with atherosclerotic renal artery stenosis should be treated first with medical management—con. *Am J Kidney Dis.* 2003;42(5):858.

Textor SC. Renovascular hypertension update. *Curr Hypertens Rep.* 2006;8:521.

Van Jaarsveld BC, Krijnen P, Pieterman H, et al. The effect of balloon angioplasty on hypertension in atherosclerotic renal-artery stenosis. Dutch Renal Artery Stenosis Intervention Cooperative Study Group. *N Engl J Med.* 2000;342:1007.

Webster J, Marshall F, Abdalla M, et al. Randomised comparison of percutaneous angioplasty vs. continued medical therapy for hypertensive patients with atheromatous renal artery stenosis. Scottish and Newcastle Renal Artery Stenosis Collaborative Group. *J Hum Hypertens.* 1998;12:329.

Cystic Diseases of the Kidney

21

Michele Cabellon

R enal cystic diseases, particularly polycystic kidney diseases, are some of the most common afflictions to lead to end-stage renal disease. Many of these are inherited and are discovered in children. There are a few that may initially be encountered in adulthood, which will be addressed here. The term *polycystic* refers to the genetic renal diseases of autosomal dominant or autosomal recessive cystic disease, whereas *pluricystic* refers to multiple cysts in both inherited and noninherited syndromes with extrarenal manifestations. *Multicystic* defines mainly sporadic cystic disease. It is important to look at several aspects of the history when evaluating a patient with cystic disease. The age of the patient may help to distinguish the etiology of the cysts. Any family history of kidney disease may give clues to a possible genetic predisposition. The location of the cysts in the tubules or the glomeruli should be determined, if possible. Any other extrarenal manifestations that may be fit into a syndrome will also be important pieces of the puzzle.

AUTOSOMAL DOMINANT POLYCYSTIC KIDNEY DISEASE

Epidemiology

The pathologic definition of the term *polycystic* refers to the genetic renal diseases of autosomal dominant polycystic kidney disease and autosomal recessive disease of the child. Autosomal dominant polycystic kidney disease, or **ADPKD**, is one of the most common inheritable diseases in humans, and the third most common cause of end-stage renal disease after diabetes mellitus and hypertension. It is present in about 1 in 400 to 1000 live births and has no predilection for gender or race. In contrast, autosomal recessive disease is present in 1 in 10,000 to 40,000 births, is associated with congenital hepatic fibrosis, and usually presents in infancy or early childhood. The following discussion focuses on ADPKD, which generally manifests with chronic kidney disease in adulthood.

Etiology and Pathogenesis

ADPKD is a genetic disease caused by a mutation in either the PKD1 or PKD2 locus on chromosome 16 or chromosome 4, respectively. A small percentage of patients have no family history of the disease. These may be instances of a new spontaneous mutation in one of loci, which can then be passed on to future generations. Polycystin-1, encoded for by PKD1, is a large integral membrane protein localized in the renal tubular epithelia, as well as the hepatic bile and pancreatic ducts. It is believed to be involved in adhesive cell–cell and cell–matrix interactions, and may play a role in inducing cell cycle arrest. Polycystin-2 is a gene product of PKD2 and may be involved in cell calcium signaling. PKD1 and PKD2 also localize to primary cilia of renal tubular cells It is hypothesized that possibly lack of perceived fluid flow of diseased cilia leads to increased fluid secretion and cell growth, and ultimately cyst formation.

It is unclear why ADPKD has such a variable clinical course and expression of the disease. Patients with the PKD1 mutation (~85%) tend to form cysts and progress to end-stage renal disease earlier. Although the genetic mutation is present in all cells, cysts only develop in a very small percentage of tubules. There is some speculation that a "second-hit" somatic mutation to the remaining normal locus is required to initiate cyst formation.

Differential Diagnosis

The diagnosis of ADPKD is not difficult when there is a positive family history for the disease. When this is absent, the possibility of alternative renal cystic disease or a syndrome that includes renal cysts must be excluded. Glomerulocystic disease often presents in adulthood but does not usually have the extrarenal manifestations of ADPKD. Medullary cystic disease of the kidney may present with renal cysts but they are often a late manifestation and kidneys are normal to small in size. Acquired cystic disease occurs in advanced kidney disease, but the kidneys and cyst size should be small. Other genetic syndromes, including tuberous sclerosis and von-Hippel Lindau must also be excluded.

Mechanism and Physiology

In ADPKD, cysts form from any segment in the nephron or collecting ducts. This leads to innumerable, variably sized cysts that are evenly distributed in the cortex and the medulla. Initially the cysts communicate with the tubular lumen but eventually become disconnected to form independent cysts. Although these cysts are present in <5% to 10% of tubules, they encroach on normal renal parenchyma, leading to early interstitial fibrosis, vascular sclerosis, and loss of glomeruli. Eventually, these glomeruli are also lost as further injury occurs, leading to decline in kidney function and end-stage renal disease.

Several mechanisms appear to contribute to cyst formation and growth. The affected tubular epithelial cells demonstrate dedifferentiation with polarization defects and increased proliferation. In addition, increased cyclic adenosine monophosphate (cAMP) and abnormal activation of transcription factors and proto-oncogenes may also play a role. Blockade of vasopressin V2 receptors decreases intracellular cAMP and inhibits cyst development.

Clinical Features

Initial diagnosis is often made in patients with a known family history of ADPKD or by screening for onset of one of the symptoms. New cases of ADPKD are sometimes discovered when a renal ultrasound is obtained for an alternate reason, such as newly diagnosed hypertension or hematuria. Delayed diagnosis occurs because disease is often asymptomatic until late in the course. Less often, patients may complain of increased abdominal girth or flank pain, leading to some form of imaging.

The **history** should include an in-depth family history, including anyone who may have required dialysis or a renal transplant and the age that they reached end-stage renal disease. Family history of a brain aneurysm or sudden death of unknown etiology should also be obtained, in addition to a personal history of severe headaches or neurological symptoms. A history of gross hematuria, nephrolithiasis, or flank pain is important. Patients may complain of pain or early satiety from large renal or hepatic cysts.

The **physical exam** is often normal in the early stages of the disease. The first presenting sign of any problem is most frequently the new onset of hypertension. As the kidneys progressively enlarge, the cysts may be palpable on abdominal exam. Hepatic enlargement with detectable cysts may also be evident. Flank tenderness may be elicited. Cardiac auscultation may reveal associated valvular abnormalities. As kidney disease progresses, worsening hypertension and peripheral edema may manifest.

Renal Manifestations

Microscopic or Gross Hematuria

Hematuria is present in up to 50% of patients at some course in the disease. Often this is due to a ruptured cyst, but it also can be secondary to an infection or nephrolithiasis. If due to cyst hemorrhage, the hematuria usually resolves in several days but can last for 1 to 2 weeks. Persistent hematuria in patients >50 years should prompt evaluation for an underlying renal cell or bladder cancer.

Nephrolithiasis

ADPKD patients are at increased risk of renal stones. More than 50% of stones are composed of uric acid. A full metabolic stone workup should be performed to look for hypocitraturia, hypercalciuria, hyperuricosuria, and low urinary volume.

Hypertension

This is thought to be partially mediated by activation of the renin-angiotensin axis through local ischemia from external compression by enlarging cysts. The onset of hypertension is often early, when GFR remains preserved. These patients are generally afflicted with larger cyst burden.

Concentrating Defect

This is generally mild and often is not clinically evident. It can become important when patients are fluid-restricted or have suffered volume loss, such as postoperatively.

Extrarenal Manifestations

Liver Cysts

These can be present in up to 80% of patients with ADPKD, but in general do not result in liver disease. Abdominal discomfort and early satiety are the main symptoms. Cysts may also be present in the pancreas and spleen.

Cerebral Aneurysms

This is the most serious extrarenal manifestation of ADPKD. Patients with ADPKD have approximately a 5% increased incidence of cerebral aneurysms over the general population. If there is a family history of a cerebral aneurysm, the incidence increases to as high as 20%. Sixty-five to 75% of patients with aneurysms are at risk of rupture, and this usually occurs in younger patients with uncontrolled hypertension. It is recommended that asymptomatic patients at high risk or with special circumstances undergo screening for aneurysms (Table 21-1). The problem with screening all patients is the possible detection of small aneurysms, which are at low risk for rupture (<7 mm) and

TABLE 21-1	INDICATIONS FOR CEREBRAL ANEURYSM SCREENING IN ADPKD PATIENTS

1. Positive family history for cerebral aneurysm or sudden death of unknown etiology
2. Suggestive neurologic symptoms
3. History of prior aneurysm rupture
4. High-risk occupation in which loss of consciousness would put patient or others at risk
5. Need for surgery that might result in hemodynamic instability
6. Need for anticoagulation

at risk for complications following elective repair. Patients with larger aneurysms should be referred for repair, whereas smaller aneurysms can be followed annually. The tests of choice are magnetic resonance angiography (MRA) or computed tomography (CT) angiography.

Colonic Diverticulosis
This appears with increased frequency in ADPKD patients with end-stage renal disease. There seems to be a higher risk of colonic perforation compared with the general population.

Valvular Disease
Mitral valve prolapse is commonly detected in patients with ADPKD, as well as aortic, mitral, and tricuspid regurgitation. Most patients are asymptomatic, and often disease is only detected by echocardiography. Antibiotic prophylaxis for invasive procedures is recommended in these patients.

Abdominal Wall Hernias
ADPKD patients have an increased frequency of abdominal and inguinal hernias, which may worsen if treatment with peritoneal dialysis is pursued.

Diagnosis and Evaluation
The diagnosis of ADPKD is made using the combination of renal cysts present on radiologic imaging, family history, and the constellation of other extrarenal manifestations. **Ultrasound diagnostic criteria** for patients with the PKD 1 gene have been established (Table 21-2). These criteria only apply to patients who have the defect at the PKD-1 locus, as the PKD-2 mutation has a more benign course of disease with later onset of cysts. **CT** and **MR imaging** are capable of detecting smaller cysts, so the diagnosis of PKD may be made at an earlier age. No diagnostic criteria are widely accepted for these modalities as of yet. Commercial **genetic testing** for the PKD1 and PKD2 mutations using bidirectional DNA sequencing is available but is not widely used. Potential reasons to use the test include excluding the disease in a possible renal transplant donor, confirming PKD if the clinical diagnosis is difficult, distinguishing between PKD1 and PKD2 mutations to establish a more clear prognosis, or for family planning in patients who may be carriers of the disease but do not yet display clinical signs. **Routine screening of family members** of patients with PKD is not recommended if they are asymptomatic, especially with children. Early diagnosis may lead to emotional anguish and possible health insurance difficulties. It is prudent for relatives of patients with PKD to obtain regular blood pressure checks and urinalyses to look for early signs of the disease, and then to pursue further evaluation if indicated.

Initial evaluation in a patient newly diagnosed with PKD should include a urinalysis looking for hematuria and proteinuria. If a large amount of proteinuria is discovered, an alternate or secondary diagnosis should be pursued, as this is not a usual characteristic of

TABLE 21-2	ULTRASOUND CRITERIA FOR DIAGNOSIS OF ADPKD WITH PKD1 DEFECT
Age	**Number of Cysts Required**
<30	At least two cysts in one or both kidneys
30–59	At least two cysts in each kidney
≥60	At least four cysts in each kidney

TABLE 21-3	CLINICAL CHARACTERISTICS OF ACUTE PYELONEPHRITIS VERSUS INFECTED CYST	
	Pyelonephritis	Infected Cyst
Urine culture	Positive	May be negative
Onset	Acute	May be insidious
Flank pain	Diffuse	May be focal or diffuse
Urine sediment	WBC casts	Bland
Lower urinary tract symptoms	Dysuria/frequency	Usually none

PKD itself. Presenting serum creatinine should be documented. A baseline renal ultrasound should be considered to determine cyst number and size, as well as kidney size. This will be useful in the future to track cyst growth as well to localize any particularly large cysts.

Evaluation of acute flank pain in a PKD patient should be directed at either infectious or noninfectious causes. Findings of fever and leukocytosis are most suggestive of an infectious etiology although cyst rupture may transiently cause these symptoms as well. Noninfectious causes of the abrupt onset of flank pain may either be secondary to acute cyst hemorrhage or a renal stone. Urinalysis should be obtained to look for hematuria. Ruptured cysts may not communicate with the tubules and the urine may be negative for blood. A CT with stone protocol is useful for stones and hemorrhagic cysts. A urine culture is prudent to rule out occult infection. Acute cyst hemorrhage is managed conservatively with fluids and bed rest.

Infectious etiologies of flank pain include pyelonephritis and an infected cyst. These may be difficult to separate clinically, but specific clues may be used to determine the source (Table 21-3). A urinalysis with Gram stain and culture and blood cultures should be obtained prior to initiation of antibiotics.

Treatment

Current treatment for ADPKD patients should focus on strict blood pressure control and complications of chronic kidney disease as the disease progresses. ACE inhibitors or angiotensin receptor blockers should be considered as first-line antihypertensive agents. Cardiovascular risk factor modification is important as heart disease is a leading cause of mortality in these patients. Anemia is not often an early issue for these patients compared with patients with other etiologies of chronic kidney disease due to erythropoietin production by cells surrounding the cysts themselves. Caffeine intake should be avoided, as in vitro studies indicate it can promote cyst growth by increasing intracellular cAMP levels. The value of vasopressin V2 receptor antagonists is currently under investigation.

Large-volume surgical cyst reduction does not affect long-term outcome on renal function. This is likely due to the fact that renal dysfunction results from interstitial fibrosis and vascular sclerosis, which has already occurred at this point. Aspiration or sclerosis of specific problematic cysts can be pursued if clinically indicated.

Gram negative enteric organisms are most commonly the source of infection. Antibiotics must enter the cysts by diffusion, so a lipid-soluble drug should be chosen for initial empiric coverage. These include the fluoroquinolones, trimethoprim-sulfamethoxazole, and chloramphenicol. Antibiotics can be tailored once urine culture

TABLE 21-4	RISK FACTORS FOR EARLY PROGRESSION OF PKD

PKD1 mutation
Hypertension
Early diagnosis at young age
Episode of gross hematuria
Male gender
Increasing renal size and cyst size

information is available, or the original regimen can be continued if the patient is clinically improving and the urine culture is negative. Duration of therapy for infected cysts should be at least 4 weeks.

Prognosis

Several risk factors have been identified that predict a more rapid deterioration of renal function in ADPKD patients (Table 21-4). History of family members can also be useful to help predict a patient's time course. Patients with the PKD1 mutation have an average age of onset of end-stage renal disease in the mid-50s, as opposed to the mid-70s with the PKD2 mutation. In addition, there appears to be a correlation between the rate of kidney and cyst size enlargement with the rate of decline of GFR.

SIMPLE RENAL CYSTS

Introduction

Simple renal cysts are common in the general population and usually are present in healthy, nondiseased kidneys. They can be solitary or present in multiples. They also can be unilocular or multilocular. The major concern with isolated renal cysts is distinguishing them from a malignancy. They are lined with a single layer of flattened epithelial cells and are confined to the renal cortex. Simple cysts can range in size from <1 cm to ≥10 cm. The etiology of why cysts form is unclear.

Presentation

Like many of the other cystic diseases of the kidneys, simple renal cysts are most often found when imaging the kidneys for an alternate purpose. Approximately 5% of the general population undergoing abdominal ultrasound will have a simple cyst. The presence of cysts is dependent on age, with cysts being very rare in healthy children and young adults. Approximately 20% of 40-year-olds and 33% of 60-year-olds or greater will have a simple cyst on renal ultrasound.

Simple cysts are usually asymptomatic and do not affect renal function. There have been rare instances of association with abdominal pain, a palpable abdominal mass, hematuria or hemorrhage, cyst infection, or hypertension. Urinary obstruction can result if the cyst is large and near the renal pelvis.

Evaluation

Simple renal cysts are usually detected by ultrasound. The three **major ultrasound criteria** to distinguish a simple cyst from a malignancy or abscess are: (a) the renal mass is

TABLE 21-5	BOSNIAK RENAL CYST CLASSIFICATION SYSTEM
Category	Description
I	**Simple benign cyst** Hairline-thin wall Measures water density No enhancement No septa, calcifications, or solid components
II	**Benign cyst with additional features** Fine calcifications Few hairline-thin septa "Perceived" enhancement Mass <3 cm with high attenuation but no enhancement
IIF	**Cysts with minimally complicated features** Multiple hairline-thin septa or smooth thickening of wall or septa Calcifications may be thick and nodular No measurable enhancement Generally well marginated Lesions >3 cm with high attenuation
III	**"Indeterminate" cystic mass** Thickened irregular or smooth walls or septa with enhancement
IV	**Mass with high likelihood of malignancy** All criteria of category III Adjacent enhancing soft-tissue components

anechoic; (b) it has a round shape with smooth walls; and (c) there is sharp definition of posterior wall with a strong echo. If all these criteria are met, no further evaluation is indicated. The Bosniak classification system has been developed to characterize renal cystic masses by CT (Table 21-5). Categories I and II describe benign cysts that do not require additional radiologic follow-up, as the likelihood of malignancy is extremely low. Category IIF requires repeat imaging in order to confirm benign nature of the cyst. Categories III and IV almost always will necessitate surgical evaluation, as the probability of malignancy is high.

Management

Almost all simple cysts are asymptomatic and do not require further therapy. Pain from a large cyst is usually managed conservatively. If clinically warranted, cysts can be aspirated and sclerosed by either percutaneous or surgical route.

ACQUIRED CYSTIC KIDNEY DISEASE

Introduction

Acquired cystic kidney disease occurs in patients with advanced chronic kidney disease or end-stage renal disease. The incidence of cysts increases with increased time on dialysis, with up to 90% of patients affected after 10 years or more. Males tend to develop the disease earlier and with more severity than females. It is thought that chronic uremia and compensatory hypertrophy of remaining nephrons leads to cellular proliferation, tubular hyperplasia, and cyst formation. Grossly, they can range from just a few millimeters in size to several centimeters in diameter. They are almost always bilateral.

Differential Diagnosis

Acquired cystic disease must be distinguished from autosomal dominant polycystic kidney disease (ADPKD). With acquired disease, kidneys are small to normal in size with smooth contour. Patients will have obvious severe chronic kidney disease or will be on dialysis. ADPKD patients will have grossly enlarged kidneys with irregular borders and cysts of varying sizes throughout.

Presentation

Most often, acquired cystic disease is asymptomatic. Cysts are detected by imaging of the kidneys, and four or more cysts need to be present to make the diagnosis to differentiate from simple cysts. The risk of cyst hemorrhage is high, and these patients may present with flank pain or hematuria. Pain may arise from an enlarging cyst itself, although this is rare.

Management

Management of these lesions is conservative. Renal cell carcinoma occurs in up to 7% of patients with acquired cystic disease after 7 to 10 years. These cancers may be multiple and bilateral. A higher proportion has papillary carcinoma compared with the more common clear cell carcinomas seen in the general population.

Screening dialysis patients for renal cell carcinoma is controversial due to the high mortality rate from alternate causes in this population. Currently, screening is recommended for patients who are generally healthy with few comorbid conditions and who have been on dialysis for more than 5 years. Ultrasound is a lower cost, effective screening modality in most cases.

GLOMERULOCYSTIC DISEASE

Introduction

Glomerulocystic kidney disease consists of the cystic dilatation of Bowman's space and the adjacent proximal tubule. The remainder of the tubule is unaffected, unlike polycystic kidney disease, in which any portion of the tubule may be involved. Most cases are in children, although this finding is sometimes seen in adults. The condition is relatively rare, and there appears to be both sporadic cases and autosomal dominant transmission in some families. Cysts form by dilatation of Bowman's space around a primitive glomerulus. Most of the cysts are subcapsular in contrast to polycystic kidney disease, in which cysts are seen throughout the cortex and medulla. Glomerular cysts are small, with most being <1 cm in diameter.

Presentation

Glomerular cysts are often found incidentally with imaging the kidney during the evaluation of new-onset hypertension or other kidney disease. Patients are most often asymptomatic. The cysts may be present in other syndromes and diseases such as tuberous sclerosis and autosomal dominant polycystic kidney disease. Thus, it is important to look for other extrarenal manifestations suggestive of another process.

Evaluation

Glomerular cysts can be seen by ultrasound, but their small size can make them hard to characterize by this modality. MRI is more sensitive as it can detect smaller cysts and confirm the subcapsular distribution. If indicated, a renal biopsy could be done to confirm the diagnosis.

Management

There is no specific treatment for glomerulocystic disease. Prognosis is variable among cases, possibly due to the number of glomeruli that are affected by cysts in each patient.

MEDULLARY CYSTIC KIDNEY DISEASE

Introduction

Medullary cystic kidney disease (MCKD) and nephronophthisis are part of a complex of disorders that manifest cyst development at the corticomedullary junction and tubulointerstitial fibrosis that invariably leads to end-stage renal disease. *Nephronophthisis* is a childhood disease, with development of renal failure within the first three decades of life. *MCKD* usually is discovered in adulthood, reaching end-stage disease in the fourth to seventh decades. Both conditions are rare, with only approximately 50 new cases of MCKD reported per year in the United States. There is no predilection for race or gender with MCKD. The disease is likely underdiagnosed due to the nonspecific clinical presentation. Family history is the key to the diagnosis.

Pathophysiology

MCKD is autosomal dominantly inherited, and there are two genetic loci thought to be responsible for the disease—MCKD1 and MCKD2. Pathologically, there is tubular basement membrane disintegration with interstitial fibrosis and tubular atrophy, along with cyst formation in the distal tubules and medullary collecting tubules. Kidneys are normal to small in overall size. Cysts are small and arise late in the course of the disease. The presence of renal cysts is actually not a prerequisite for diagnosis of MCKD.

Presentation

Patients usually present in the fifth decade with an elevated serum creatinine of unclear etiology. Mild hypertension may be present and there is an association with hyperuricemia and gout. Family history of end-stage renal disease is important to elicit as a clue to diagnosis, as many of the manifestations are nonspecific. Extrarenal involvement is not present. Although a mild concentrating defect in the kidney may be present, polyuria is generally not seen, as opposed to nephronophthisis, in which this is common.

Evaluation

The urinary sediment is usually bland. MRI may be more sensitive for detection compared with ultrasound. Often a renal biopsy is indicated to confirm the diagnosis. Genetic testing is available for the MCKD2 mutation but not for MCKD1.

Management

There is no specific treatment for MCKD. Strict control of blood pressure and management of the complications of chronic kidney disease are the mainstays of therapy. End-stage renal disease usually occurs by the fifth decade.

MEDULLARY SPONGE KIDNEY

Introduction

Medullary sponge kidney (MSK) is a disorder involving diffuse ectatic or cystic dilatation of collecting ducts within the medullary pyramids of the kidney. The incidence is thought to be approximately 1 in 20,000 with no predilection for race or gender. It is thought to be underdiagnosed as it is not easily detectable by ultrasound and it is often asymptomatic. Up to 0.5% of patients undergoing IV urography for various reasons are found to have MSK.

Pathophysiology

The pathogenesis of MSK is unknown. Only the inner papillary portions of the medulla are affected with cystic dilatation. Most cysts communicate directly with the dilated collecting ducts, and they connect proximally with collecting tubules of normal diameter. Cysts are very small and range from 1 to 7 mm in size. Patients with MSK are at high risk for renal stones, and stones themselves as well as concretions may be located within the cysts. Medullary calcinosis may also be present. Congenital hemihypertrophy and Beckwith-Wiedemann syndrome are also associated with MSK.

Presentation

MSK alone is usually asymptomatic. Complications usually present by the second or third decade. Up to 20% of patients will experience gross **hematuria**. This may be an isolated event or in association with a renal stone or urinary tract infection. Isolated hematuria is not detrimental to renal function, unless it results in large blood clots that are at risk of obstructing the urinary tract. **Urinary tract infections** seem to be more frequent in MSK patients than in the general population. This is especially true in female patients who form stones. There is a special concern for urease-forming bacteria in this population due to the threat of staghorn calculi, so prompt urinary culture and treatment is prudent upon onset of possible urinary tract infection symptoms. **Nephrolithiasis** is the most common complication of MSK. The prevalence of MSK in all stone formers is up to 25% and the number of episodes of stone formation is higher. Urinary stasis in the ectatic collecting ducts leading to a high concentration of pooled solutes is a major risk factor. The majority of stone episodes are benign, but severe cases can lead to obstruction, pyelonephritis, and in worst cases, renal failure.

Diagnosis

The gold standard for making the diagnosis of MSK is IV excretory urography. Dilated collecting ducts appear as linear striations, causing a classic "paintbrushlike" effect. Ectatic areas are described as bouquets of flowers or bunches of grapes. Medullary calcinosis and stones are readily apparent. Ultrasound is not usually helpful for diagnosis due to inability to detect the small cysts. Use of CT for MSK is not defined.

Treatment

Treatment of MSK patients should focus on adequate fluid intake to avoid urinary stasis. For frequent stone formers, a search for modifiable risk factors should be done with a metabolic stone evaluation and stone analysis. Hematuria is usually benign, but urinary tract infection should be considered with each episode. Persistent hematuria in persons over 50 years of age should prompt evaluation for malignancy or other causes.

KEY POINTS TO REMEMBER

- It is important to look at clinical and family history, any extrarenal manifestations, and the location and size of cysts in the kidneys when evaluating a patient with renal cystic disease.
- ADPKD is one of the most common inheritable diseases and a frequent cause of end-stage renal disease.
- Simple renal cysts are very common in healthy patients without renal disease, and their frequency increases with age. The main consideration is distinguishing the lesion from a malignancy.

REFERENCES AND SUGGESTED READINGS

Belibi FA, et al. The effect of caffeine on renal epithelial cells from patients with autosomal dominant polycystic kidney disease. *J Am Soc Nephrol.* 2002;13:2723.

Bisceglia M, Galliani CA, Senger C, et al. Renal cystic diseases: a review. *Adv Anat Pathol.* 2006;13(1):26–56.

Bosniak MA, Israel GM. An update of the Bosniak renal cyst classification system. *Urology.* 2005;66:484.

Chapman AB, Guay-Woodrord LM, Grantham JJ, et al. Renal structure in early autosomal-dominant polycystic kidney disease (ADPKD):The Consortium for Radiologic Imaging Studies of Polycystic Kidney Disease (CRISP) cohort. *Kidney Int.* 2003;64:1035–1045.

Choyke PL. Acquired cystic kidney disease. *Eur Radiol.* 2000;10:1716.

Fick-Brosnahan GM, Ecder T, Schrier RW. Polycystic kidney disease. In: Schrier RW, ed. *Diseases of the Kidney and Urinary Tract.* Philadelphia: Lippincott Williams & Wilkins; 2001:547.

Gambaro G, Feltrin GP, Lupo A, et al. Medullary sponge kidney (Lenarduzzi-Cacchi-Ricci disease): A Padua Medical School discovery in the 1930s. *Kidney Int.* 2006;69:663–670.

Grantham JJ, Torres VE, Chapman AB, et al. Volume progression in polycystic kidney disease. *New Engl J Med.* 2006;354(20):2122.

Jennette JC, Olsen JL, Schwartz, MM, et al., eds. *Heptinstall's Pathology of the Kidney.* Philadelphia: Lippincott Williams & Wilkins; 2007.

Kiser RL, Wolf MTF, Martin JL, et al. Medullary cystic kidney disease type 1 in a large Native-American kindred. *Am J Kidney Dis.* 2004;44:611–617.

Liapis H, Winyard P. Cystic diseases and developmental kidney defects. In: Jennette JC, Olsen JL, Schwartz, MM, et al., eds. *Heptinstall's Pathology of the Kidney.* Philadelphia: Lippincott Williams & Wilkins; 2007:1257.

PKD Foundation. www.pkdcure.org.

Ravine D, Gibson RN. Evaluation of ultrasonographic diagnostic criteria for autosomal dominant polycystic kidney disease 1. *Lancet.* 1994;343:824.

Schrier RW, ed. *Diseases of the Kidney and Urinary Tract.* Philadelphia: Lippincott Williams & Wilkins; 2001:547.

Wang X, et al. Effectiveness of vasopressin V2 receptor antagonists OPC-31260 and OPC-41061 on polycystic kidney disease development in the PCK rat. *J Am Soc Nephrol.* 2005;16:846.

Renal Diseases in Pregnancy

22

Drew C. Heiple

INTRODUCTION

Pregnancy is associated with predictable anatomic and physiologic changes of the kidney. Hypertension and proteinuria are common medical complications of pregnancy and the presence of these findings must lead to consideration of preeclampsia or other conditions. Women with mild kidney disease have a somewhat higher risk of complications for the mother and fetus but are generally successful. More advanced kidney disease is associated with lower fertility rates and higher complication rates.

NORMAL RENAL CHANGES IN PREGNANCY

Anatomic Changes

Kidney size increases by 1.0 to 1.5 cm during pregnancy in response to increased renal blood flow and interstitial volume. Dilation of the ureters, renal pelvis, and renal calyces is attributed to the hormonal effects of progesterone during the gravid state as well as some degree of mechanical obstruction caused by the enlarging uterus. This physiologic hydronephrosis makes the diagnosis of pathologic obstruction difficult and is more often pronounced on the right side. The urinary collecting system can hold an additional 200 to 300 cc of urine, making 24-hour urine collections less accurate and predisposing to ascending infection of the urinary tract.

Physiologic and Hemodynamic Changes

Pregnancy is characterized by substantial changes in systemic and renal hemodynamics. Cardiac output increases 50% by the 24th week of pregnancy due to a 10% to 20% increase in heart rate and stroke volume. Plasma volume increases by around 1.25 liters; however, by the end of the first trimester, the **systolic blood pressure** often decreases by 10 mm Hg due to systemic vasodilatation. Renal plasma flow increases by 70% and the glomerular filtration rate (GFR) increases by 50% due to the increase in cardiac output and plasma volume combined with renal vasodilatation. **Creatinine** concentration subsequently falls from average nonpregnant levels of 0.7 to 0.8 mg/dL to 0.4 to 0.5 mg/dL. Increased GFR and increased metabolism of vasopressin in the gravid state cause increased urinary frequency. During pregnancy, total body water is 6 to 8 L higher than baseline and an additional 900 mmol of salt is retained. This increase in plasma volume is responsible for the "physiologic anemia of pregnancy." Women experience a 10-mOsm/kg drop in **plasma osmolality** to around 270 to 275 mOsm/kg due to a reset osmostat. This inappropriate ADH release leads to an average decline in **sodium** concentration by 5 mmol/L. Aldosterone levels increase significantly during pregnancy to help maintain blood pressure by facilitating salt retention in the face of systemic vasodilatation. Administration of

TABLE 22-1	EXPECTED LABORATORY VALUES IN PREGNANCY	
	Nonpregnant	Pregnant
Hematocrit (vol/dL)	41	33
Plasma creatinine (mg/dL)	0.7–0.8	0.4–0.5
Plasma osmolality (mOsm/kg)	285	275
Plasma sodium (mmol/L)	140	135
Arterial P CO_2 (mm Hg)	40	30
pH	7.40	7.44
Bicarbonate (mmol/L)	25	22
Uric acid (mg/dL)	4.0	3.2 early in pregnancy, increases to 4.2 in third trimester
Plasma protein (g/dL)	7.0	6.0

ACE/ARBs during pregnancy may disturb this balance and precipitate dangerous drops in blood pressure. Stimulation of the central respiratory receptors by progesterone causes a **mild respiratory alkalosis** (average partial pressure of CO_2 of 30 mm Hg) and compensatory decrement in serum bicarbonate concentration to an average of 20 to 22 mEq/L. **Protein excretion** is increased during pregnancy with pathologic proteinuria defined as a level of >300 mg of urine protein. Renal excretion of calcium, uric acid, and glucose increases during pregnancy but is not of pathologic significance. Table 22-1 summarizes the normal laboratory values during pregnancy.

HYPERTENSIVE DISORDERS OF PREGNANCY

Hypertension occurs in 8% to 10% of all pregnancies and is the most common medical condition found. Pregnancies complicated by hypertension have increased risk of placental abruption, preeclampsia, preterm delivery, intrauterine growth retardation, and second-trimester fetal death. The presence of hypertension during pregnancy is usually indicative of one of the following:

- *Chronic hypertension:* hypertension prior to pregnancy, diagnosed prior to the 20th week of gestation, or continuing longer than 12 weeks postpartum
- *Preeclampsia:* presence of hypertension and proteinuria after the 20th week of gestation
- *Gestational hypertension:* hypertension appearing after the 20th week without proteinuria
- *Preeclampsia superimposed on chronic hypertension:* usually with worsening hypertension and new onset proteinuria. This can be difficult to differentiate from chronic hypertension.

Chronic Hypertension in Pregnancy

The treatment goal for blood pressure in a pregnant female with uncomplicated hypertension is 130 to 150 mm Hg systolic and 80 to 100 mm Hg diastolic. Tight control of patients with hypertension does not improve outcomes and is associated with decreased

TABLE 22-2	DRUG OPTIONS FOR HYPERTENSION THERAPY IN PREECLAMPSIA/ECLAMPSIA
Subacute Antihypertensive Therapy	**Acute Antihypertensive Therapy**
Nifedipine; slow-release formulation: 30 mg/day PO; maximum dose, 120 mg/day	Labetalol: 20 mg IV; can be repeated at 15-minute intervals (with escalating doses, i.e., 40 mg, 60 mg, and so forth) to a total cumulative dose of 220 mg
Labetalol: 100 mg PO b.i.d.; maximum dose, 2400 mg/day	Hydralazine: 5 mg IV; can be repeated at 15-minute intervals to a maximum cumulative dose of 30 mg
Alpha-methyldopa: 250 mg PO b.i.d.–t.i.d.; usual dose, 1.0–1.5 g/day; maximum dose, 3 g/day	Diazoxide: 1–3 mg/kg (maximum, 150 mg in a single injection)

fetal growth. Treatment of severe hypertension (systolic >160 mm Hg or diastolic >105 mm Hg) is warranted to reduce the risk of cerebral hemorrhage. Subgroups of women with medical risk factors are likely to benefit from more aggressive blood pressure goal. This includes women with diabetes mellitus, hypercholesterolemia, renal dysfunction, congestive heart failure, history of stroke, maternal age >40, and history of perinatal loss. Early in pregnancy, these patients should have a screening urinalysis, urine culture, serum chemistries, and EKG. They should be assessed frequently for worsening hypertension, proteinuria, and intrauterine growth retardation.

Treatment of Severe Hypertension in Pregnancy

If intravenous therapy is required for severe hypertension, labetalol is often considered as first-line therapy (Table 22-2). Hydralazine may also be used but has a greater risk of causing maternal hypotension. Oral therapy is generally begun using the alpha/beta blocker, labetalol, or the alpha-2 agonist, methyldopa. Calcium channel blockers, such as long-acting nifedipine, are another option. Initiation of thiazide diuretics should be avoided during pregnancy due to the risk of volume depletion, but can be continued if used prior to pregnancy. **ACE inhibitors and angiotensin receptor blockers should not be used in pregnancy.**

PREECLAMPSIA

Preeclampsia complicates 3% to 5% of all pregnancies and is a leading cause of fetal and maternal morbidity and mortality. The most common characteristics include hypertension and proteinuria after the 20th week of pregnancy. If the syndrome progresses to seizures, the process is called **eclampsia.** Risk factors for preeclampsia are listed in Table 22-3.

Etiology of Preeclampsia

Although is poorly understood, preeclampsia is believed to be the result of abnormal placentation, leading to endothelial cell dysfunction. *Placentation* involves the invasion of the myometrium and spiral arteries by specialized cells called *cytotrophoblasts,* resulting in dilated, tortuous vessels and a shared maternal-fetal circulation. In preeclampsia, the

TABLE 22-3	RISK FACTORS FOR PREECLAMPSIA
Age ≥40	Multiple pregnancy
Nulliparity	Diabetes mellitus
History of preeclampsia	Preexisting hypertension
Family history of preeclampsia	Renal disease
Time between pregnancy >10 years	Connective tissue disorder
Obesity	Thrombophilia, esp. antiphospholipid
Molar pregnancy	

cytotrophoblastic invasion is incomplete, and the spiral arteries remain constricted, causing diminished uteroplacental perfusion. Endothelial cell dysfunction results in:

- Systemic vasoconstriction causing hypertension and end-organ underperfusion
- Increased vascular permeability resulting in proteinuria and pulmonary edema
- Activation of platelets and the coagulation cascade leading to coagulopathy
- The primary finding in the kidney is swollen, hypertrophied endothelial cells otherwise known as *glomerular capillary endotheliosis*.

Clinical Features

Although preeclampsia usually occurs after the 32nd week of pregnancy, it may present sooner in women with underlying hypertension or renal disease. Rarely, it may present during labor or in the immediate postpartum period. The initial symptoms of preeclampsia may be nonspecific. An increase in blood pressure, however, is often the first definitive harbinger of preeclampsia. It may begin to increase in the second trimester; however, values exceeding 140/90 mm Hg typically occur in the third trimester. As the disease progresses, many patients report a sudden weight gain and edema of the hands and face (Table 22-4). The GFR is expected to increase during pregnancy, but the vasoconstriction seen in preeclampsia causes a drop in creatinine clearance. The expected low uric acid level in pregnancy is often found to be elevated in preeclampsia. Proteinuria ranges from mild to the overtly nephrotic range. Liver dysfunction ranges from mild elevations in liver function tests to the development of fatty liver.

TABLE 22-4	FINDINGS IN PREECLAMPSIA

Neurologic: seizures, headache, scotoma, cerebral edema, cerebral hemorrhage, blurred vision, blindness, hyperreflexia, clonus
Renal: proteinuria (>300 mg), acute renal failure—often secondary to acute tubular necrosis, hyperuricemia, azotemia (average GFR decrease 30%–40%)
Hematologic: microangiopathic hemolytic anemia, thrombocytopenia, disseminated intravascular coagulation
Cardiovascular: hypertension, decreased cardiac output
Gastrointestinal: epigastric/right upper quad pain, elevated liver enzymes, capsular hemorrhage, liver rupture
Other: pulmonary edema, edema—often facial and lower extremity, petechiae, hyperuricemia

HELLP SYNDROME

Certain hematologic and hepatic abnormalities may occur with preeclampsia, and the constellation of these findings is referred to as the **HELLP syndrome:** *H*emolysis *E*levated *L*iver enzymes and *L*ow *P*latelets. HELLP is a devastating complication with significant mortality and morbidity. Preeclampsia may involve the nervous system as manifested by headaches, jitteriness, and increased deep-tendon reflexes. These findings may be followed by seizures, heralding eclampsia. Intracerebral hemorrhage may occur in severe cases and is the leading cause of maternal mortality in preeclampsia.

Management

Women with new onset hypertension and proteinuria after 20 weeks are generally considered to have preeclampsia. Women with *mild preeclampsia* should have close follow-up with scheduled laboratory and fetal well-being testing. They can often remain outpatients but should be admitted if they have neurological symptoms, renal failure, uncontrolled blood pressure, symptoms consistent with HELLP syndrome, or if the fetus is in danger. Management of women with *severe preeclampsia* includes immediate hospitalization. They are usually given corticosteroids to decrease the risk of respiratory distress syndrome in infants and seizure prophylaxis with magnesium sulfate. Women at >34 weeks' gestation with severe preeclampsia should be promptly delivered. Several studies have shown that expectant management of preterm preeclamptic pregnancies between weeks 25 and 34 are associated with improved perinatal survival, decreased neonatal ICU admissions, decreased neonatal complications and increased birth weight without differences in maternal survival. With severe and progressive manifestations of the syndrome, delivery of the fetus is the only recourse and is the definitive treatment of this disease. Some absolute indications for delivery include:

- Inability to control blood pressure despite adequate therapy
- Progressive organ system failure (kidney, liver, deranged hematologic parameters, neurologic dysfunction)
- Fetal distress

ACUTE RENAL FAILURE IN PREGNANCY

Acute renal failure during pregnancy, although uncommon, is challenging in both diagnosis and treatment. In early in pregnancy, acute renal failure is usually due to prerenal azotemia from hyperemesis gravidum or acute tubular necrosis from complications of septic abortion. In late pregnancy, the more likely causes of acute renal failure are thrombotic thrombocytopenic purpura and hemolytic uremic syndrome, acute fatty liver of pregnancy, renal cortical necrosis, and obstructive uropathy. Table 22-5 summarizes key diagnostic points differentiating several of these causes.

THROMBOTIC THROMBOCYTOPENIC PURPURA (TTP) AND HEMOLYTIC UREMIC SYNDROME (HUS)

TTP and HUS are thrombotic microangiopathies that can present with the features from the classic pentad of fever, anemia, thrombocytopenia, renal failure, and neurological symptoms. Fifteen percent of cases of TTP-HUS initially present during pregnancy or in the immediate postpartum period. These women present with azotemia, microangiopathic hemolytic anemia, and thrombocytopenia, which can be difficult to differentiate from severe preeclampsia and acute fatty liver of pregnancy.

TABLE 22-5	DISTINCTIONS BETWEEN CAUSES OF RENAL FAILURE IN PREGNANCY		
Differentiating Factors	TTP/HUS	Severe Preeclampsia	Acute Fatty Liver of Pregnancy
Time of onset	Anytime during pregnancy	After 20 weeks	Third trimester
Hepatic involvement	None	Seen with HELLP	Always
Prolongation of coagulation	None	Mild DIC can occur with abruptio placentae or liver failure	Common prolongation of PTT without DIC
Renal dysfunction	ARF common	ARF is rare even with severe preeclampsia, although some creatinine increase common	ARF occurs in 60% cases
ADAMTS-13	Severely reduced	Mild/moderate reduction	Mild/moderate reduction
Therapy	Plasmapheresis	Improves with delivery	Improves with delivery

ACUTE FATTY LIVER OF PREGNANCY

Acute fatty liver of pregnancy is a rare complication of pregnancy that is due to microvesicular fatty infiltration of hepatocytes. Patients often present with symptoms of anorexia, jaundice, nausea, and emesis. Hypotension is commonly seen. Laboratory values show elevated transaminase values with AST usually below 1000 as well as hypoglycemia, hypofibrinemia, and prolonged PTT. Acute renal failure is seen in 60% of cases. Roughly 50% of patients with acute fatty liver of pregnancy have preexisting preeclampsia, which may confuse the clinical picture. Making a correct diagnosis is critical in selecting the proper treatment.

RENAL CORTICAL NECROSIS

Renal cortical necrosis can cause acute renal failure in such conditions as abruptio placenta, amniotic fluid embolism, placenta previa, severe preeclampsia, and fetal demise with retained fetus. Disseminated intravascular coagulation and severe renal ischemia are initiating events. Patients typically present with flank pain, gross hematuria, oliguria/anuria, and hypotension. Cortical necrosis should be considered when renal recovery is prolonged. Ultrasound and CT scanning show a hypoechoic hypodense renal cortex. If needed, the diagnosis can be confirmed by renal biopsy or arteriogram. Prognosis is poor, although 20% to 40% of patients initially started on dialysis often recover enough to be dialysis independent.

OBSTRUCTIVE UROPATHY

Due to ureteral relaxation causing physiologic hydronephrosis of pregnancy, it is unusual to have an obstruction sufficient enough to cause renal failure. Keys to the diagnosis are the findings of more significant obstruction of the left kidney (because the right kidney is often more affected by physiologic hydronephrosis) and findings of oliguria or anuria. Obstructing large uterine fibroids or stones can be seen on ultrasound. Renal function may improve when the patient lies in the lateral recumbent position. No improvement with position changes may necessitate stent placement in the affected ureter.

PROTEINURIA IN PREGNANCY

During pregnancy, GFR and capillary permeability increase, resulting in mild proteinuria ($\sim$200 mg/day). If proteinuria exceeds this level, then three important possibilities are **worsening preexisting chronic renal disease**, **impending preeclampsia**, or **de novo renal disease** during pregnancy. The treatment of proteinuria in pregnancy depends on the cause and magnitude of the proteinuria. The most common renal diseases in pregnancy are those that most often occur in women of childbearing age, including FSGS, membranous, minimal change disease, IgA nephropathy, and congenital causes. Diagnosis is generally made from the first urinalysis or prior to the 20th week of gestation. Patients with lupus or other systemic disease with renal involvement will usually have other symptoms. Some diagnoses are not made until after pregnancy when the proteinuria fails to resolve. Proteinuria alone does not seem to affect pregnancy outcomes.

Treatment

Management of edema should consist of a low-salt diet and bed rest in the recumbent position. In intractable edema, judicious use of loop diuretics can achieve the aim of careful fluid loss. Kidney biopsy can be considered if there is sudden deterioration in kidney function without good explanation (especially with active urine sediment), when the diagnosis of severe preeclampsia is in doubt or with symptomatic nephrotic syndrome. Biopsy should not be attempted after 32 weeks of gestation.

NEPHROLITHIASIS IN PREGNANCY

The incidence of kidney stones in pregnant women is no different than in women in the nonpregnant state and the stones are usually calcium containing. In gravid women, the stones are more often ureteral, usually in the distal ureter. Clinical signs are flank pain, hematuria, and dysuria. Treatment is often supportive, as most stones pass spontaneously. Hydration and analgesics are helpful.

Although a majority of stones pass without complication, obstruction can cause hydronephrosis or pyonephrosis and may lead to renal failure. In such scenarios, invasive removal of the stone may be required. Lithotripsy is usually not an option during pregnancy. Cystoscopic or ureteroscopic removal of the stones may be attempted. The urinary system may need to be decompressed temporarily using percutaneous nephrostomy.

PREEXISTING CHRONIC KIDNEY DISEASE AND PREGNANCY

Chronic kidney disease was once thought to be incompatible with a successful pregnancy; outcomes now appear to be improving for both the mother and fetus. Pregnancy in women with worsening kidney disease is less common than in the general population due to increased rates of amenorrhea, anovulatory menstrual cycles, and decreased libido from hyperprolactinemia and disturbed hypothalamic-pituitary axis. Therefore, most pregnancies occur in women with only mild disease with GFR >50 mL/minute and creatinine <1.4 mg/dL. Fetal prognosis is not affected by the type of renal disease. The most significant causes of poor prognosis in pregnant women with renal disease are the presence of severe impairment of renal function, uncontrolled hypertension, and severe proteinuria.

Predictably, patients with mild renal insufficiency (creatinine <1.4 mg/dL) tend to do better than those with higher degrees of renal dysfunction. Most patients with mild renal insufficiency experience a slight decline in renal function that resolves postpartum. For patients with moderate (creatinine 1.4–2.5 mg/dL) or severe (creatinine >2.5 mg/dL) renal insufficiency, the deterioration of renal function can be much more significant. In moderate renal insufficiency, 2% to 33% will progress to end-stage renal disease. Patients with prepartum serum creatinine >2 mg/dL have the worst outcomes. Little data exist on women with severe renal insufficiency due to their relative inability to conceive. A recent study shows that women with GFR <40 mL/minute and proteinuria >1 g/day are at particular risk of pregnancy complications and renal deterioration.

Both mother and child experience the consequences of renal disease. **Maternal complications** include chronic hypertension, increased risk of preeclampsia, and permanently diminished renal function and increased proteinuria. **Fetal complications** include premature delivery, growth restriction, and an overall increase in mortality. Patients with moderate to severe kidney disease have a much higher percent of premature births (52% with moderate dysfunction, 68% with severe dysfunction) and growth retardation (30% with moderate, 52% with severe) but still have a comparable live birth rate of 88% and 86% respectively versus 90% with mild disease. Women should be counseled that they have a good chance of a live birth, but risk high rates of complications that would endanger both mother and child. It may be beneficial to advise women with mild renal insufficiency who desire children to not delay pregnancy to a time when their renal function may become worse.

Management of women with chronic kidney disease should include:

- Good blood pressure control <130/80 mm Hg
- Early detection and treatment of bacteriuria
- Monthly monitoring of maternal renal function
- Close follow-up for detection of preeclampsia
- Frequent fetal surveillance including serial fetal growth ultrasounds and biophysical testing

SYSTEMIC LUPUS ERYTHEMATOSUS AND PREGNANCY

The ability of pregnancy to precipitate lupus flares remains controversial. Women with quiescent lupus for at least 6 months have the same relapse rate during pregnancy as those that are nonpregnant. The risk factors for worse outcomes include severe proteinuria, hypertension, and renal dysfunction and are similar to other types of renal disease. The presence of antiphospholipid antibody syndrome carries a high risk of abortion, severe hypertension, fetal growth restriction, and maternal thrombotic events. Pregnant women with lupus should be tested for antiphospholipid antibody and if positive should receive preventive therapy with aspirin. In women with a history of thrombosis, heparin should be added to aspirin for treatment. Children of pregnant mothers are at risk for neonatal lupus, which is the primary cause of neonatal heart block. These patients should be screened for SSA and SSB antibodies. Women who wish to conceive are encouraged to wait 6 months from their last flare before attempting to conceive. They can be continued on maintenance therapy with low to moderate doses of steroids to prevent recurrence. Other drugs that are considered relatively safe during pregnancy include NSAIDs (during the late first and second trimester), antimalarials, Glucocorticoids, and azathioprine.

Diagnosis and Treatment

Lupus nephritis can occur during pregnancy and have the typical features seen in the nonpregnant state. However, lupus nephritis must be differentiated from preeclampsia as both can present with thrombocytopenia or can occur simultaneously. Some important distinctions are low complement levels and active urine sediment seen with lupus. The therapy for lupus nephritis should consist of high-dose prednisone, hypertension control, and azathioprine if necessary.

DIABETIC NEPHROPATHY

This is one of the most common underlying causes of kidney disease during pregnancy. As with other renal disorders those with mild dysfunction have the fewest complications and lowest risk of progression of disease. Microalbuminuria is associated with increased frequency of adverse pregnancy outcomes. General treatment principles include blood pressure control to <140/90 mm Hg, discontinuation of ACE inhibitors or angiotensin receptor blockers, and glycemic control to reduce risk of congenital defects.

PREGNANCY IN DIALYSIS PATIENTS

Pregnancy is a rare event in dialysis patients, occurring in only 1.5% of all women of childbearing age. The live birth rate is around 50% with prematurity (86%), fetal growth retardation (30%), polyhydramnios (40%–60%), and congenital abnormalities (9%). Maternal complications include severe hypertension in 85% and increased mortality rate. Peritoneal dialysis and hemodialysis have both been used successfully but attention must be given to dialysis adequacy and other medical management issues (Table 22-6). Early pregnancy is difficult to diagnose because beta HCG is not reliable.

PREGNANCY AFTER RENAL TRANSPLANT

In order to avoid an unplanned pregnancy, women of childbearing age should be aware that they may have resumption of menstrual cycles as early as 1 month following renal transplantation. The general recommendations are to wait at least 1 and preferably 2 years following transplantation for a planned pregnancy. This time period allows for appropriate posttransplant monitoring and adjustments, and decreases the likelihood of cytomegalovirus (CMV) disease during pregnancy. All pregnancies in transplant recipients should be considered high risk and appropriately monitored. Prior to a planned pregnancy, renal function should be stable with serum creatinine <1.5 to 2mg/dL, blood pressure controlled with a minimal number of medications, stable proteinuria <1 g/day, and no recent episodes of rejection or other transplant-related complications. Risk of worsening allograft function or graft increases with prepregnancy serum creatinine values >1.5 mg/dL.

TABLE 22-6	GENERAL MANAGEMENT PRINCIPLES OF PREGNANT DIALYSIS PATIENTS
Dialysis	Hemodialysis • ≥20 hours/week • Keep BUN <50 mg/dL • Adjust dialysate calcium to maintain normal level • Minimize heparinization Peritoneal dialysis • Decrease fill volume should be decreased later in pregnancy to decrease abdominal girth • Increased exchanges
Anemia	Maintain hemoglobin level at least 10 g/dL Iron and folic acid supplementation
Nutrition	Protein intake 1.8 g/kg/day supplemented with vitamins Expect weight gain of 1–2 kg early in pregnancy and 0.5 kg/week after first trimester
Blood pressure	Maintain DBP 80–90 mm Hg
Obstetric	High-risk obstetric care and serial US,? fetal monitoring during dialysis

Immunosuppressive Drug Management

Calcineurin inhibitors and azathioprine are associated with intrauterine growth retardation, but are acceptable to continue during pregnancy, as is standard maintenance-dose prednisone. Calcineurin inhibitor levels may decrease during pregnancy without a change in dosage as a result of an increased volume of distribution. It is generally not necessary to increase the dose in response. There is limited human data with mycophenolate or sirolimus use during pregnancy, but animal data suggest these agents should be discontinued at least 6 to 8 weeks prior to attempts to conceive. Other medications commonly given to transplant recipients such as sulfamethoxazole/trimethoprim and ACE inhibitors should be discontinued. In addition, immunosuppressive agents are present in breast milk at variable levels, and breastfeeding is not recommended.

Complications

With acceptable prepregnancy renal function, serum creatinine should initially decrease by 20% to 30% and increase slightly above this nadir late in pregnancy. Proteinuria may increase during pregnancy, but usually returns to previous levels in the setting of stable graft function. Preeclampsia is more common in renal transplant recipients, and close monitoring of blood pressure and proteinuria is mandatory. Blood pressure goals should be similar to those of pregnant nontransplant recipients, with knowledge of the prepregnancy readings. Graft dysfunction during pregnancy requires immediate evaluation and biopsy should be performed if necessary. Preterm delivery and low birth weight are more common with pregnancy following transplantation and long-term effects of in-utero exposure to immunosuppressive agents remains unknown. Despite this, babies born to transplant recipient mothers have complication rates similar to the nontransplant population and pregnancy should not be discouraged in the appropriate clinical setting.

KEY POINTS TO REMEMBER

- In the physiology of pregnancy, blood pressures within the normal range may signify hypertension.
- ACE inhibitors and angiotensin receptor blockers are contraindicated during pregnancy. Blood pressure should not be aggressively controlled in patients with hypertension in pregnancy.
- Delivery of the fetus is the primary treatment for preeclampsia.
- Significant proteinuria (>200 mg/day) is not an expected finding during pregnancy and should be thoroughly evaluated.
- Asymptomatic bacteriuria during pregnancy merits antibiotic therapy to prevent complications of pyelonephritis.
- Pyelonephritis during pregnancy is a medical emergency.
- Women with renal disease can have successful pregnancies, especially if the disease is mild, but those with moderate to severe renal disease have significant risk of complications to the mother and fetus as well as risk of progression of renal dysfunction.

REFERENCES AND SUGGESTED READINGS

American College of Obstetricians and Gynecologists. *Antimicrobial Therapy for Obstetric Patients. ACOG Educational Bulletin 245.* Washington, DC; 1998.

American College of Obstetricians and Gynecologists. *Diagnosis and Management of Preeclampsia and Eclampsia. ACOG Practice Bulletin 33.* Washington, DC; 2002.

Bar, OB, Hackman, R, Einarson, J. et al. Pregnancy outcome after cyclosporine therapy during pregnancy: a meta-analysis. *Transplantation.* 2001;71:1051–1055.

Baumwell, S, Karumanchi, SA. Pre-eclampsia: clinical manifestations and molecular mechanisms. *Nephron Clin Pract.* 2007;106:c72–81.

Delzell JE Jr, Lefevre ML. Urinary tract infections during pregnancy. *Am Fam Physician.* 2000;61:713.

Ekbom P, Damm P, Feldt-Rasmussen B, et al. Pregnancy outcome in type one diabetic women with microalbuminuria. *Diabetes Care.* 2001;24:1739.

Greenberg, A. *Primer on Kidney Disease.* 4th ed. Philadelphia: WB Saunders; 2005: 426–435.

Hou, SH. Frequency and outcome of pregnancy in women on dialysis. *Am J Kidney Dis.* 1994;23:60.

Imbasciati E, Gregorini G, Cabiddu G, et al. Pregnancy in CKD stages 3 to 5: fetal and maternal outcomes. *Am J Kidney Dis.* 2007;49:753–762.

Johnson, RJ, Feehally, J, ed. *Comprehensive Clinical Nephrology.* 2nd ed. Spain: Elsevier; 2003:559–565.

Jones DC. Pregnancy complicated by chronic renal disease. *Clin Perinatol.* 1997;24:483.

Kuller JA, D'Andrea NM, McMahon MJ. Renal biopsy in pregnancy. *Am J Obstet Gynecol.* 2001;184:1093.

Martin JN Jr, Thigpen BD, Moore RC, et al. Stroke and severe preeclampsia and eclampsia: a paradigm shift focusing on systolic blood pressure. *Obstet Gynecol.* 2005;105: 246.

Odendaal HJ, Pattinson RC, Bam R, et al. Aggressive or expectant management for patients with severe preeclampsia between 28–34 weeks' gestation: a randomized controlled trial. *Obstet Gynecol.* 1990;76:1070.

Okundaye I, Abrinko P, Hou S. Registry of pregnancy in dialysis patients. *Am J Kidney Dis.* 1998;31:766.

Ruano R, Fontes RS, Zugaib M. Prevention of preeclampsia with low dose aspirin—a systemic review and meta-analysis of the main randomized controlled trials. *Clinics.* 2005;60(5):407–414.

Stanley CW, Gottlieb R, Zager R, et al. Developmental well-being in offspring of women receiving cyclosporine post-renal transplant. *Transplant Proc.* 1999;31:241–242.

Stratta P, Canavese C, Quaglia M. Pregnancy in patients with kidney disease. *J Nephrol.* 2006;19:135–143.

Strauch BS, Hayslett JP. Kidney disease and pregnancy. *Brit Med J.* 1974;4:578.

Von Dadelszen P, Magee LA. Fall in mean arterial pressure and fetal growth restriction in pregnancy hypertension: an updated meta regression analysis. *J Obstet Gynaecol Can.* 2002;24:941.

Nephrolithiasis: Physicochemical Principles and General Management

Sreedhara B. Alla

23

INTRODUCTION

Kidney stones are crystalline structures in the urinary tract that have achieved sufficient size to cause symptoms or be visible by radiographic imaging techniques. Most kidney stones in Western countries are composed of calcium salts and occur in the upper urinary tract. Conversely, in developing countries, the majority of stones are composed of uric acid and occur in the urinary bladder. It is believed that a protein-rich Western diet and lifestyle is responsible for this difference. The economic impact of kidney stones relates to surgical extraction or fragmentation of stones, loss of productivity, and need for preventive treatment.

Epidemiology

Nephrolithiasis is one of the most common diseases in Western countries. In the United States, the prevalence of nephrolithiasis is 5.2%, with an annual incidence of 1 to 2 per 1000. Prevalence is influenced by age, sex, race, body size, and geographic distribution. The peak age of onset is the third decade, with increasing prevalence until the age of 70 years. In women, there is a second peak at age 55. Historically, men have had a 2 to 3 times greater risk than women. More recently, an increasing rate of nephrolithiasis in females has been attributed to more obesity, narrowing the gender ratio to 1.3:1(M:F). Lifetime risk of developing a kidney stone is approximately 12% for men and 6% for women. Whites are affected more frequently than blacks, Hispanics, or Asian Americans. Two large epidemiological studies have demonstrated that larger body mass index (BMI) is associated with an increased risk of nephrolithiasis. The southeastern states have the highest incidence of nephrolithiasis which is attributed to higher average temperatures and greater sun exposure resulting in oversaturation of stone-forming salts in the urine.

CHEMICAL COMPOSITION OF STONES

Chemical composition of stones can be determined in specialized laboratories. Based on chemical composition, urinary stones can be classified in the following manner:

- **Stones composed of calcium salts.** In Western societies, 80% of all kidney stones are composed of calcium salts. Of these, 35% are composed exclusively of calcium oxalate; 40% are mixed (i.e., composed of calcium oxalate and calcium phosphate), whereas 5% of stones are composed exclusively of calcium phosphate (hydroxyapatite or brushite).
- **Uric acid stones and struvite stones.** These form roughly 10% to 20% of all stones in the urinary tract. Uric acid stones are radiolucent.

- **Cystine stones.** The hereditary disorder *cystinuria* (not to be confused with *cystinosis*) accounts for approximately 1% of all cases. Cystinuria is characterized by an amino acid transport defect in the proximal renal tubule, resulting in a urinary loss of dibasic amino acids.
- **Other.** Rarely, stones can be formed by poorly soluble drugs (e.g., triamterene, indinavir), xanthine, hypoxanthine, or ammonium urate.

PHYSICAL CHEMISTRY OF NEPHROLITHIASIS

One can infer from the variety of stones observed that several pathophysiologic mechanisms are responsible for stone formation. Nevertheless, a common pathway leading to stone formation is urinary supersaturation. Crystals form when the amount of solute in the urine exceeds its solubility limits.

Stone Formation
Three steps are necessary to form a stone:

1. Formation of a small initial crystal, or *nidus*.
2. Retention of a nidus in the urinary tract. If washed away by urine flow, crystal formation would remain a mere physiologic curiosity.
3. Growth of a nidus to a size at which it either becomes symptomatic or visible by imaging techniques.

Solubility Product, Formation Product, and Nucleation
Solubility Product
Solubility product describes the level of a solution's saturation with solute at which solid-phase material exists in equilibrium with liquid-phase material. Imagine a calcium oxalate crystal immersed in a calcium oxalate solution. The solubility product describes such concentrations of calcium and oxalate when the product is so high that it does not allow the crystal to dissolve. At the same time, the product is too low to permit crystal growth; the size of the calcium oxalate crystal remains unchanged. Concentrations lower than solubility products are called *undersaturated.* Concentrations higher than the solubility product are called *supersaturated.*

Formation Product
Formation product is the level of supersaturation at which a solute can no longer remain in a solution and precipitates out spontaneously (*homogeneous nucleation*). *Nucleation* can take place at a lower level of supersaturation if a solid phase is already present (*heterogeneous nucleation*). Even normal urine is often supersaturated with calcium oxalate. Urinary calcium oxalate product can exceed its solubility three to four times. Calcium oxalate crystalluria occurs in both stone formers and non–stone formers. Studies suggest that calcium oxalate crystal formation occurs by heterogeneous nucleation. Potential nucleating agents are calcium phosphate crystals, uric acid crystals, and cellular debris. Indeed, calcium phosphate is commonly present in stones composed primarily of calcium oxalate. By a similar mechanism of heterogeneous nucleation, hyperuricosuria contributes to calcium oxalate stone formation.

Urinary Saturation
Urinary saturation levels are influenced by the amount of solute and urine volume. The importance of the absolute amount of solute and urine volume is obvious: The more solute is excreted in a lower volume, the higher levels of saturation are achieved.

Urine pH
Urinary pH has a variable effect depending on the solutes involved. *Low urine pH* significantly lowers the solubility of *uric acid*. This effect is a result of different solubilities of the protonated and dissociated forms of uric acid. Solubility of the undisassociated form in acidic urine is very poor. Low urine pH makes uric acid supersaturation easy to achieve, even at normal uric acid excretion rates of 600 to 800 mg/day (3.6–4.8 mM/day). Uric acid crystals not only form into uric acid stones but also can nucleate out calcium oxalate (heterogeneous nucleation). Hence, low urine pH is a risk factor for uric acid and calcium oxalate stones. *Alkaline urine* pH predisposes to formation of crystals containing *phosphates: calcium phosphate and struvite (ammonium magnesium phosphate) stones*. Calcium phosphate nephrolithiasis is most commonly observed in patients with distal renal tubular acidosis (RTA), a condition leading to a persistently high urine pH. Struvite stones form in the presence of a urinary tract infection (UTI) caused by urease-producing bacteria. Urease-producing bacteria split abundant urinary urea into ammonia and carbon dioxide. Ammonia alkalinizes the urine and, together with magnesium, combines with phosphate to form struvite crystals.

Amount of Inhibitors of Crystallization
Citrate, the main inhibitor of crystallization of calcium salts, complexes with calcium to form a soluble calcium citrate compound. By doing so, it makes calcium unavailable to precipitate out as calcium oxalate or calcium phosphate. Hypocitraturia is a common finding among calcium stone formers. *Magnesium* also inhibits crystallization of calcium salts, although its effect is not as important as that of citrate.

PATHOGENESIS OF CALCIUM OXALATE AND CALCIUM PHOSPHATE NEPHROLITHIASIS

Hypercalciuria
Hypercalciuria is the most common metabolic derangement among stone formers. The amount of calcium excreted in the urine varies with body size and dietary calcium intake. The upper limit of normal calcium excretion in the urine is 4 mg/kg/day ($\approx$280 mg/day for men, 240 mg/day for women) for patients consuming 1000 mg of elemental calcium. For patients consuming only 400 mg, the upper value becomes only approximately 200 mg/day. Hypercalciuria can be classified as either idiopathic or secondary to hypercalcemia (Table 23-1).

TABLE 23-1	DIFFERENTIAL DIAGNOSIS OF HYPERCALCIURIA

Normal serum calcium
Idiopathic hypercalciuria
PTH-dependent elevated serum calcium
Primary hyperparathyroidism: adenoma or hyperplasia
PTH-independent elevated serum calcium
Malignancy: squamous cell carcinoma, breast cancer, bladder cancer, multiple myeloma, lymphoma
Granulomatous disease: sarcoidosis, tuberculosis, berylliosis
Hypervitaminosis D
Hyperthyroidism

PTH, parathyroid hormone.

Hypercalciuria Due to Hypercalcemia

Hypercalcemia imposes an increased filtered load of calcium and results in an overflow hypercalciuria. The causes and approach to hypercalcemia are discussed in Chapter 8.

Idiopathic Hypercalciuria

Idiopathic hypercalciuria, by definition, is not a consequence of hypercalcemia. It is currently believed that most cases of idiopathic hypercalciuria are caused by excessive calcium absorption from the GI tract (absorptive hypercalciuria). This disorder has a strong familial component. The pathophysiology of this disorder is not clear, but vitamin D receptor polymorphisms have been implicated. The degree of hypercalciuria can also be influenced by dietary sodium intake. Excessive sodium intake causes extracellular fluid volume expansion and diminished sodium resorption along the nephron. Volume expansion results not only in natriuresis but in calciuresis as well. Hence, dietary salt restriction can be an effective method of lowering hypercalciuria. Thiazide diuretics reduce hypercalciuria predominantly through reduction in extracellular fluid volume, leading to enhanced proximal and distal reabsorption of calcium.

Hyperoxaluria

Hyperoxaluria is divided into dietary, enteric, or primary forms (Table 23-2).

Dietary Hyperoxaluria

Normal daily urinary excretion of oxalate is <40 mg/day. Excessive dietary intake of oxalate-rich foods can result in a mild form of dietary hyperoxaluria (urinary oxalate excretion of 50–60 mg/day). Oxalate-rich foods include nuts, sunflower seeds, spinach, rhubarb, chocolate, Swiss chard, lime peel, star fruit, peppers, and tea.

TABLE 23-2 CAUSES OF HYPEROXALURIA		
Dietary Hyperoxaluria	**Enteric Hyperoxaluria**	**Primary Hyperoxaluria**
Cause: excessive dietary oxalate intake	*Cause:* small bowel malabsorption, Crohn disease, jejunoileal bypass, celiac sprue, short bowel syndrome, chronic pancreatitis, biliary obstruction	*Type I:* deficiency of alanine glyoxylate aminotransferase
Foods rich in oxalate: cocoa, chocolate, black tea, green beans, beets, celery, green onions, leafy greens (spinach, rhubarb), Swiss chard, mustard greens, berries, dried figs, orange and lemon peel, summer squash, nuts, peanut butter	Moderate to severe elevation of urinary oxalate excretion; may result in nephrocalcinosis and renal failure	*Type II:* D-glycerate dehydrogenase or glyoxylate reductase deficiency Severe hyperoxaluria, resulting in nephrocalcinosis and renal failure
Mild elevation in urinary oxalate excretion		

Enteric Hyperoxaluria

Fat malabsorption and saponification of calcium in the gut by free fatty acids result in increased colonic absorption of oxalate. Detergent bile acids nonselectively increase the permeability of colonic mucosa to a number of substances, including oxalate. The resultant hyperoxaluria is more severe than in a dietary form. Urinary oxalate excretion often exceeds 100 mg/day. Thus, small bowel resection, jejunal bypass surgery, and inflammatory bowel disorders can lead to hyperoxaluria, calcium oxalate nephrolithiasis, and even chronic renal failure due to nephrocalcinosis. In addition to hyperoxaluria, malabsorption has several other consequences that predispose to stone formation, including:

- Low urine volumes due to diarrheal loss of water
- Low urine pH due to colonic loss of bicarbonate
- Hypocitraturia due to chronic metabolic acidosis and hypokalemia
- Hypomagnesuria due to magnesium malabsorption

Primary Hyperoxaluria

Primary forms of hyperoxaluria result from well-described metabolic defects. These are characterized by excessive endogenous production of oxalate, resulting in profound hyperoxaluria (135–270 mg/day). Stone formation often begins in childhood. Deposition of calcium oxalate in the tubulointerstitial compartment of the kidneys (renal oxalosis) often leads to progressive loss of renal function. Deposition of calcium oxalate also occurs in the heart, bone, joints, eyes, and other tissues. Two major defects are worth mentioning: **Type I primary hyperoxaluria** is an autosomal-recessive disorder that results from reduced activity of hepatic peroxisomal alanine glyoxylate aminotransferase. This increases the availability of glyoxylate, which is irreversibly converted to oxalic acid. **Type II primary hyperoxaluria** is a much rarer form of the disease due to D-glycerate dehydrogenase or glyoxylate reductase deficiency.

Hypocitraturia

Hypocitraturia is defined as a urinary citrate excretion <250 mg/day. It is observed in approximately 40% of patients with nephrolithiasis. The presence of hypocitraturia should arouse suspicions of a disorder associated with chronic metabolic acidosis, such as distal RTA or a GI disorder. The eubicarbonatemic form of distal RTA should be suspected in patients with persistently high urine pH but normal or near-normal plasma bicarbonate concentrations. Such patients may develop overt metabolic acidosis only when challenged with an acid load. Patients with complete or incomplete distal RTA make stones composed predominantly of calcium phosphate (apatite).

Hyperuricosuria

Hyperuricosuria is a common finding noted in 10% to 26% of calcium stone formers. The amount of uric acid in the urine is determined by daily production of uric acid and is not necessarily associated with hyperuricemia. Studies have demonstrated that allopurinol, a xanthine oxidase inhibitor, significantly reduces the rate of calcium oxalate stone recurrences. The benefits are attributed to a decreased urinary excretion of uric acid.

Urinary Proteins

Although a number of urinary proteins have been implicated in the pathogenesis of calcium nephrolithiasis, their role remains to be further elucidated. Uropontin and nephrocalcin both inhibit crystal growth. Their role in nephrolithiasis is still not fully established.

Medullary Sponge Kidney

Medullary sponge kidney is a radiologic diagnosis of dilated distal collecting ducts seen on an IV pyelogram. When filled with contrast, dilated collecting ducts have an appearance

TABLE 23-3	NONSPECIFIC AND SPECIFIC TREATMENT OPTIONS FOR CALCIUM STONE FORMERS

Nonspecific treatment options:

Adequate oral liquid intake to maintain UOP of 2 L/day
Restrict salt intake to <100 mEq/day
Restrict protein consumption to <12 oz of beef/poultry/fish per day

Specific treatment options:

Hypercalciuria	*Hypocitraturia*
Eliminate dietary excess	K citrate
Thiazides	Neutral phosphates
No-added-salt diet	
Hyperoxaluria	*Hyperuricosuria*
Low-oxalate diet	Dietary purine restriction
Oral calcium	Allopurinol
Cholestyramine	K citrate if pH is low
Pyridoxine	

of a brush emanating from a renal papilla. Medullary sponge kidney is probably not a disease per se, but it is a result of damage to the collecting ducts by the process that causes calcium oxalate nephrolithiasis in the first place—most commonly, hypercalciuria.

PATHOGENESIS OF URIC ACID NEPHROLITHIASIS

Uric acid is a product of purine metabolism and is primarily derived from endogenous sources with dietary purines generally providing little substrate. Four abnormalities have been strongly associated with uric acid stones: persistently low urine pH, hyperuricemia, hyperuricosuria, and low urine volume.

Persistently Low Urine pH

The pK_a of uric acid is 5.35. Hence, low urine pH makes urinary saturation with uric acid easy to achieve even at normal excretion rates of 600 to 800 mg/day (3.6–4.8 mM/day). Patients with gout, obesity, diabetes, or metabolic syndrome are at greater risk of forming uric acid stones, presumably secondary to excretion of abnormally acidic urine. A linear drop in urine pH with increase in BMI has been demonstrated, which is thought to be the link between obesity and risk of forming uric acid stones.

Hyperuricemia and Hyperuricosuria

Hyperuricosuria can be secondary to an increased production of uric acid with an increased burden of excretion; alternatively, it can result from enhanced renal excretion of uric acid in the absence of hyperuricemia. Increased uric acid production can be either congenital or acquired. Congenital causes of uric acid overproduction are typically diseases of single-gene defects such as hypoxanthine guanine phosphoribosyltransferase (HPRT) deficiency and other similarly rare diseases. Acquired uric acid overproduction is common in myeloproliferative disorders, such as polycythemia vera, or after chemotherapy for certain cancers resulting in large-scale cell death (tumor lysis syndrome). Hyperuricosuria with normal uric acid levels can occur due to uricosuric agents such as probenecid and high-dose salicylates. Other commonly used medications have uricosuric effects. Several examples include losartan (increases uric acid excretion by $\approx$10%), fenofibrate (increases uric acid excretion by 20%–30%), and atorvastatin.

Low Urine Volume

Low urine volume is not a specific risk factor for uric acid nephrolithiasis, but increases the risk of all stone types by increasing the urinary supersaturation, as mentioned above.

PATHOGENESIS OF STRUVITE NEPHROLITHIASIS

Struvite stones are also referred to as *magnesium ammonium phosphate, triple phosphate, urease,* or *infection stones.* Each synonym provides insight into the pathogenesis of these stones. Struvite stones form only during a urinary tract infection caused by urease-producing bacteria, such as *Proteus* species, *Providencia* species, *Pseudomonas,* and *Enterococcus.* These bacteria cleave ammonia from urea, causing an elevation of urinary pH >7.0. Abundant ammonium and magnesium combine with phosphates to give rise to struvite stones. Sometimes, calcium phosphate (apatite) may become incorporated into stones. Mixed struvite and calcium stones can occur in cases in which primary calcium stones cause a UTI by one of the urea-splitting organisms. Mixed struvite and calcium stones occur more often in men with idiopathic hypercalciuria, in which calcium stones become secondarily infected or when alkaline urine becomes supersaturated for calcium phosphate. Pure struvite stones occur more commonly in women and are not associated with other metabolic derangements leading to calcium stone formation.

Factors that predispose one to recurrent UTIs, such as urinary retention, increase the likelihood of struvite stone formation (neurogenic bladder, indwelling bladder catheters, ileal conduit, urethral stricture, BPH, bladder and caliceal diverticuli, cystocele). Patients with history of diabetes mellitus or laxative or analgesic abuse are at increased risk for struvite stones. Struvite stones are often large and can fill the entire renal pelvis to form staghorn calculi. They often cause bleeding and obstruction and, as a rule, do not pass spontaneously. Chronic obstruction and infections may result in renal parenchymal damage and chronic kidney disease. The definitive diagnosis of struvite stones is made by chemical analysis of the stone or by finding typical "coffin-lid" ammonium magnesium phosphate crystals in the urine.

CLINICAL PRESENTATION OF NEPHROLITHIASIS

The clinical presentation of nephrolithiasis ranges from incidental diagnosis of otherwise asymptomatic disease to presentation with severe symptoms, such as abdominal or flank pain (renal colic), macroscopic or microscopic hematuria, UTIs, or even renal failure resulting from bilateral urinary tract obstruction.

Asymptomatic Disease

Patients with nephrolithiasis may remain asymptomatic for years. They usually become symptomatic if a calculus or its fragments begin to move along the urinary tract or cause obstruction. However, even chronic obstruction can be asymptomatic but may eventually result in a permanent loss of renal function.

Renal Colic

In renal colic, the pain is usually abrupt in onset, colicky in nature, and located in the flank area. It often loops around and radiates down along the path of the affected ureter; sometimes, it migrates anteriorly and inferiorly into the groin and testicles or labia majora. Usually, hematuria, urinary frequency, urgency, nausea, and vomiting accompany the pain.

Hematuria

Trauma to the urinary tract incited by passage of gravel or a stone leads to hematuria. It may be gross or microscopic and can occur even in completely asymptomatic patients.

APPROACH TO THE DIAGNOSIS OF RENAL COLIC

In its classic form, the clinical presentation of renal colic is quite suggestive of the diagnosis. However, it is imperative to consider other serious conditions that can masquerade as renal colic in the differential diagnosis: Ectopic pregnancy, intestinal obstruction, acute appendicitis, diverticulitis, and many other abdominal catastrophes have been confused with renal colic. The presence of hematuria is suggestive of the diagnosis but not conclusive proof; an imaging study is required to make a positive diagnosis.

Imaging Modalities
Plain Abdominal Radiograph
Approximately 90% of renal stones are radiopaque and can be seen on plain radiographs of the abdomen. However, the plain x-ray provides no information concerning presence or absence of urinary obstruction, and it may not add significant insight to the differential diagnosis of acute abdominal pain. Thus, plain abdominal x-rays have limited use in the evaluation of acute renal colic.

IV Urography and CT Scan
IV urography used to be the preferred test of choice for evaluation of these patients. The application of helical noncontrast CT has largely replaced it as the initial step in evaluation of suspected renal colic. It allows nephrolithiasis to be excluded or confirmed expeditiously and without administration of potentially nephrotoxic radiocontrast material.

Renal Ultrasound
Ultrasound is useful to rule out significant hydronephrosis or hydroureter; however, it may not detect stones until they are relatively large. At times, the exact site of obstruction may also not be clearly delineated. Ultrasound remains very useful for evaluation of patients who cannot receive radiation, such as pregnant women.

Radiographic Appearance of Stones
The radiographic appearance of stones on a plain abdominal radiograph may help identify stone type and guide further evaluation. Calcium phosphate and calcium oxalate stones are radiodense. Struvite stones (magnesium ammonium phosphate), when complexed with calcium carbonate or phosphate, are also visible as large, irregular stones. They sometimes take the shape of the calyces and are referred to as *staghorn calculi*. A plain x-ray of the abdomen (kidneys, ureter, and bladder) may miss radiolucent uric acid or poorly visible cystine stones. Xanthine and hypoxanthine stones are also radiolucent, but occur very rarely.

TREATMENT OF RENAL COLIC

The treatment of acute renal colic consists of pain management, relief of obstruction, and control of infection if present. If the stone is <5 mm, conservative management is adequate, as 80% to 90% of these stones pass spontaneously. The urine must be strained to retrieve the stone for analysis. Stones 5 to 7 mm only pass spontaneously 50% of the time, and stones >7 mm rarely pass spontaneously. If the stone is <7 mm, there is no obstruction, the urine is sterile, and the pain is controlled, conservative management is warranted. Fluid replacement should be designed to obtain a urine output of 2.5 L/day to assist with the passage of the stone. If the stone is passed but the patient had evidence of hydronephrosis or evidence of multiple stones, a follow-up imaging study, such as helical CT, within 2 weeks is warranted.

Indications for expedient stone removal are complete obstruction, UTI, urosepsis, or uncontrollable colic. Treatment modalities include extracorporeal shockwave lithotripsy (ESWL), percutaneous nephrostolithotomy (PCN), ureteroscopic removal, surgery, and chemolysis. The selection of treatment modality is determined by the size, composition, and anatomic location of the stone, anatomy of the collecting system, health status, and patient preference. Stones that are lodged in the proximal ureter above the iliac vessels are treated with ESWL or a combination of cystoscopy to push the stone upward into the renal pelvis followed by ESWL. Stones lodged distal to the iliac vessels are preferably treated by ureteroscopic removal given the high success rate of this procedure. Brushite and cystine stones are less responsive to ESWL. Stones that are >2 cm are usually treated with PCN. Surgical intervention is preferred for large staghorn calculi.

FOLLOW-UP OF NEPHROLITHIASIS

Subsequent imaging studies are recommended at 1 year for evaluation of recurrence. The study may be a kidneys/ureter/bladder x-ray, ultrasound, or helical CT. If there is no evidence of new stones, then imaging studies may be repeated every 5 years. Recurrent nephrolithiasis may mandate more frequent imaging. All patients with nephrolithiasis deserve a screening evaluation for common problems that can lead to stone formation, although there is no consensus of how extensive evaluation should be after the first episode. Patients with recurrent nephrolithiasis deserve a thorough metabolic evaluation, which should be done once the acute episode has resolved and the patient has returned to his or her daily routine.

MEDICAL TREATMENT OF NEPHROLITHIASIS

Medical prevention based on appropriate evaluation and treatment of metabolically active stone disease could save nearly $2200 per year per patient in related treatment costs. An understanding of the factors leading to stone formation and a structured patient evaluation are the basis for effective metabolic prevention.

Essential Diagnostic Evaluation

All stone formers should have a basic evaluation that includes history and physical examination, laboratory evaluation, and radiological studies. **History and physical examination** should be directed at identification of various risk factors such as inflammatory bowel diseases, bowel surgeries, recurrent UTIs, family history of stones, fluid and diet, and so forth. **Laboratory evaluation** includes urine and blood chemistries and chemical analysis of the stone, which can be used to identify the principal drivers of stone formation. Whenever available, chemical analysis of the stone should be performed. This provides not only the diagnosis but also some clues to the pathophysiologic mechanisms contributing to stone formation in a given patient. For example, presence of a uric acid crystal nidus should suggest that hyperuricosuria plays a cardinal role in that patient. Stones predominantly composed of calcium phosphate should raise suspicions for distal RTA. **Blood chemistries** should include determinations of sodium, potassium, chloride, bicarbonate, BUN, creatinine, plasma calcium, uric acid, magnesium, phosphorus, intact parathyroid hormone (PTH), and 1,25 (OH)2 D_3 levels. A **24-hour urine** sample should be collected on at least two occasions and approximately 4 weeks after the acute event has resolved and the patient has returned to his or her usual lifestyle. The drugs prescribed for stone disease, as well as vitamin supplements, should be stopped 5 days before urine collection.

The following **urinary parameters** are routinely determined when performing **stone risk evaluation:**

- Total urine volume: It is desirable to achieve urinary volume >2.5 L/day.
- Urine pH.
- Creatinine: Urinary excretion of creatinine is determined to assure adequacy of the collection. It is expected that in a 24-hour period, men excrete approximately 20 mg/kg and women 15 mg/kg of creatinine.
- Calcium: normal 50 to 250 mg/day.
- Uric acid: normal <750 mg/day.
- Citrate: normal >250 mg/day.
- Oxalate: normal <40 mg/day.
- Sodium: <100 mmol/day is consistent with low dietary sodium intake.
- Phosphorus: normal <1100 mg/day.
- Magnesium: normal 18 to 130 mg/day.
- Ammonia: normal 25 to 50 mmol/day.
- Sulfate: normal 4 to 35 mmol/day.

A number of commercial urine collection kits, quantitating urinary salt composition and saturations, are widely available. To account for day-to-day variability in urinary salt excretion, several 24-hour urinary collections may be necessary.

TREATMENT OF CALCIUM OXALATE AND CALCIUM PHOSPHATE NEPHROLITHIASIS

High Urine Volume

The first tenet of prevention of nephrolithiasis is maintenance of high urine volume. Nephrolithiasis patients should achieve a **daily urine volume of** ≥2.5 L. High urine volumes lower urine saturation with all salts. There are several helpful hints to assist patients in increasing urine volume. They can be instructed to drink sufficient amounts of fluids to a point that the urine appears clear. It is crucial to make sure they drink enough fluids in the evening to the point of nocturia to avoid excessive urinary concentration during the night. Patients may take metered quantities of water to work to remind them to drink plenty of water throughout the day. This is particularly important for those patients who suffer from chronic diarrheal disorders resulting in excessive fluid loss from the GI tract. Adequate fluid intake is also very important for patients who demonstrate significant hyperuricosuria, as urine can become easily saturated with uric acid even at normal levels of uric acid excretion.

Diet

Dietary intervention plays a cardinal role in the preventive treatment of calcium nephrolithiasis. Studies have shown that a low-protein, low-salt diet significantly reduces nephrolithiasis recurrence rates in patients with idiopathic hypercalciuria. Long-term dietary compliance with a low-protein, low-salt diet has been shown to be superior to a low-calcium diet in prevention of nephrolithiasis. A low-calcium diet may increase the intestinal absorption of oxalate, reducing the effectiveness of this therapy. Therefore, low-calcium diets are not recommended. Diets containing 700 to 800 mg of calcium are adequate for patients with idiopathic hypercalciuria. Low-protein diets reduce purine intake resulting in reduced systemic acid and uric acid loads. Low-sodium diets reduce the amount of calcium in the urine by the mechanisms described previously.

Thiazide Diuretics

Thiazide diuretics have long been the mainstay in treatment of idiopathic hypercalciuria, with metabolic abnormality noted with more than half of calcium oxalate nephrolithiasis. They lower urinary excretion of calcium by at least two mechanisms. The main mechanism is contraction of the extracellular fluid volume. By reducing the extracellular volume, thiazide diuretics increase proximal reabsorption of calcium. Thiazides also directly increase calcium reabsorption in the distal nephron. However, the effects of thiazide diuretics can be completely negated by high dietary salt intake. Urinary sodium excretion of ≥ 120 mEq/day suggests nonadherence to a low-sodium diet. If calcium excretion is not reduced, compliance with thiazide treatment and sodium intake should be questioned. Hypokalemia and hypocitraturia may complicate long-term therapy with thiazide diuretics and can be prevented by adding oral potassium citrate. Sometimes, to enhance the effect of thiazides and conserve potassium, amiloride may be added. The optional treatment regimens that have been studied include: chlorthalidone 12.5 to 25 mg every day to a maximum of 100 mg every day; hydrochlorothiazide 25 to 50 mg b.i.d.; hydrochlorothiazide 50 mg with amiloride (Moduretic) ½ tablet b.i.d.

Oral Phosphate

Patients with urinary phosphate wasting and hypophosphatemia may benefit from phosphate replacement therapy. **Neutral potassium phosphate** (Neutraphos) divided into three to four doses (total daily dose 1500 mg) can lower urinary calcium excretion in some patients and as one study has shown, may be as effective as thiazide diuretics. However, compliance is difficult to achieve due to the frequent doses and side effects, such as diarrhea and bloating.

Hypocitraturia

Citrate therapy is the principal intervention for a large number of calcium stone formers. In particular, hypocitraturia often occurs in patients with small bowel malabsorption syndromes and distal renal tubular acidosis. As an added advantage, in these patients with chronic acidosis, citrate serves as a source of alkali (citrate is metabolized in the liver to bicarbonate). Citrate is administered in divided doses throughout the day; the starting dose is usually 10 mEq PO 2 or 3 times daily. Administration of an excessive amount of citrate can result in a persistently alkaline urinary pH, which may increase the risk of calcium phosphate stone formation in some patients.

Hyperoxaluria

Dietary hyperoxaluria is treated by dietary restriction of oxalate-rich foods. Treatment of the enteric form of hyperoxaluria should be directed toward correction of metabolic derangements resulting in stone formation and nephrocalcinosis. Thiazide diuretics are usually ineffective because patients with small bowel malabsorption demonstrate hypocalciuria. Absorptive hyperoxaluria is most often treated with a dietary restriction of oxalate-rich foods and administration of intestinal oxalate binders, such as calcium carbonate, which form nonreabsorbable compounds in the GI tract. If calcium carbonate is ineffective, bile sequestrants, such as cholestyramine, could be added.

Other Management Issues

Metabolic Acidosis and Hypocitraturia

Metabolic acidosis and hypocitraturia can be corrected either with potassium citrate or sodium bicarbonate. The dose of base needed to correct acidosis may vary from 20 to several hundred mEq/day depending on the severity of GI losses of bicarbonate. Magnesium deficits and hypomagnesuria are treated by administering magnesium supplements. Rarely, in cases of small bowel bypass surgery, a reversal of the surgical procedure may be necessary to correct the metabolic defects.

Type I Primary Hyperoxaluria

Type I primary hyperoxaluria occasionally can respond to pyridoxine supplements. However, no good medical treatment short of liver transplantation exists. Increasing urinary volume to 3 L/day is beneficial. Liver transplantation restores the enzymatic defects responsible for the disease. Renal transplantation in patients who have developed end-stage renal disease due to primary hyperoxaluria requires a special protocol to avoid accelerated renal oxalosis in the allograft; the ideal approach is combined liver and kidney transplantation.

TREATMENT OF URIC ACID NEPHROLITHIASIS

Treatment of uric acid nephrolithiasis is based on attempts to increase the solubility of uric acid and to decrease its excretion. All patients should maintain urine volume >2.5 L/day. **Dietary counseling** about low purine and low protein intake is paramount. Alkalinization of urine to a pH >6.5 markedly increases the solubility of uric acid. **Potassium citrate** (10–20 mEq PO t.i.d.; maximum, 100 mEq/day) is the preferred alkalinizing agent because, unlike sodium salts, it does not augment urinary calcium excretion. However, urinary alkalinization alone is rarely sufficient. It is very difficult to avoid temporary episodes of urinary acidification throughout the entire day (e.g., during the night). **Allopurinol**, a xanthine oxidase inhibitor that blocks the conversion of xanthine to uric acid, is well tolerated and very effective in reducing urinary uric acid excretion. The benefits of allopurinol are attributed to its ability to treat hyperuricosuria and reduce uric acid crystal–induced nucleation of calcium oxalate. The dose of allopurinol should be adjusted to achieve a target excretion of uric acid of <600 mg/day. The success of the treatment should be monitored by repeated 24-hour urinary collections for stone risk assessment.

TREATMENT OF STRUVITE STONES

Surgical intervention is usually needed to remove struvite stones. Open surgical removal (kidney-splitting surgery) is no longer the treatment of choice for staghorn struvite calculi. A combination of PCN and ESWL—referred to as *sandwich therapy*—is currently the preferred treatment of choice. All staghorn calculi should be cultured after extraction as urine cultures are not always representative of organism(s) present in the stone. Once patients are free of stones, they benefit from antibiotic therapy directed against the predominant urinary organism. Most patients with residual stone fragments progress despite treatment with antibiotics. Reducing the bacterial population with antibiotics often slows stone growth but stone resolution with antibiotics is unlikely. **Acetohydroxamic acid** (AHA), a urease inhibitor is effective in reducing and even reversing struvite stone formation by decreasing the urinary supersaturation with struvite. However its usefulness is limited by side effects including dose-related hemolytic anemia, thrombophlebitis, and nonspecific neurological symptoms (disorientation, tremor, and headache). AHA should not be used in patients with creatinine clearances <40 mL/minute or serum creatinines >2.5 mg/dL, as impaired renal function prolongs its half life and increases toxicity. It is also teratogenic.

CYSTINE STONES

Cystinuria is a hereditary disorder of dibasic amino acid transport in the proximal renal tubule. The defect rests in a common dibasic amino acid transporter located on the apical membrane of the proximal tubular cell (Fig. 23-1). A genetic defect of this transporter results in urinary wasting of the dibasic amino acids cystine, ornithine, arginine, and lysine. Approximately 1% to 2% of patients attending renal stone clinics exhibit this hereditary defect. Cystinuria should not be confused with *cystinosis*, a lysosomal disorder resulting in Fanconi syndrome and chronic renal failure.

Cystine is a poorly soluble disulfide of the amino acid cysteine. The solubility of cystine is approximately 300 mg/L (1.25 mmol/L). Normal urinary cystine excretion is only 30 to 50 mg/day (0.12–0.21 mmol/day). Patients with cystinuria often excrete as much as 480 to 3,600 mg/day (2–15 mmol/day), easily achieving urinary supersaturation status. The other three dibasic amino acids are soluble, and their loss in the urine is inconsequential.

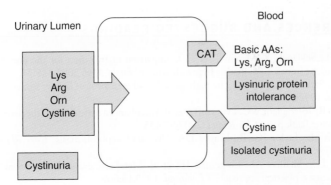

FIGURE 23-1. Schematic representation of the dibasic amino acid (AA) transport in the proximal renal tubule. Cystinuria results from a defect in the dibasic AA transporter on the apical side of the membrane. Hence, cystinuria is also attended by elevated urinary excretion of lysine (Lys), arginine (Arg), and ornithine (Orn). CAT, cationic amino acid transporter. (Data from Lopez-Nieto CE, Brenner BM. Molecular basis of inherited disorders of renal solute transport. *Curr Opin Nephrol Hypertens.* 1997;6:411–421.)

Cystine stones are opaque on abdominal radiographs. Microscopic urinalysis often reveals hexagonal cystine crystals. The diagnosis of cystinuria can be made by a chemical analysis of a retrieved stone or by a demonstration of excessive amount of cystine in the urine. Cystine stones can become very large and form staghorn calculi. Once formed, cystine stones often require surgical removal. Preventive medical therapy is directed toward reducing urinary cystine concentration below its solubility limits. High fluid intake can prevent stones only in some patients with low levels of cystine excretion. Most patients require treatment with penicillamine, tiopronin, or captopril. By forming soluble disulfides, both of these drugs reduce urinary saturation with cystine. However, side effects may limit their use. Dietary restriction of the essential amino acid methionine, a cystine precursor, is impractical. Urinary alkalinization to a pH >7.5 increases cystine solubility. However, persistently alkaline urine is difficult to attain.

KEY POINTS TO REMEMBER

- Eighty percent of kidney stones consist of calcium salts.
- Hypercalciuria (idiopathic or secondary to hypercalcemia) is the most common abnormality in stone patients.
- Helical noncontrast CT scans have largely replaced IV urography as the imaging modality of choice for stone patients.
- Stones may result in renal failure with no prior warning signs such as renal colic and so forth.
- Maintenance of adequate urine volume is essential in managing recurrent nephrolithiasis
- Very-low-calcium diets may be counterproductive in the treatment of calcium stones.
- Low-sodium, low-protein diets are useful in preventing recurrences of calcium stones.
- Hypocitraturia must be identified and aggressively treated.

REFERENCES AND SUGGESTED READINGS

Borghi L, Schianchi T, Meschi T, et al. Comparison of two diets for the prevention of recurrent stones in idiopathic hypercalciuria. *N Engl J Med.* 2002;346:77.

Coe FL, Parks JH, Asplin JR. The pathogenesis and treatment of kidney stones. *N Engl J Med.* 1992;327:1141.

Colistro R, Torreggiani WC, Lyburn ID, et al. Unenhanced helical CT in the investigation of acute flank pain. *Clin Radiol.* 2002;57:435.

Liebman SE, Taylor JG, Bushinsky DA. Uric acid nephrolithiasis. *Curr Rheum Rep.* 2007;9:251.

Lifshitz DA, Shalhav AL, Lingeman JE, et al. Metabolic evaluation of stone disease patients: a practical approach. *J Endourol.* 1999;13:669.

Pearle MS, Roehrborn CG, Pak CY. Meta-analysis of randomized trials for medical prevention of calcium oxalate nephrolithiasis. *J Endourol.* 1999;13:679.

Portis AJ, Sundaram CP. Diagnosis and initial management of kidney stones. *Am Fam Physician.* 2001;63:1329.

Ramello A, Vitale C, Marangella M. Epidemiology of nephrolithiasis. *J Nephrol.* 2000; 13[Suppl 3]:S45.

Rodman JS. Struvite stones. *Nephron.* 1998;81[Suppl 1]:50.

Smith CL. Renal stone analysis: is there any clinical value? *Curr Opin Nephrol Hypertens.* 1998;703:709.

Smith CL, Berkseth R, Lee J, et al. Calculous disease. In: Cass AS, ed. *Imaging of Urologic Disorders.* New York: Futura Publishing; 1992.

Smith CL, Davis M, Berkseth RO. Dietary factors in calcium nephrolithiasis. *J Renal Nutr.* 1992;2:146.

Management of Chronic Kidney Disease

Daniel O. Young

INTRODUCTION

Scope of the Problem

Chronic kidney disease (CKD) is a diagnosis given to any patient with evidence of kidney damage, even those with a normal or increased glomerular filtration rate (GFR). However, the term CKD is typically applied to patients with a glomerular filtration rate (GFR) <60 mL/minute. Estimates suggest that more than 8 million Americans have CKD as evidenced by a GFR below this cutoff. Identification of kidney damage is critical because the progression of CKD has been associated with increased rates of death, cardiovascular events, and hospitalization. This chapter focuses primarily on management of the CKD patient not yet requiring renal replacement therapy.

Staging of Chronic Kidney Disease

In 2003, a National Kidney Foundation (NKF) work group released guidelines for the classification and stratification of patients with CKD. Table 24-1 reviews the NKF stages of CKD. As previously noted, although patients with a GFR >60 mL/minute may have kidney damage, the focus of this chapter is limited primarily to patients with a GFR between 15 and 60 mL/minute. Patients with a GFR between 30 and 59 mL/minute are classified as having stage 3 CKD and are assumed to have a moderately decreased GFR. Appropriate treatment for these patients includes treatment of CKD complications that either manifest or worsen at this level of kidney function. Patients with a GFR between 15 and 29 mL/minute are classified as having stage 4 CKD and are assumed to have a severely decreased GFR. Treatment for these patients includes treatment as noted above for stage 3 patients as well as consideration and planning for initiation of renal replacement therapy. Table 24-2 presents some recommended and select testing for patients with stage 3 or 4 CKD. Patients with stage 5 CKD are considered those with a GFR <15 mL/minute or those already requiring dialysis.

Limitations of the Modification of Diet in Renal Disease Equation

A discussion on GFR estimates can be found elsewhere in this manual, but a brief mention of some important limitations of the Modification of Diet in Renal Disease (MDRD) equation is pertinent. The MDRD equation is a creatinine-based equation used to estimate GFR. The estimated GFR as calculated by the MDRD equation can only be interpreted when the creatinine level is stable. Thus the equation should not be applied to patients with acute kidney injury nor should it be applied to CKD patients with an acute or chronic kidney insult. Additionally, in adults more than 70 years old or those with reduced muscle mass, and especially in elderly females, a 24-hour urine collection for the average of creatinine and urea clearances may more accurately estimate an individual's true level of kidney function.

TABLE 24-1	NATIONAL KIDNEY FOUNDATION STAGES OF CHRONIC KIDNEY DISEASE		
Stage	Description	GFR ml/minute per 1.73 m^2	Action
1	Kidney damage with normal or increased GFR	≥90	Diagnosis and treatment; slow progression
2	Kidney damage with mildly decreased GFR	60–89	Estimate progression
3	Moderately decreased GFR	30–59	Evaluate and treat complications
4	Severely decreased GFR	15–29	Prepare for kidney replacement therapy
5	Kidney failure	<15 or dialysis	Kidney replacement (if uremia present)

Adapted from Levey AS, Coresh J, Balk E, et al. National Kidney Foundation practice guidelines for chronic kidney disease: evaluation, classification, and stratification. *Ann Intern Med.* 2003; 139(2):137–147.

HYPERTENSION

Pathophysiology

In patients with a reduced GFR, the pathophysiology of hypertension relates to inappropriate sodium reabsorption. The positive sodium balance with resultant volume expansion is the primary mechanism for elevated blood pressure in the CKD population although several other mechanisms (e.g., activation of the renin-angiotensin-aldosterone system) undoubtedly contribute. The Seventh Report of the Joint National Committee on Prevention, Detection, Evaluation, and Treatment of High Blood Pressure (JNC 7) recognized CKD as not only an identifiable cause of hypertension, but also reiterated that the kidney is an organ subject to target damage from high blood pressure.

Blood Pressure Goal

In patients with CKD, the JNC 7 recommends a blood pressure goal of <130/80 mm Hg. Lifestyle recommendations such as decreasing dietary sodium intake, weight loss, regular exercise, and smoking cessation are important, but frequently insufficient to attain this goal. Most patients with CKD will require two or more antihypertensives to achieve a blood pressure goal of <130/80 mm Hg. CKD represents one high-risk condition with a compelling indication for initial use of an angiotensin-converting enzyme (ACE) inhibitor or an angiotensin-receptor blocker (ARB). Not only do these medication classes result in reduced systemic blood pressure, but classically they also lower intraglomerular pressure thus protecting the kidneys from more severe disease progression. These principles apply best to CKD patients with proteinuria, such as those with diabetic nephropathy, but also

TABLE 24-2	INITIAL WORKUP OF THE CHRONIC KIDNEY DISEASE PATIENT

Initial Tests and Diagnostics	Significance and/or Goal
Blood pressure	<130/80 mm Hg; use of an ACE inhibitor or ARB
Serum creatinine	Used to estimate GFR; historical values assist in determining acuity and progression of disease
Urinalysis with microscopy	Presence of RBCs, RBC casts, and/or proteinuria suggests additional workup is necessary
Serum electrolytes (sodium, potassium, bicarbonate)	Useful as a crude surrogate of renal disease, may help guide use of antihypertensives, may help identify patients in need of medical nutrition education
Calcium, phosphorus, intact PTH, 25-OH vitamin D	Assists in treatment of metabolic bone disease
Renal ultrasound with or without arterial Dopplers	Characterizes kidney number and size, echogenicity of kidneys, rules out presence of obstruction or renovascular disease
Complete blood count	Evaluate for anemia
Cholesterol panel	Especially useful for patients with nephrotic proteinuria
Hepatitis serology	Negative Hepatitis B testing mandates vaccination
SPEP and UPEP	Reasonable for adults with renal disease
Random urine protein and random urine creatinine	Ratio approximates values obtained by 24-hour collection; check urine dipstick first
HIV	Warranted for select populations with risk factors
Antinuclear antibody	Warranted for adults with proteinuria and/or evidence for systemic lupus erythematosus
TSAT and ferritin	Useful in the evaluation of iron stores
Kidney biopsy	Indicated for individuals with hematuria and/or proteinuria and lack of evidence for systemic disease

apply to other causes of renal disease. In a patient with CKD, the serum creatinine and potassium should be checked within 1 to 2 weeks after starting an ACE inhibitor or an ARB and up to a 30% increase in serum creatinine is usually acceptable. It may be necessary to repeat these measurements with dose increases, especially in patients prone to hyperkalemia as an elevated potassium can limit use of these agents. Also, given the pathophysiology of hypertension in CKD (sodium retention with volume expansion), diuretics are also frequently appropriate as second-line antihypertensive therapy. Thiazide-type diuretics become less efficacious once the GFR falls below 30 to 40 mL/minute, whereas loop diuretics remain effective at lower GFRs as long as albumin levels do not fall too low and there is minimal proteinuria. A reasonable starting dose for a loop diuretic in a patient with CKD is **furosemide 40 mg PO b.i.d. or bumetanide 1 mg PO b.i.d.** A new steady state will be reached within 1 to 2 weeks. Both classes of diuretics can help ameliorate the hyperkalemia seen with ACE inhibitors and ARBs. Additional options to consider as second- and third-line agents include beta-blockers, calcium channel blockers, alpha blockers, alpha-2 agonists, and vasodilators. Control of blood pressure is of utmost importance in the CKD population because it is one of the most easily identifiable and treatable risk factors for cardiovascular disease (CVD) and because most CKD patients will die from cardiovascular causes well before ever needing dialysis. Patients should be educated about the importance of recording blood pressure measurements and encouraged to perform home monitoring of blood pressure.

Renin-Angiotensin-Aldosterone System Interruption Is Renoprotective

Several studies have demonstrated the benefit of interruption of the renin-angiotensin-aldosterone system (RAAS). Even in advanced CKD, ACE-inhibitor therapy has been demonstrated to slow progression to combined endpoints including end-stage renal disease (ESRD). Combination ACE-inhibitor and ARB therapy or "dual-blockade" therapy has been shown to be effective in reducing blood pressure, is well tolerated, and may result in better control of proteinuria. Recently, there has been interest in aldosterone receptor blockade as an antifibrotic strategy to lower blood pressure, reduce proteinuria, and abrogate the progression of renal disease. However, additional long-term studies are necessary before endorsing this additional promising therapy.

ANEMIA

Pathophysiology

The kidneys typically receive 20% to 25% of cardiac output. The oxygen-carrying capacity of this output far exceeds normal oxygen demand and utilization by the kidneys. Thus, the kidneys are well suited to serve as oxygen sensors for the body. The kidneys produce and secrete *erythropoietin,* a hormone that stimulates red blood cell production by the bone marrow. With advancing kidney damage, the kidneys are less able to produce adequate amounts of erythropoietin necessary to maintain normal or near-normal hemoglobin levels. Resistance to the action of erythropoietin also plays a role in the development and maintenance of anemia. Often erythropoietin replacement becomes necessary once hemoglobin levels fall to <10 g/dL but may be necessary at higher values. Frequently, these patients are concurrently iron deficient and require iron replacement. Further, not all CKD patients with anemia will have a renal-related pathophysiologic mechanism for their reduced hemoglobin level. Hemodialysis patients lose blood and hence iron from the dialysis procedure and frequent blood draws. This iron loss scenario does not apply to non–dialysis-dependent CKD patients. Therefore, an iron deficient stage 3 CKD patient may require an anemia workup including age-appropriate cancer screening measures to rule out an occult malignancy. Other patients may have a systemic illness such as systemic lupus erythematosus or multiple myeloma, which may explain both the CKD and the anemia.

Erythropoiesis-Stimulating Agents

Currently approved erythropoiesis-stimulating agents (ESAs) include epoetin alfa and darbepoetin alfa. There is no well-defined critical threshold for initiating an ESA in CKD patients. In the opinion of the Kidney Disease Outcomes Quality Initiative (KDOQI) anemia management work group, initial starting doses for the above approved ESAs are not defined and should be determined according to clinical circumstances and the patient's starting hemoglobin. Our clinic practice is to generally start **epoetin alfa** at a dose of **50 to 100 units/kg SC every week** or **darbepoetin alfa 40 mcg SC every 2 weeks**. The subcutaneous route is preferred in stage 3 and 4 CKD patients. We recommend—and current evidence supports—a target hemoglobin range of 11.0 to 12.0 g/dL. The FDA also recommends an upper target hemoglobin limit of 12.0 g/dL. Because of recently completed studies, the FDA has issued a "black box" warning for ESAs in that targeting persons with CKD to an upper limit of 13.0 g/dL may result in increased rates of blood clots, heart attacks, strokes, and death. The complete blood count (CBC) should be monitored at least monthly while administering an ESA.

Iron Deficiency

The KDOQI work group recommends a ferritin level >100 ng/mL and a transferrin saturation (TSAT) >20% in nondialysis CKD patients. It is our practice to begin iron replacement in a CKD patient once the hemoglobin has fallen to <11.0 g/dL and evidence for iron deficiency has been demonstrated. If no contraindications exist, iron replacement can begin via the oral route which is the preferred first line of treatment. We recommend **ferrous sulfate 325 mg PO b.i.d.–t.i.d**. Iron is best absorbed on an empty stomach and in an acid environment. Patients treated with antireflux medications will not absorb the iron as efficiently as patients not taking these drugs. If after 6 months the response has been less than optimal to oral iron as measured by the hemoglobin level and iron parameters or if a patient has been unable to tolerate oral iron, we typically prescribe **iron dextran** via an intravenous (IV) route. A 25-mg test dose should be administered and the patient monitored for any adverse events. If the patient tolerates the test dose without difficulty, a 500-mg to 1000-mg dose of iron dextran can then be given. Other IV iron formulations such as **iron sucrose** and **sodium ferric gluconate complex** are available and have significantly less potential for adverse effect, but are more costly and require a greater number of IV administrations.

RENAL OSTEODYSTROPHY

Secondary Hyperparathyroidism

Retention of phosphates due to decreased GFR and hypocalcemia due to reduced synthesis of active vitamin D (via reduced activity of 1 alpha hydroxylase in the kidney) result in elevated parathyroid hormone (PTH) levels. This secondary hyperparathyroidism (SHPT) can lead to a state of high bone turnover called *osteitis fibrosa* placing CKD patients at high risk for bone fractures. Treatment of SHPT is aimed initially at reducing phosphorus levels and later replacing vitamin D as necessary. For most nondialysis CKD patients, the first tenet of decreasing phosphorus levels is to reduce dietary phosphorus intake. In later stages of CKD, it may become necessary to provide patients with phosphate binders with meals such as calcium carbonate, calcium acetate, or lanthanum carbonate. It may be advisable to limit the amount of elemental calcium administered each day to no more than 2000 mg. As an example, a 500-mg tablet of calcium carbonate provides 200 mg of elemental calcium. Active vitamin D (1,25-dihydroxycholecalciferol also known as *calcitriol*) provides a feedback mechanism to the parathyroid gland to reduce PTH production and secretion. However, this therapy often leads to unacceptable increases in calcium and phosphorus levels via its action on the small intestine. Some active vitamin D analogs, such as paricalcitol, retain the PTH-lowering effect of calcitriol with less hypercalcemia and hyperphosphatemia. For patients with stage 3 CKD, the KDOQI clinical guidelines for bone metabolism recommend an opinion-based target of an intact PTH level between 35 and 70 pg/mL. Measurement of intact PTH is recommended every 12 months for patients not taking vitamin D. For patients with stage 4 CKD, the recommended target range is 70 to 110 pg/mL and measurement should occur every 3 months in patients not receiving vitamin D. Whether therapy is instituted with calcitriol or an analog such as paricalcitol, the calcium, phosphorus, and intact PTH should be checked in about 2 weeks. Additionally, for both stage 3 and 4 CKD patients, the KDOQI work group recommends maintaining a corrected calcium in the "normal" range for the laboratory used and a phosphorus value between 2.7 and 4.6 mg/dL. The typical starting dose for **calcitriol** is **0.25 mcg PO daily** and for **paricalcitol** is **1 mcg PO daily or 2 mcg PO three times a week.**

Vitamin D Deficiency/Insufficiency

The KDOQI bone metabolism work group recommends replacement of 25-hydroxy vitamin D, the storage form, once levels fall to <30 ng/mL. For levels <5 ng/mL, **ergocalciferol 50,000 IU** orally should be given weekly for 12 weeks and then monthly thereafter. For CKD patients with milder deficiency (5–15 ng/mL), the same dose of ergocalciferol is given weekly for 4 weeks and then monthly thereafter. For CKD patients with insufficiency (16–30 ng/mL), the work group recommends monthly ergocalciferol. For patients with deficiency (levels <16 ng/mL), the work group recommends repeating the blood measurement of 25-hydroxy vitamin D after 6 months of treatment, whereas others can have levels checked annually.

Acidosis in Chronic Kidney Disease

With advancing CKD and decreasing GFR, the ability of the kidney to effectively eliminate the total acid load is reduced. A large percentage of patients with stage 4 CKD have an overt nonanion gap metabolic acidosis. In clinical practice, we measure the bicarbonate as a crude measure of this acidosis. The KDOQI bone metabolism work group guidelines recommend maintaining a total CO_2 ≥22 mEq/L (22 mmol/L). Alkali salts can be administered to improve the bicarbonate concentration in the blood. It is our practice to administer **sodium bicarbonate 650 to 1300 mg PO b.i.d.–t.i.d.** A 650-mg tablet contains 7.6 mEq bicarbonate. An individual typically generates 1 mEq H^+ (acid) per kg body weight daily. The maintenance of higher bicarbonate levels may help preserve bone histology, lessen the impact of acidosis on protein catabolism, and avoid chronic metabolic acidosis from further contributing to renal osteodystrophy.

LIPID MANAGEMENT

Cholesterol Targets and Treatment in CKD

The updated NCEP ATP III guidelines for cholesterol management recommend an LDL-C goal of <100 mg/dL for high-risk patients defined as those with established coronary heart disease (CHD) or coronary heart disease risk equivalents. This population is assumed to have a 10-year risk of coronary heart disease events of >20%. For patients at moderate to moderately high risk for CHD, an LDL-C level of <130 mg/dL is recommended. A recent review has concisely summarized the role, safety, initial dosing, and potential benefits of statins in patients with CKD and ESRD. In brief, statins are safe in the CKD population and although they demonstrate similar relative risk reductions for cardiovascular events as compared with non-CKD patients, the absolute risk reductions are greater in the CKD population given the high rates of underlying disease and the greater number of cardiovascular events. Most patients with CKD will die prior to reaching the need for renal replacement therapy, with the most common cause of mortality related to a cardiovascular event. Therefore, patients with CKD represent a group with increased cardiovascular risk and a select population for lipid-modifying therapy. The optimal LDL-C target has not been defined for the CKD population and the presence of traditional CHD risk factors in the CKD patient should help guide the physician in deciding when to start a statin and what the target LDL-C should be.

IMMUNIZATIONS

Hepatitis B

The Advisory Committee on Immunization Practices (ACIP) publishes an annual recommended adult immunization schedule for adults in the United States. It can be found online at: http://www.cdc.gov/Nip/recs/adult-schedule.htm. The three-dose Hepatitis B immunization is recommended for all patients with CKD. Assuming the patient is Hepatitis B surface antibody negative, the immunization is typically administered as 3 doses (0, 1–2, 4–6 months). However, unlike the general population, there is a special formulation indication for the CKD and ESRD population. **These patients should receive the higher dose of 40 μg/mL for each of the three administered doses.** Surface antibody immunity can be checked 1 to 6 months after the vaccination has been completed.

Pneumococcal Vaccination

The ACIP recommends Pneumococcal polysaccharide vaccination for all patients with CKD. Current guidelines recommend a one-time revaccination 5 years after the initial vaccination. It may be important to educate patients that this particular immunization does not protect against Pneumococcal pneumonia, rather it protects against the life-threatening complications of Pneumococcal pneumonia such as bacteremia.

Influenza Vaccination

Influenza vaccination is recommended annually for all individuals age 50 and older. The ACIP also recommends annual influenza vaccination (inactivated vaccine) for all younger patients with CKD.

REFERRAL FOR DIALYSIS ACCESS AND TRANSPLANTATION

Referral for Dialysis Access

Patients with stage 4 CKD rapidly approaching stage 5 should be referred for vascular access if hemodialysis is the preferred renal replacement modality and for peritoneal dialysis (PD) catheter placement if PD is preferred. The NKF also has KDOQI practice guidelines detailing recommendations for vascular access. These guidelines were last updated in July 2006. An arteriovenous fistula (AVF) is the most preferred access for hemodialysis patients, however an arteriovenous graft (AVG) is preferred over long-term dialysis catheters. Although it is difficult to anticipate exactly when a patient will need to initiate renal replacement therapy, an AVF should ideally be placed 6 months prior to the start of hemodialysis and an AVG placed at least 3 to 6 weeks prior to the start of hemodialysis. The PD catheter should be placed at least 2 weeks prior to the anticipated start of PD. Early referral to a vascular surgeon is prudent so that preoperative studies (e.g., vein mapping) can be completed. Further, the nondominant upper extremity is the preferred site for AVF placement. This arm should be protected from IV access including peripheral IVs and PICC lines, and from blood pressure measurements. We recommend avoiding subclavian central lines in CKD patients because of the enhanced risk of central vein stenosis.

Referral for Transplantation

Suitable candidates with stage 4 CKD should be referred for evaluation by a multidisciplinary kidney transplant clinic. Typically, patients cannot be listed for transplantation until the GFR has fallen to <20 mL/minute. This GFR is higher than the level at which the initiation of maintenance dialysis is typically indicated in the United States.

EDUCATION

Nutritional Issues in CKD

We offer to all our stage 3 and 4 CKD patients the opportunity to meet with a renal dietician to discuss nutritional issues relevant to the CKD patient. The most common indication for referral is generally hyperkalemia, however, patients are also given education about high phosphorus-containing foods and guidelines for appropriate protein intake. Patients should be counseled about the consequences of a high-protein diet including the generation of extra solute (i.e., urea) that will need to be eliminated and the enhanced production of an acid load that will also need to be excreted. Specific recommendations are summarized in Table 24-3. Current recommendations include a sodium intake of <2,000 mg/day (87 mEq sodium), a protein intake of 0.60 to 0.75 g/kg/day, a daily energy intake of 35 kcal/kg/day (slightly less for patients over 60 years of age), dietary phosphorus restriction to 800 to 1000 mg/day, and a target potassium intake of <2 to 3 g/day (~50–75 mEq potassium). Although current recommendations suggest reducing dietary protein intake to minimize the need for urea and acid excretion, a risk of malnutrition does exist and malnutrition in the setting of a GFR higher than normally recommended for initiating renal replacement therapy should influence the decision to begin dialysis earlier in patients who could otherwise delay starting. Serum albumin is a strong prognostic indicator in ESRD patients and a low level can prohibit an individual from starting PD because of the ongoing and substantial protein losses with this particular renal replacement modality. The KDOQI Nutrition guidelines recommend checking serum albumin every 1 to 3 months in patients with a GFR <20 mL/minute as an assessment of nutritional status. Although the values provided above are presented as absolutes, individualizing the dietetic therapy may ultimately prove to be the most appropriate strategy for CKD patients. For example, a daily energy intake of 35 kcal/kg body weight may not be appropriate for the obese nor for the malnourished. Therefore, a nutrition evaluation referral to a renal dietician can best assist patients in optimizing metabolic parameters of interest.

TABLE 24-3	STANDARD NUTRITIONAL GOALS FOR STAGE 3 AND 4 CKD PATIENTS[a]	
Nutritional Item	**Significance and/or Goal**
Sodium	2,000 mg/day (87 mEq)
Total caloric intake	35 kcal/kg/day
Protein	0.6–0.75 g/kg/day
Phosphorus	800–1000 mg/day
Potassium	2–3 g/day (51–77 mEq)

[a]Individualized patient therapy is often more appropriate than the absolute numbers provided in the table above.

Living with Chronic Kidney Disease

Our practice involves offering all stage 3 and 4 CKD patients the opportunity to partici-
pate in classes that educate individuals about the consequences of living with CKD.
Importantly, these classes educate patients about anemia and bone disease as well as high
blood pressure and cardiovascular disease.

Renal Replacement Therapies

We recommend to all appropriate stage 4 CKD patients attendance at dialysis education
classes. This is particularly important for patients who may not be aware of the different
modalities (i.e., hemodialysis versus PD) available. Unfortunately, some patients with stage
4 CKD may not be interested in dialysis or may not be suitable candidates. The responsibility of the treating physician is to address the appropriateness of dialysis initiation with
these patients and often their family members and then to plan accordingly.

INITIATION OF RENAL REPLACEMENT THERAPY

Referral to a nephrologist is almost always indicated once the GFR has fallen to <30
mL/minute and is appropriate in earlier stages of CKD (i.e., GFR <60 mL/minute) when
progression of renal disease is anticipated, especially because the nephrology clinic is often
better prepared to coordinate the care of the CKD patient with anemia, difficult-to-control
hypertension, significant proteinuria, or primary renal disease. Late nephrology referral is
associated with poorer outcomes and increased cost. However, a more difficult question to
answer with absolute certainty is when to initiate dialysis in a patient. In practical terms,
it is advisable to initiate dialysis in patients with diabetic CKD once the GFR falls to <15
mL/minute. In patients with nondiabetic CKD, dialysis should be initiated once the GFR
falls to <10 mL/minute. Although the values presented here are convenient, they are not
absolute. Additional considerations should be contemplated including the level of nutrition as noted above. Malnutrition in the setting of a GFR higher than the cutoff points
recommended above can be an indication to proceed with initiation of dialysis. Signs and
symptoms of uremia such as poor appetite, nausea, vomiting, restless legs, volume overload
refractory to diuretics, and high blood pressure should also contribute to the decision making as to when to favor initiating renal replacement therapy.

KEY POINTS TO REMEMBER

- The blood pressure goal for CKD patients is <130/80 mm Hg.
- ACE inhibitors and ARBs slow progression of kidney disease. Up to a 30% increase in
  the serum creatinine is generally acceptable after initiating therapy with an ACE inhibitor
  or ARB.
- Optimal treatment for stage 3 CKD patients entails management of the complications of
  CKD and modification of cardiovascular disease risk factors.
- Optimal treatment for stage 4 CKD patients includes treatment as above for stage 3 CKD
  patients and preparation for renal replacement therapy.
- In CKD patients with anemia, the target hemoglobin level should be 11 to 12 g/dL and
  the goal of iron stores repletion should be to achieve a TSAT of >20% and a ferritin of
  >100 ng/mL.
- Timely referral to a nephrologist for renal replacement planning and education has been
  shown to predict superior outcomes and delay the need for initiating dialysis.

REFERENCES AND SUGGESTED READINGS

Baber U, Toto RD, de Lemos JA. Statins and cardiovascular risk reduction in patients with chronic kidney disease and end-stage renal failure. *Am Heart J.* 2007;153(4):471–477.

Bianchi S, Bigazzi R, Campese VM. Long-term effects of spironolactone on proteinuria and kidney function in patients with chronic kidney disease. *Kidney Int.* 2006;70(12):2116–2123.

Cheng S, Coyne D. Paricalcitol capsules for the control of secondary hyperparathyroidism in chronic kidney disease. *Expert Opin Pharmacother.* 2006;7(5):617–621.

Chobanian AV, Bakris GL, Black HR, et al. The Seventh Report of the Joint National Committee on Prevention, Detection, Evaluation, and Treatment of High Blood Pressure: the JNC 7 report. *JAMA.* 2003;289(19):2560–2572.

Clinical practice guidelines and clinical practice recommendations for anemia in chronic kidney disease in adults. *Am J Kidney Dis.* 2006;47[5 Suppl 3]:S16–85.

Clinical practice guidelines for vascular access. *Am J Kidney Dis.* 2006;48[Suppl 1]:S176–247.

Drueke TB, Locatelli F, Clyne N, et al. Normalization of hemoglobin level in patients with chronic kidney disease and anemia. *N Engl J Med.* 2006;355(20):2071–2084.

Go AS, Chertow GM, Fan D, et al. Chronic kidney disease and the risks of death, cardiovascular events, and hospitalization. *N Engl J Med.* 2004;351(13):1296–1305.

Grundy SM, Cleeman JI, Merz CN, et al. Implications of recent clinical trials for the National Cholesterol Education Program Adult Treatment Panel III guidelines. *Circulation.* 2004;110(2):227–239.

Hou FF, Zhang X, Zhang GH, et al. Efficacy and safety of benazepril for advanced chronic renal insufficiency. *N Engl J Med.* 2006;354(2):131–140.

KDOQI clinical practice guidelines for bone metabolism and disease in chronic kidney disease. *Am J Kidney Dis.* 2003;42[4 Suppl 3]:S1–201.

Levey AS, Bosch JP, Lewis JB, et al. A more accurate method to estimate glomerular filtration rate from serum creatinine: a new prediction equation. Modification of Diet in Renal Disease Study Group. *Ann Intern Med.* 1999;130(6):461–470.

Levey AS, Coresh J, Balk E, et al. National Kidney Foundation practice guidelines for chronic kidney disease: evaluation, classification, and stratification. *Ann Intern Med.* 2003;139(2):137–147.

Mogensen CE, Neldam S, Tikkanen I, et al. Randomised controlled trial of dual blockade of renin-angiotensin system in patients with hypertension, microalbuminuria, and non-insulin dependent diabetes: the candesartan and lisinopril microalbuminuria (CALM) study. *BMJ.* 2000;321(7274):1440–1444.

Singh AK, Szczech L, Tang KL, et al. Correction of anemia with epoetin alfa in chronic kidney disease. *N Engl J Med.* 2006;355(20):2085–2098.

Toto RD. Treatment of hypertension in chronic kidney disease. *Semin Nephrol.* 2005;25(6):435–439.

Hemodialysis

25

Steven Cheng

INTRODUCTION

The loss of kidney function in end-stage renal disease (ESRD) results in uremia and an impairment in the regulation of fluids and electrolytes. Without intervention, ESRD is inevitably fatal. Therapeutic options include hemodialysis, peritoneal dialysis, transplantation, and supportive/palliative care. Hemodialysis (HD) is the most commonly utilized form of renal replacement therapy. Of the 490,000 patients with ESRD in the United States, more than 300,000 are currently on HD. Like the general ESRD population, the prevalent HD population is predominately white (55% white, 38% black, 4% Asian, 3% Native American/Other) with a slightly higher proportion of males (54%). Diabetes is the most common underlying diagnosis, followed by hypertension, glomerulonephritis, and congenital and cystic kidney diseases. The largest age group of HD patients is between 70 and 79 years old. This differs from the generalized ESRD population, whose mean age is 58 years, and reflects a younger and generally healthier cohort undergoing transplant and peritoneal dialysis. Despite advances in care, the mortality rate in HD patients is startling. Cardiovascular disease is clearly the leading cause of death among patients on HD, followed by septicemia. The probability of death in the 5 five years after starting HD is 63%. Among diabetics on HD, this probability rises to 71%. Dialysis patients over the age of 65 have a mortality rate seven times higher than the general Medicare population. Dialysis patients between the ages of 20 and 64 have a mortality rate 8 times higher.

INITIATING DIALYSIS: WHO NEEDS TO START?

Given the poor outcomes for patients on HD, every effort should be undertaken to preserve residual renal function. Early nephrology referrals, patient education, and serious consideration of transplant options may be helpful in attenuating the progression to ESRD. But even with aggressive early medical care, dialysis may become necessary to relieve uremic symptoms, electrolyte imbalances, or fluid accumulation due to declining renal function.

The vast majority of patients who require HD have chronic kidney diseases with a gradual but progressive loss of renal function over time. These patients usually develop uremic symptoms and require dialysis initiation as their estimated glomerular filtration rate (GFR) falls below 10 mL/minute/1.73 m^2. Those with significant co-morbidities, particularly diabetes, may require dialysis initiation at an earlier stage, usually near an estimated GFR of 15 mL/minute/1.73 m^2. Uremic symptoms develop due to the accumulation of toxic metabolites that are no longer adequately cleared by the failing kidney. This may manifest in a variety of ways, including nausea, vomiting, poor energy levels, decreased appetite, lethargy, pruritus, and a metallic aftertaste. Motor neuropathies may be elicited on physical exam, while asterixis, tremor, and myoclonus suggest uremic encephalopathy. Uremic pericarditis manifests as a pericardial friction rub or pericardial effusion and is a clear indication for urgent initiation of dialysis therapy.

Acute kidney injury may also require dialysis support, particularly in those who develop pulmonary edema, hyperkalemia, or metabolic acidosis. Acute indications for the initiation of dialysis can be remembered with the mnemonic AEIOU:

- Acidosis: life-threatening metabolic acidosis with a pH <7.2, not responsive to conservative treatments
- Electrolyte abnormalities: life-threatening hyperkalemia associated with ECG changes and symptomatic hypermagnesemia and hypercalcemia
- Intoxications: there are a limited number of intoxications for which HD is indicated. It should be considered in patients with deteriorating medical status, those whose measured levels of a substance are indicative of poor outcomes, or those with metabolic derangements (e.g., metabolic acidosis caused by intoxication). Substances that are effectively cleared with dialysis have the following characteristics: (a) low molecular weight (<500 Da), (b) high water solubility, (c) low degree of protein binding, (d) small volumes of distribution (<1 L/kg), and (e) high dialysis clearance relative to endogenous clearance. The following substances can be cleared with dialysis: barbiturates, bromides, chloral hydrate, alcohols, lithium, theophylline, procainamide, salicylates, atenolol, and sotalol.
- Overload: fluid overload or pulmonary edema not responsive to aggressive diuresis
- Uremia: mental status changes attributable to uremia, uremic pericarditis or neuropathy, bleeding diatheses or vomiting associated with uremia.

MODALITIES: HOW CAN IT BE ADMINISTERED?

Choosing the appropriate HD modality is an important decision that should be made with the consideration of both patient preference and a practical assessment of patient resources and capabilities. The primary variables that differentiate the various modalities are: location, independence, duration, and cumulative dialysis dose.

Intermittent in-center HD is the most common form of HD. This form of HD typically involves treatments three times per week, with each session averaging between 3 and 4 hours in duration. Patients receive HD at an in-center location, where trained staff are able to set up and supervise each treatment. For patients new to HD, this is often the modality of choice to acclimate patients to a supervised and controlled HD session.

Intermittent home HD is similar to intermittent in-center HD in frequency and duration of treatments. The key difference is location, giving patients the greater freedom of undergoing treatments at their own homes. The home environment must be carefully evaluated and both water supply and electricity must be able to accommodate the dialysis system. Furthermore, patients need to demonstrate sufficient responsibility over their treatments and the ability to cannulate their own arteriovenous accesses with a safe and sterile technique.

Short daily HD exposes patients to more frequent treatments (usually 6 times/week), albeit with a shorter duration of each session. The cumulative weekly dose of dialysis is similar to that obtained on intermittent HD. However, dividing the treatments into frequent, shorter treatments may prevent intradialytic complications, particularly hypotension and cramping. This modality is predominately performed at home, although some in-center locations are able to accommodate the daily treatments.

Nocturnal HD is different in that it offers a larger cumulative dose of dialysis each week. Patients who undergo nocturnal HD at home typically have longer treatment times, averaging 6 to 8 hours, performed 6 nights per week. It is still uncertain whether more dialysis leads to better patient outcomes. However, this modality does have the added convenience of allowing the patient greater freedom during the day. Like short daily HD, nocturnal HD is predominately done at home, although in-center locations are available. In-center nocturnal HD typically offers 8-hour treatments, 3 nights per week.

The decision to dialyze patients with acute renal failure is often performed based on acute indications, and the selection of modalities is often done in consideration of the patient's hemodynamic status. A full description of dialysis options, including continuous dialysis modalities, is addressed in Chapter 15.

Dialysis Access

For HD to be efficient, there must first be an effective system of blood delivery from the patient to the machine, and vice versa. This is referred to as a *dialysis access*. There are three types of access: arteriovenous fistulas (AVF), arteriovenous grafts (AVG), and dialysis catheters. Fistulas and grafts are vascular conduits that can support a high flow of blood. They are cannulated at each dialysis treatment with two needles—one through which arterial blood is pumped through the dialyzer, and one through which blood is returned into the venous system. Catheters are placed in a central venous position, typically in the internal jugular location, with flow through separate luminal ports to simulate arterial output and venous return. Specific characteristics of each type of access are described below.

The *arteriovenous fistula (AVF)* is the most desirable form of vascular access. It is created by the surgical manipulation of a patient's native vasculature. Construction is performed under regional anesthesia by an experienced vascular surgeon and can consist of either a side-to-side anastomosis between an artery and vein, or a side-of-artery to end-of-vein anastomosis. The goal is to provide an access site that can withstand repeated cannulation with large-bore needles, and can sustain the high flow of blood necessary for dialysis. Flow through an AVF averages between 600 and 800 cc/minute and may be able to maintain patency at flows of 200 cc/minute. Complications with thrombosis, infection, and vascular steal are lower in comparison with the AVG. However, placement of an AVF requires foresight, as they can take 3 to 4 months to mature. Furthermore, the construction of an adequate AVF may be impossible if the patient lacks healthy vasculature. In particular, patients with advanced diabetes or peripheral vascular disease may not have vessels that are amenable to the creation of a fistula.

The *arteriovenous graft (AVG)* can be placed in patients for whom an AVF cannot be created. In lieu of the patient's native vasculature, a synthetic graft (frequently created from polytetrafluoroethylene) is placed for the arteriovenous connection. Long-term patency rates are less impressive than those obtained with AVF. However, the AVG does have a few advantages, including a large surface area for cannulation and a maturation time of only 3 to 4 weeks. Flow rates through an AVG are typically 1000 to 1500 cc/minute with thrombosis occurring at flows <600 to 800 cc/minute.

A *catheter* is the least desirable form of vascular access for HD. Cuffed tunneled dialysis catheters are typically placed in the right internal jugular vein with a tunneled exit site just below the ipsilateral clavicle. These can be placed in patients requiring HD who do not yet have a site for a permanent vascular access. However, given variable success with flows, difficulties with recirculation, catheter dysfunction, and significant risk of infection, the catheter should not be used except as an access of last resort.

Access Complications

Poor flow, recirculation, infection, hemodynamic complications, and the development of aneurysms and pseudoaneurysms are some of the major issues that may arise with vascular access.

Hemodynamic Complications

Poor flow due to a stenosis of an AVG or AVF can affect both arterial and venous flow. It should be suspected in patients with a decreased rate of blood flow on dialysis, declining dialysis adequacy, or elevated venous pressures on dialysis. Prolonged bleeding times from the access after needle removal may also indicate vascular congestion as a result of a venous outflow obstruction. Patients with a suspected stenosis should have an evaluation of their access with a fistulogram. A percutaneous transluminal angioplasty or surgical revision is warranted in lesions that are >50% of the luminal diameter. If angioplasty is required more than two times within a 3-month period, the patient should be referred back to vascular surgery for a possible revision. Stents are sometimes placed for surgically inaccessible lesions, limited access, or patients with surgical contraindications.

Thrombosis can be detected by the absence of a bruit or thrill and should be addressed promptly to salvage the access. Evaluation with a fistulogram is necessary to exclude the possibility of stenosis. Thrombectomies can be performed to treat AVG thrombosis, though they have limited success in AVF. Thrombosis of a fistula may require referral to the access surgeon for re-evaluation. If extensive surgical revision or new fistula placement is necessary, the patient may require a tunneled catheter for access until the new access is ready.

Poor flow from a catheter can result from malpositioning, kinking, thrombus formation, and central venous stenosis. Early malfunction, preventing successful use shortly after catheter placement, may require positional adjustments or an exchange over a guide wire. Thrombosis and stenosis should be suspected in previously functional catheters that are now unable to sustain flows >300 mL/minute. Intraluminal thrombosis is a common complication that can be treated by instilling the catheter with a thrombolytic agent, such as alteplase. A dwell time of 30 minutes is usually sufficient to restore flow, although a repeated trial for 30 to 60 minutes is warranted if suspected catheter thrombosis does not respond to the initial treatment. Persistent tunneled catheter failure warrants a contrast study to evaluate for a fibrin sheath. These can be removed or disrupted via fibrin sheath stripping or balloon angioplasty. The placement of stiff, nonsilicone catheters—particularly in the subclavian position—also increases the risk of central stenosis. While this may remain clinically silent during catheter use, it can cause dysfunction in subsequent AV accesses. For this reason, subclavian catheters should be avoided for HD unless absolutely necessary.

Recirculation. During a normal HD treatment, uremic blood leaves the patient's circulation through the arterial needle, is pumped through the dialysis system, and then returns to the patient's venous circulation. Recirculation is a phenomenon by which blood returning to the patient through the venous needle is taken back up by the arterial needle and recirculated through the dialysis mechanism (Fig. 25-1). Recirculation adversely affects the efficiency and adequacy of dialysis. Recirculation can occur from different mechanisms. Stenosis at the venous end of an access can impair flow and allow blood to be pulled back through the extracorporeal circuit. This can also occur if the site of venous return is in close proximity to the arterial outflow. Correction of stenosis, proper needle placement, and repositioning of dialysis catheters are all useful in decreasing the likelihood of access recirculation.

Ischemia and high flow. Any vascular access creates a pathway of extremely high blood flow. As a result, patients may experience symptoms of vascular steal or venous congestion. Limb ischemia as a result of a steal syndrome is an important complication of vascular access. Patients with mild symptoms, such as coldness or paresthesias, can be followed conservatively. However, pain and poor wound healing require surgical evaluation and motor/sensory loss is considered a surgical emergency. The high flows through vascular access may also be problematic for patients with cardiovascular disease. High output failure may be exacerbated due to the placement of an AVG and may require ligation to restore hemodynamic stability.

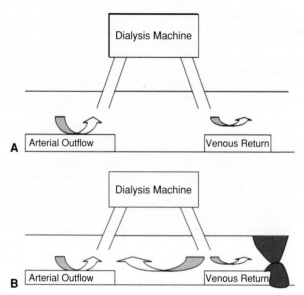

FIGURE. 25-1. **A:** Normal blood flow on dialysis. **B:** Access recirculation.

Infectious Complications

Infections represent the second most common cause of mortality in ESRD patients and are an important part of management in dialysis patients. Dialysis catheters are particularly susceptible to infection. Exit site infections are identified by wound cultures at the site of an erythematous or tender catheter. Infected sites should be cleaned thoroughly and topical antibiotics should be applied. In the presence of an exudate or discharge, wound cultures should be sent and IV antibiotics initiated. If there is discharge from the actual tunnel site, the catheter should be removed.

Catheter-related bacteremia is identified by constitutional symptoms along with growth from blood cultures and stigmata associated with catheter infection (purulence, erythema, tenderness). Initial antibiotic coverage should include gram-positive organisms, particularly Staphylococci, as well as gram-negative organisms. Dual coverage with vancomycin and gentamicin is recommended as empiric therapy. Blood culture growth, speciation, and antibiotic sensitivities should guide continued therapy. Removing an infected catheter is more successful than attempts to salvage catheters with antibiotics alone. However, as dialysis patients require regular access for treatment sessions, some find it impractical to remove all catheters. In a stable patient who demonstrates prompt clinical improvement and has no indications of a tunneled infection, immediate removal of the catheter may not be necessary and the patient should be started on a 3-week course of antibiotics. However, once blood cultures are negative, a catheter exchange is recommended. Patients who demonstrate a poor clinical response after 36 hours of antibiotic therapy or show any deterioration of clinical status should have the catheter promptly removed. If dialysis is necessary prior to clinical improvement, a temporary dialysis catheter can be placed for individual treatment sessions. Catheters should also be removed as soon as possible for all catheter-related infections with *Staphylococcus aureus* or gram-negative organisms.

Infections of grafts or fistulas are less common. Both should be treated aggressively with antibiotics. Areas of fluctuance should be evaluated with ultrasound for evidence of an abscess. Extensive graft infections may require partial or complete graft excisions. Infections of AVFs are rare and require a 6-week course of antibiotics. There should be a cautious examination for septic emboli or metastatic infections, particularly endocarditis and osteomyelitis. Occasionally, fistula resection is required.

Aneurysms and Pseudoaneurysms

Aneurysms and pseudoaneurysms can develop in fistulas and grafts, stimulated by the trauma of repetitive cannulation. Generally, these can be managed with observation and by avoiding cannulation at the site of aneurysmal dilation. However, in patients who demonstrate rapid growth of the aneurysm, poor eschar formation, or spontaneous bleeding, surgical evaluation should be made urgently. Rupture of an aneurysm or pseudoaneurysm can result in prompt exsanguination and imminent death.

BASIC MECHANISM OF HEMODIALYSIS: HOW DOES IT WORK?

The goal of HD is to replace the basic functions of the failing kidney. To approximate normal kidney function, HD must clear uremic solutes, adjust serum electrolytes, and remove accumulated fluid. During HD, blood from a uremic patient is passed through a dialyzer, a complex system of hollow fibers constructed from semipermeable membranes. While blood flows through the fibers in one direction, a prescribed dialysate solution flows through the adjacent space in the opposite direction. The difference in solute concentration and hydrostatic pressure drives the movement of fluid and solute from one compartment to another. The purified blood is eventually returned to the patient, while fluid from the dialysate compartment, which has absorbed uremic solutes and excess fluid, is discarded. **Diffusion** and **convection** are the mechanisms responsible for the balance of solutes and electrolytes. **Ultrafiltration** is the mechanism responsible for the removal of fluid.

It is no surprise that patients with renal failure need assistance with mechanical fluid removal. As patients become anuric, all fluid consumed becomes fluid retained. Fluid accumulation in the interstitial compartment can manifest as edema, ascites, or pleural effusion. HD must, therefore, be able to remove fluid volume from patients to avoid perpetual volume overload. Ultrafiltration utilizes a hydrostatic pressure gradient to move fluid from blood into the discarded dialysate. While ultrafiltration is primarily responsible for the alleviation of volume retention, the removal of fluid also contributes to the clearance of small- and middle-sized molecules that are carried through the pores of the dialysis membrane by the efflux of fluid from the blood to dialysate compartments. This mechanism of clearance is referred to as *convection* and is often described as a "solvent drag." Despite the ability of convection to remove uremic particles, it is not sufficient for the HD mechanism as it is unable to fine tune the electrolyte composition of the cleansed blood. Diffusion offers further clearance of uremic solutes while controlling the influx and efflux of electrolytes based on the concentration difference between the blood and the prescribed dialysate. While any molecule smaller than the membrane pore is capable of moving between compartments, diffusion favors the movement of smaller molecules, as they possess a higher particle velocity and a greater likelihood of contact with the membrane surface.

Dialysis Prescription

The dialysis prescription allows the physician to adjust the specifications of the dialysis treatment to the individual patient. The dialysis prescription should be tailored to the goals of attaining adequate clearance of toxins, correction of electrolyte abnormalities, and removing an appropriate volume of fluid. The variables that can be adjusted to achieve this are the constitution of the dialysate, the duration of treatment, the desired flow rate for both blood and dialysate, the surface area of the dialyzer, and the amount of ultrafiltration (Table 25-1). This section discusses these variables and how they can be adjusted to attain specific goals of therapy.

Attaining Dialysis Adequacy: Time, Flow, and Choice of Dialyzer

For chronic HD, the adequacy of dialysis dose is modeled by two equations, the Kt/V and the urea reduction ratio. Both can be measured with dialysis treatments and reflect the clearance of urea. Urea is not the sole toxin that accumulates in renal failure; however, studies have shown that urea removal is useful in predicting mortality rates on dialysis, and thus serves as a practical surrogate for dialysis adequacy.

Kt/V is a ratio that relates the volume of cleared plasma (Kt) to the volume of urea distribution (V). K is the dialyzer clearance—a variable affected by the rate of blood flow, dialysate flow rate, and the KoA (a manufacturer-predicted efficiency of a given dialysis membrane). V represents the volume of distribution, often estimated to be 55% of body weight, and t represents the time on dialysis in minutes. In practice, this figure is often reported as a single-pool Kt/V (spKt/V), reflecting this model's assumption that urea is removed from a single pool, or single compartment, of body water through which urea is distributed. In reality, the body is not comprised of one single pool of water, but numerous compartments. Because of this, there is typically a rebound in urea concentration after dialysis, which lowers the actual attained Kt/V by approximately 15%. Accordingly, the guidelines instituted by the National Kidney Foundation's Kidney Disease Outcomes Quality Initiative (KDOQI) set the *minimal* Kt/V for a patient dialyzed thrice weekly at 1.2 for each dialysis treatment. However, the *target* goal is 15% higher, a spKt/V of 1.4.

The **urea reduction rate (URR)** similarly reflects the removal of urea and is calculated by the simpler equation:

$$URR = (predialysis\ BUN - postdialysis\ BUN)/predialysis\ BUN$$

A Kt/V of 1.3 roughly correlates to a URR of 70%. KDOQI guidelines recommend the attainment of a minimal URR of 65% and a target URR of 70%.

When writing a prescription for a maintenance HD treatment, it should be realized that each variable contributes to a specific goal. For the goal of attaining adequate spKt/V and URR values, the principle variables are: duration of treatment, blood flow, dialysate flow, and dialyzer size. A **typical dialysis treatment** is between 3 and 4 hours in length, administered thrice weekly. Blood flow rate is largely dependent on the access used. Most grafts and fistulas can support blood flow between 400 and 500 cc/minute. Catheters are less predictable, and, on average, support flows of 350 to 400 cc/minute. Dialysate flow rate is generally between 500 and 800 cc/minute.

If a patient is not attaining target Kt/V or URR values, these variables should be evaluated and modified. Time is perhaps the easiest variable to increase and can be raised in 15-minute increments to improve dialysis clearances. But it is the least palatable option for patients and will ultimately be rendered ineffective if patients are unwilling to stay for the added duration. High-efficiency dialyzers, with a larger exposed surface area, can also be used to help improve adequacy. The availability of various dialyzers is institution dependent, though most dialysis facilities are stocked with high-efficiency dialyzers. Adjusting the dialysate flow rate is an option, particularly in those with a prescribed dialysate flow under 800 cc/minute, but it is unlikely that increasing the rate beyond 800 cc/minute will contribute significantly to improved clearance. In contrast, maximizing blood flows can be extremely helpful in attaining target goals. Patients with decreasing dialysis adequacy and poor blood flows from their access should be evaluated for vascular stenosis or thrombosis. Correction of flow-limiting complications or changing the type of access from a catheter to an AVG/AVF permits higher blood flows and improves dialysis adequacy.

TABLE 25-1	GUIDELINES FOR MAINTENANCE HEMODIALYSIS PRESCRIPTION		
Goal	**Variable**	**Typical Prescription**	**Comments**
Kt/V >1.2 (target Kt/V = 1.4)	Time	3–4 hours	Can be adjusted in 15-minute increments
	Frequency	3 times/week	Consider adding weekly treatments for large volumes of distribution.
OR			
URR >65% (target URR = 70%)	Dialyzer	Variable by institution	High-efficiency dialyzers have larger surface areas.
	Blood flow	350–450 mL/minute	AV grafts and fistulas: 400–500 mL/minute Catheters: 350–400 mL/minute
	Dialysate flow	500–800 mL/minute	Little benefit for dialysate flow rates >800 mL/minute
Electrolyte balance	Dialysate [K]	2–3 mEq/L	0 or 1 mEq/L can be used for severe hyperkalemia but requires monitoring of serum [K] at 30- to 60-minute intervals.
	Dialysate [Na]	140–145 mEq/L	Should be no more than 15–20 mEq/L higher than serum [Na] in patients with chronic hyponatremia.
	Dialysate [Ca]	2.5 mEq/L	Consider higher Ca content in ARF or hypocalcemia.
	Dialysate [HCO3]	35–38 mEq/L	Can be lowered to 28 mEq/L for alkalotic patients.
Volume regulation	Ultrafiltration	Based on EDW; typically 2–3 L	UF >4 L during a single treatment may lead to uncomfortable fluid shifts and hypotension.

ARF, acute renal failure; AV, arteriovenous; EDW, estimated dry weight; Kt/V, volume of cleared plasma (Kt) to the volume of urea distribution (V); UF, ultrafiltration; URR, urea reduction rate.

Attaining Electrolyte Balance: The Dialysate Composition

The choice of dialysate is the key variable for the balance of serum electrolytes and the correction of conditions such as hyperkalemia. As such, it is important to prescribe a dialysate that will be appropriate to the clinical scenario. Potassium, sodium, calcium, and bicarbonate levels are the primary electrolytes that can be controlled in the choice of a dialysate solution.

Potassium. Potassium concentration in the dialysate can vary widely depending on the patient's pre-HD potassium concentration. For a patient potassium ≥ 5.5 mEq/L, a dialysate potassium concentration of 2 or 3 mEq/L is appropriate. In those with a propensity toward arrhythmias, the 3-mEq/L bath is preferred to avoid precipitating hypokalemia. A dialysate potassium concentration of 4 mEq/L is appropriate for patients with hypokalemia or persistent serum potassium concentrations of <3.5 mEq/L. In those with a potassium concentration of >6.5 to 7.0 mEq/L or EKG changes concerning for hyperkalemia, a 0- or 1-mEq/L potassium bath may be required for a rapid correction. However, as this can cause a rapid fall in potassium levels, serum potassium levels should be monitored every 30 to 60 minutes. It is important to also acknowledge that there is a rebound in potassium levels 1 to 2 hours after dialysis. Further supplementation of potassium based on labs drawn immediately after a dialysis treatment is unwise unless there are extenuating circumstances.

Sodium. A dialysate sodium concentration of 140 to 145 mEq/L is appropriate in most circumstances, but can be adjusted in patients with pre-existing dysnatremias to prevent overcorrection. Low serum sodium levels in dialysis patients are often indicative of excessive free water intake in the context of limited, or absent, capacity for renal water handling. The majority of these patients can be managed through the enforcement of a fluid restriction. However, initiating dialysis on patients with chronic hyponatremia requires caution. When dialyzing patients with a chronic serum sodium concentration of <130 mEq/L, the dialysate sodium concentration should be no >15 to 20 mEq/L above the serum levels. Patients with hypernatremia should also be corrected slowly. Dialysate sodium should be between 3 and 5 mEq/L lower than serum levels.

Calcium. Most dialysate preparations are available with calcium concentrations of 2.5, 3, or 3.5 mEq/L. A 2.5-mEq/L calcium concentration is equivalent to an ionized calcium concentration of 5 mg/dL. In chronic HD patients, there are concerns about positive calcium balance contributing to vascular calcification and cardiovascular morbidity and mortality. Because of this, a 2.5-mEq/L Ca bath is generally recommended. In patients with persistent hypocalcemia, such as in patients who have had a parathyroidectomy, this may need to be increased to maintain serum calcium levels in a safe range. A higher calcium bath of 3 or 3.5 mEq/L is also used in patients who undergo HD acutely or have a significant concurrent acidosis, as the correction of acidosis on dialysis further lowers the plasma calcium concentrations.

Bicarbonate. Most chronic dialysis centers use dialysate solutions containing bicarbonate levels 35 to 38 mEq/L. This is usually sufficient to correct the metabolic acidosis associated with chronic renal failure. There are patients who are susceptible to alkalosis, particularly those who are receiving total parenteral nutrition, have vomiting or nasogastric suction, have poor protein intake, or have respiratory alkalosis. To avoid detrimental effects of alkalemia, including arrhythmias, headaches, or soft tissue calcifications, a lower bicarbonate bath of 20 to 28 mEq/L can be used.

Attaining Appropriate Volume Status: Prescribing Ultrafiltration

The goal of volume removal in dialysis patients is to attain the patient's estimated dry weight (EDW). The dry weight refers to a weight in which the patient is clinically euvolemic and does not demonstrate symptomatic volume contraction (particularly cramping). Ultrafiltrating fluid to the EDW allows physicians to remove fluid weight that is gained between dialysis treatments. Ideally, dialysis patients should restrict fluid intake to limit intradialytic weight gains to <4 kg, as excessive fluid gains may exceed the capacity to ultrafiltrate during a single treatment. This is particularly true in patients on intermittent HD who may go through a 3-day weekend period prior to their next dialysis treatment. Attempts to remove >4 to 5 L of fluid during a standard 3- to 4-hour treatment may cause uncomfortable fluid shifts and intradialytic hypotension. In patients who are well over their dry weight with evidence of edema, aggressive volume removal can be paired with additional treatments to continue ultrafiltration.

It is also important to acknowledge that a patient's dry weight is not a fixed number. As a result of improved or worsened nutritional status, a patient's dry weight may increase or decrease. This is a result of true weight that is gained, and not merely fluid retention. With this in mind, the clinical volume status of patients should be reviewed regularly. Patients with limited intradialytic fluid gains and no edema who note hypotension, lightheadedness, or severe cramping should be considered for an increase in their EDW. Patients who are attaining their usual EDW but develop worsening edema or shortness of breath should be challenged with fluid removal to a lower EDW to prevent florid volume retention.

Anticoagulation

Heparin administration during HD minimizes clotting of the dialysis circuit during the treatment. Clotting is particularly problematic among patients with high hemoglobin and hematocrit values, a high rate of ultrafiltration, and a low blood flow on dialysis. In the United States, **unfractionated heparin** is most commonly used to prevent this, although low-molecular-weight heparins can also be used. Heparin may be given as a bolus of 1000 to 2000 units, followed by a constant infusion of 1000 to 1200 units/hour. Alternatively, a bolus can be followed by repeated bolus dosing as necessary to maintain target clotting times.

COMPLICATIONS OF HEMODIALYSIS

Complications of Urea Clearance

Dialysis disequilibrium syndrome occurs in response to an acute reduction of uremic solutes in patients with chronic kidney disease. This is typically seen after the initiation of dialysis, when aggressive treatment prescriptions result in a rapid reduction of uremic solutes. Cells that have accommodated to the uremic milieu may not be able to rapidly respond to the dramatic osmolal change, resulting in symptoms of dialysis disequilibrium. This may manifest with nausea, restlessness, confusion or, in the most serious cases, seizure and coma. As a result, the goal of the first dialysis treatment is limited to a reduction of urea by no more than 30% to avoid a dramatic shift in solute concentration.

Uremia also contributes to nausea, malnutrition, and pruritus. The differential for these symptoms is broad, but special attention should be paid to the adequacy of dialysis. **Pruritus** may also result from concurrent disorders of mineral metabolism, particularly the deposition of mineral salts and hyperphosphatemia. Adherence to dietary restriction, compliance with phosphorus binders, and control of the parathyroid-bone-mineral axis are required. Symptoms of pruritus may also be amenable to diphenhydramine or other antihistamines, although oral administration is preferred due to the addictive potential of IV diphenhydramine.

Skin Diseases

Patients on HD are susceptible to all the common skin findings of the general population, such as rashes, acne, eczema, fungal infections, and venous stasis. However, there are two conditions unique to patients on dialysis.

Calcific uremic arteriolopathy, previously known as *calciphylaxis,* is caused by arteriolar mineralization and subsequent tissue ischemia. A number of factors thought to promote the underlying process of ectopic mineralization have been reported, including elevated phosphorus and parathyroid hormone levels and the administration of calcium-containing agents and the anticoagulant warfarin. Lesions often begin as erythematous or subcutaneous nodular lesions which can be very painful. Progression to poorly healing ulcerative lesions is associated with a high mortality rate, especially when located centrally. Treatment options are limited, but proper wound care is crucial to avoid infectious sequelae and subsequent amputations. Once the diagnosis is made, calcium-based supplements, vitamin D analogs, and warfarin should be stopped while non–calcium-based phosphorus binders are titrated for aggressive control of serum phosphorus levels. Sodium thiosulfate, which improves the solubility of calcium, has been used with variable success. In patients with refractory hyperparathyroidism or persistent hypercalcemia and hyperphosphatemia, parathyroidectomy can considered, though this does not guarantee an improvement in wound healing or a survival benefit.

Nephrogenic systemic fibrosis is a newly recognized condition characterized by progressive fibrosis and induration of skin, as well as other soft tissues. It tends to progress proximally, resulting in joint contractures and progressive immobility. Lesions typically have a "woody" texture. As of yet, there are no curative options. Cumulative exposure to gadolinium contrast agents have been associated with the development of nephrogenic systemic fibrosis and thus should be avoided if possible in patients with ESRD. If such a contrast study is necessary, most agree that immediate HD after contrast exposure is warranted.

Dialyzer Reactions

Dialyzer reactions are divided into **type A reactions** (in which severe dyspnea, pruritus, abdominal cramping, and angioedema occur in the first 30 minutes of treatment) and **type B reactions** (characterized by mild back pain and chest pain and occurring in the first hour of dialysis). Type A reactions have variously been attributed to ethylene oxide used in device sterilization, contaminated dialysate, latex allergy, and bradykinins, particularly in patients taking ACE inhibitors in conjunction with exposure to the AN69 dialysis membrane. Treatment of suspected type A reactions includes cessation of dialysis, diphenhydramine (25 mg IV for pruritus), oxygen as needed, and 200 mL normal saline if hypotensive. Blood should not be returned. To prevent subsequent reactions, an alternate sterilant may be tried, and dialyzers should be thoroughly rinsed before use. In type B reactions, one may attempt to treat through symptoms with supplemental oxygen and antihistamine therapy, as needed. Symptoms should diminish during the remainder of therapy. As the etiology of type B reactions is uncertain, methods for prevention are also uncertain, although trial of an alternate membrane may help.

Cardiovascular Complications

Cardiovascular disease is by far the largest cause of mortality in patients with ESRD. As patients are at great cardiovascular risk, chest pain should not be treated lightly in the dialysis units. While a high suspicion for coronary disease should be considered, a broad differential should be entertained, including musculoskeletal causes, dialyzer reactions, reflux disease, and pulmonary edema. In suspected angina, patients should be placed on nasal oxygen, ultrafiltration should be held, an ECG should be obtained, and nitroglycerin should be considered if tolerated by the blood pressure. If chest pain persists, dialysis should be discontinued and further workup afforded.

Both **hypotension** and **hypertension** are commonly seen in patients on dialysis. Hypotension may be a product of excessive volume removal and ultrafiltration should be stopped with saline return administered as necessary to maintain hemodynamic stability.

However, it is also important to rule out cardiovascular etiologies as well as infection or sepsis. Febrile patients who develop hypotension during dialysis treatments should have blood cultures drawn and empiric antibiotics dosed after treatment. The management of hypertension in patients with chronic kidney disease is discussed elsewhere in this book.

KEY POINTS TO REMEMBER

- HD is the most commonly utilized form of renal replacement therapy in the growing ESRD population.
- Cardiovascular disease is the most important cause of morbidity and mortality in the HD population.
- The placement of a successful dialysis access requires foresight and adequate planning to avoid catheter-related complications.
- The dialysis prescription should be tailored toward the specific goals of adequate clearance, electrolyte balance, and volume adjustment.

REFERENCES AND SUGGESTED READINGS

Bradbury BD, Fissell RB, Albert JM, et al. Predictors of early mortality among incident us hemodialysis patients in the Dialysis Outcomes and Practice Patterns Study (DOPPS). *Clin J Am Soc Nephrol.* 2007;2:89–99.

Brouns R, De Deyn PP. Neurological complications in renal failure: a review. *Clin Neurol Neurosurg.* 2004;107(1):1–16.

Cheung AK, Levin NW, Green T, et al. Effects of high-flux hemodialysis on clinical outcomes: results of the HEMO study. *J Am Soc Nephrol.* 2003;14(12):3251–3263.

Clase CM, Crowther MA, Alistair JI, et al. Thrombolysis for restoration of patency to haemodialysis central venous catheters: a systemic review. *J Thromb Thrombolysis.* 2001;11(2):127–136.

Daugirdas JT, Blake PG, Ing TS. *Handbook of Dialysis.* Baltimore: Lippincott Williams & Wilkins; 2007.

Daugirdas JT, Green T, Depner T, et al. Relationship between apparent (single-pool) and true (double-pool) urea distribution volume. *Kidney Int.* 1999;56(5):1928–1933.

Germain MJ, Cohen LM, Davison SN. Withholding and withdrawal from dialysis: what we know about how our patients die. *Semin Dial.* 2007;20(3):195–199.

Gotch FA. Evolution of the single-pool urea kinetic model. *Semin Dial.* 2001;14(4):252–256.

Jaber BL, Pereira JG. Dialysis reactions. *Semin Dial.* 1997;10:158–165.

Karnik JA, Young BS, Lew NL, et al. Cardiac arrest and sudden death in dialysis units. *Kidney Int.* 2001;60:350–357.

Katneni R, Hedayati SS. Central venous catheter-related bacteremia in chronic hemodialysis patients: epidemiology and evidence-based management. *Nat Clin Pract Nephrol.* 2007;3(5):256–266.

Korevaar JC, Jansen MA, Dekker FW, et al. When to initiate dialysis: effect of proposed US guidelines on survival. *Lancet.* 2001;358(9287):1046–1050.

Maya ID, Oser R, Saddekni S, et al. Vascular access stenosis: comparison of arteriovenous grafts and fistulas. *Am J Kidney Dis.* 2004;44(5):859–865.

National Kidney Foundation. *KDOQI Clinical Practice Guidelines.* Available at: http://www.kidney.org/professionals/kdoqi/guidelines.cfm. Accessed August 22, 2007.

Obrador GT, Arora P, Kausz AT, et al. Level of renal function at the initiation of dialysis in the U.S. end-stage renal disease population. *Kidney Int.* 1999;56(6):2227–2235.

Parnes EL, Shapiro WB. Anaphylactoid reactions in hemodialysis patients treated with the AN69 dialyzer. *Kidney Int.* 1991;40:1148.

Pierratos A. New approaches to hemodialysis. *Annu Rev Med.* 2004;55:179–189.

Rogers NM, Teubner D, Coates TH. Calcific uremic arteriolopathy: advances in pathogenesis and treatment. *Semin Dial.* 2007;20(2):150–157.

Roy-Chaudhury P, Spergel LM, Besarab A, et al. Biology of arteriovenous fistula failure. *J Nephrol.* 2007;20:150–163.

Saab G, Cheng S. Nephrogenic systemic fibrosis: a nephrologist's perspective. *Hemodial Int.* 2007;11:S2–S6.

Schanzer H, Eisenberg D. Management of steal syndrome resulting from dialysis access. *Semin Vasc Surg.* 2004;17(1):45–49.

U.S. Renal Data System. *USRDS 2006 Annual Data Report.* Bethesda, MD: National Institutes of Health, National Institute of Diabetes and Digestive and Kidney Diseases; 2006.

Xue JL, Dahl D, Ebben JP, et al. The association of initial hemodialysis access type with mortality outcomes in elderly Medicare ESRD patients. *Am J Kidney Dis.* 2003;42(5):1013–1019.

Peritoneal Dialysis

26

Seth Goldberg

INTRODUCTION

In the 1970s, the widening availability of peritoneal dialysis (PD) made this a viable alternative for patients with end-stage renal disease requiring renal replacement therapy. However, the more recent trend in the United States has been in the opposite direction. Approximately 10% to 15% of dialysis patients in the United States utilize PD. While the treatment costs of PD and hemodialysis are similar, the overall cost of care for hemodialysis patients is higher when vascular access problems are considered. PD patients generally require fewer hospitalizations and shorter durations of hospital stay. Although neither dialysis modality conveys a survival advantage, greater satisfaction and convenience are qualities frequently promoted by patients on PD as compared with their counterparts on hemodialysis.

PATIENT SELECTION

Success of any dialysis modality depends heavily on patient characteristics. This is especially true regarding PD. Patients offered this modality need to be highly motivated to perform regular treatments in a home environment. Either the patient or a suitable assistant must be able to learn and perform the physical tasks required to set up the PD apparatus. Typically, patients starting on PD are those who prefer PD over hemodialysis or who are not able to tolerate hemodialysis secondary to congestive heart disease, vascular problems, or access difficulty.

Several **contraindications** for PD exist. A recent abdominal operation or the presence of uncorrectable mechanical defects, such as an irreparable abdominal hernia, would exclude PD as an option. Relative contraindications include a recent aortic vascular graft, frequent episodes of diverticulitis, abdominal wall cellulitis, or history of repeated abdominal operations with adhesion formation. Patients who are physically unable to perform their own exchanges or who lack a suitable caregiver at home are also poor candidates for this modality.

As with other forms of renal replacement therapy, early patient discussion and planning is important to facilitate a smooth transition from chronic disease to end-stage disease. In the chronic setting, renal replacement therapy is indicated when the estimated glomerular filtration rate drops to <10 to 15 mL/minute. The decision is typically made when conservative measures are unable to control electrolyte abnormalities, volume overload, or uremic symptoms. As PD catheters may take several weeks to fully mature, anticipation of their need is required as the patient approaches this threshold.

PHYSIOLOGY OF PERITONEAL DIALYSIS

As in conventional hemodialysis, PD involves solute and water transport across a semi-permeable membrane separating two fluid-filled compartments. The compartments consist of blood in the peritoneal capillaries and the dialysis solution in the peritoneal cavity. Urea, creatinine, potassium, and other waste products of metabolism are present in higher concentrations in the blood. Three transport processes occur simultaneously during PD.

- **Diffusion**: As in conventional hemodialysis, uremic solutes and potassium diffuse down their concentration gradients from the peritoneal capillaries to the dialysis solution. Glucose diffuses in the opposite direction, also along its concentration gradient. Calcium also diffuses into the capillaries, although to a lesser extent given the lower concentration now used in dialysis solutions.
- **Ultrafiltration**: Water is removed from the peritoneal capillaries as it primarily travels down the osmotic gradient into the relatively hyperosmolar dialysis solution. This differs from convection utilized in hemodialysis, which relies on a transmembrane pressure to force water across the membrane.
- **Absorption**: This process, by which solutes and water return to the circulation either directly into the capillaries or through abdominal wall lymphatics, counteracts their removal. Some of the protein that diffuses into the peritoneal cavity is reclaimed by this process.

PERITONEAL DIALYSIS SYSTEM

There are three major components in the PD system. These include the dialysis catheter, dialysis solution, and the peritoneal membrane.

Dialysis Catheter and Transfer Sets

Most centers use a typical two-cuff silastic Tenckhoff catheter. The intra-abdominal portion contains multiple perforations to allow fluid to more easily enter and leave the peritoneal cavity. When surgically placed, approximately 10 to 14 days should elapse prior to initiating PD. This allows the wound to heal and reduces the incidence of leaks and early infection. The patient should avoid submerging the catheter in water during this period. Catheter modifications have been developed to attempt to reduce the incidence of exit-site infections or of peritonitis. The bent, or swan-neck, catheters allow for easier creation of a downward exit-site, which may reduce the rate of infectious complications. Tunneled presternal catheters are advantageous in patients in whom body habitus makes the placement of an abdominal exit-site difficult.

The Y-set is the standard setup used in manual PD (Fig. 26-1). Here, a fill-bag and a drain-bag are connected to the stem attached to the patient, each tube with its own clamp. Patients should use the flush-before-fill technique, in which the stem is clamped and a small volume of dialysis solution is allowed to pass into the drain bag in order to flush out the air in the tubing. The drain bag is then clamped and the stem opened, to allow the solution to fill the peritoneal cavity via gravity (10–15 minutes). The bags are clamped and the apparatus disconnected to allow the patient to continue with daily activities. Once the dwell time is completed, a new transfer set is connected and the stem and drain bag are unclamped. The peritoneal cavity is emptied via gravity (20–25 minutes) into the drain bag. The stem is then clamped and a new exchange can be initiated, again with the flush-before-fill technique.

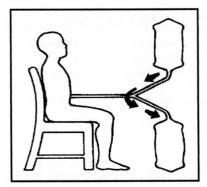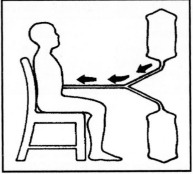

FIGURE 26-1. The Y set for peritoneal dialysis (PD), with demonstration of the "flush-before-fill" technique.

Dialysis Solutions

Standard PD solutions contain sodium, chloride, lactate, magnesium, calcium, and varying concentrations of dextrose (Table 26-1). Most commercial solutions contain a sodium concentration of 132 mEq/L, allowing sodium to move down its concentration gradient from the blood into the peritoneal solution. This protects against hypernatremia that might otherwise occur with ultrafiltration, particularly with the more hypertonic solutions. Potassium is not present in standard solutions. Phosphorus is also absent, but its removal with PD is usually insufficient to fully account for the dietary load. In the present era of widespread use of calcium-containing phosphate binders, a PD solution with a lower calcium concentration (2.5 mEq/L) is considered standard. Lactate has been used as the primary acid-base buffer due to technical problems with bicarbonate in the preparation of solutions. Lactate and the acidic pH (5.5) can be damaging to the mesothelium and may partially account for the inflow pain experienced by some patients. Newer dual-chamber bags with bicarbonate are becoming available and can be mixed at the time of use, avoiding the caramelization of dextrose that occurs during the autoclaving process.

The relatively hyperosmolar dialysis solution allows ultrafiltration to occur. The dextrose concentration is typically 1.5%, 2.5%, or 4.25%, with the higher concentrations

TABLE 26-1	STANDARD PERITONEAL DIALYSIS SOLUTION COMPONENTS
Sodium	132 mEq/L
Potassium	0 mEq/L
Chloride	Variable (95–105 mEq/L)
Calcium	2.5 mEq/L (1.25 mmol/L) or 3.5 mEq/L (1.75 mmol/L)
Phosphorus	0 mEq/L
Magnesium	1.5 mEq/L or 0.5–0.75 mEq/L
Lactate	35 mEq/L or 40 mEq/L
Dextrose	Variable (1.5%, 2.5%, 4.25%)

TABLE 26-2 DEXTROSE-CONTAINING DIALYSIS SOLUTIONS

Dextrose	Glucose	Osmolarity	Color Code
1.5% (1.5 g/dL)	1.36 g/dL	346 mOsm/L	Yellow
2.5% (2.5 g/dL)	2.27 g/dL	396 mOsm/L	Green
4.25% (4.25 g/dL)	3.86 g/dL	485 mOsm/L	Red

providing a stronger osmotic gradient to achieve a greater degree of ultrafiltration. Some commercially available solutions have color-coded tabs with which patients may be more familiar rather than the percent of dextrose (Table 26-2). One major drawback with the use of dextrose is that as much as 60% to 80% can be absorbed, thereby dissipating the osmotic gradient and limiting the total ultrafiltration that can be achieved, particularly with longer dwells. A newer solution with icodextrin, a glucose-polymer preparation, has the added advantage of not being significantly absorbed, and thus has a more sustained osmotic effect. This effect is more pronounced in longer dwell times, and can sustain an ultrafiltration equivalent to a 2.5% dextrose solution in a dwell of up to 18 hours. However, in the shorter cycled dwells, this osmotic effect is less pronounced. Of note, the icodextrin can falsely elevate glucose levels on some test strips and such results must be interpreted cautiously.

Mixtures of amino acids have been studied as an alternative to high dextrose concentrations in generating an osmotic gradient. While the ultrafiltration capacity is somewhat reduced (equivalent to 1.5% dextrose solutions), there is the potential to avoid some of the metabolic complications associated with hyperglycemia. With reduced glucose degradation products, there may be better peritoneal membrane preservation. There is also the theoretical advantage in improving nutritional parameters, although this has yet to be conclusively demonstrated to justify the significantly higher cost of amino acid solutions. Drawbacks include a mild degree of acidosis and elevations in the serum urea concentration.

Peritoneal Membrane

The PD interface consists of multiple layers separating the blood from the peritoneal fluid: the vascular endothelium, basement membrane, interstitium, and peritoneal mesothelium, as well as unstirred fluid layers on both sides (blood and peritoneal fluid). The peritoneal membrane has a total surface area of approximately 2 m² in adults, consisting of both the parietal and visceral layers. The three-pore model describes large pores (>25 nm) through which proteins and other macromolecules pass, small pores (4–6 nm) for electrolytes and other small solutes such as urea and creatinine, and ultrasmall pores (0.3–0.5 nm), which serve much like aquaporins allowing only solute-free water to pass. The peritoneal cavity can usually accommodate 2 to 3 L of fluid without patient discomfort or respiratory compromise.

Peritoneal Equilibration Test

There is considerable variability in the composition and character of the peritoneal membrane among patients. Knowing this is important because the membrane type determines the efficiency of solute transport and quality of ultrafiltration. Four classes of transporters are defined, based on the degree of creatinine diffusion: high, high-average, low-average, and low (Table 26-3). In order to determine the type of membrane present, a peritoneal equilibration test (PET) is performed. A 2-L infusion of 2.5% dextrose solution is allowed to dwell for 4 hours, then a dialysate-to-plasma ratio of creatinine (D/P) is calculated. Higher values correlate with more efficient movement of solutes. While this allows for better clearance of uremic solutes, there is also greater absorption of dextrose, dissipating

TABLE 26-3 PERITONEAL MEMBRANE TYPES

Membrane Type	D/P Creatinine Ratio	Characteristics
High	>0.81	Transports solutes quickly, poor ultrafiltration and problems with protein loss
High average	0.65–0.81	Transports solutes well, with adequate ultrafiltration
Low average	0.50–0.64	Transports solutes somewhat slowly, with good ultrafiltration
Low	<0.50	Transports solutes slowly, with excellent ultrafiltration

D/P, dialysate-to-plasma.

the osmotic gradient and limiting ultrafiltration. The Canada-USA (CANUSA) Study Group found a greater risk of technique failure or death in patients with high transport membranes undergoing CAPD. The underlying mechanism for this increased risk is thought to involve poorer ultrafiltration as well as increased albumin loss and malnutrition.

PERITONEAL DIALYSIS MODALITIES AND PRESCRIPTIONS

Continuous Ambulatory Peritoneal Dialysis (CAPD)

CAPD involves patient-operated manual exchanges performed throughout the day. Fluid volumes of 2 to 3 L are typically used, with dwell times ranging from 4 to 8 hours. Most patients are educated and trained in CAPD prior to learning other modalities, as this can be used as a backup or emergency modality in the event of machine malfunction or power outage. Patients admitted overnight to the hospital can also resort to CAPD if nurse staffing or machine availability is limited. A sample prescription would be 2 L of 2.5% dextrose solution with four exchanges of approximately 6 hours each (or can be spaced unevenly at more convenient times of day such as awakening, noon, dinner, and bedtime).

Continuous Cycling Peritoneal Dialysis (CCPD)

In CCPD, the patient undergoes automated exchanges overnight, with three or more cycles (2 hours each, for example). The final exchange remains in the peritoneal cavity, and the patient disconnects from the machine and is free to go about daily activities. The "continuous" label in the name of this modality refers to the retained daytime dwell that allows for solute transfer to take place around the clock. A manual exchange is sometimes added to this regimen during the daytime if required for solute or fluid issues. A sample prescription would have four dwells of 2 hours each, with 2.5 L of 2.5% dextrose solution as well as a final fill (daytime dwell) of 2 L of icodextrin.

Nocturnal Intermittent Peritoneal Dialysis (NIPD)

NIPD is an automated modality similar to CCPD except that the final nighttime cycle is fully drained and the patient's peritoneal cavity remains "dry" throughout the day. Solute clearances tend to be lower without the continuous daytime dwell, but with fewer mechanical complications. Patients with good residual renal function may prefer this option.

Prescriptions

In choosing a PD modality, the patient's membrane type should be known, as determined from the results of a PET described above. Patients at either end of the spectrum require special consideration. Those with high transport membranes dissipate their osmotic gradients more rapidly, and thus may require short dwell times to achieve adequate ultrafiltration. These patients tend to fare better on cycled dialysis without a long daytime dwell. Those with low transport membranes require long dwell times to achieve adequate solute clearance. Therefore, the long, evenly spaced dwells of CAPD are preferred in this subgroup. Patients with either high-average or low-average transporter membranes can usually achieve solute removal and ultrafiltration targets regardless of modality; thus selection can generally depend on patient preference.

DIALYSIS ADEQUACY

As with hemodialysis, a specific clearance target is defined in measuring the adequacy of PD. The updated National Kidney Foundation's Kidney Disease Outcomes Quality Initiative (KDOQI) guidelines from 2006 recommend a weekly clearance of urea (Kt/V_{urea}) of at least 1.7. This value should reflect the combined contribution from PD and residual renal function in patients making >100 mL of urine per day. Prior targets based on the calculated weekly creatinine clearance have been dropped as they demonstrated no survival advantage.

The weekly Kt/V_{urea} should be measured within the first month after initiating therapy. Thereafter, it is usually measured at 4-month intervals unless there has been a prescription change or a significant change in the clinical status of the patient. The urea clearance is calculated from the 24-hour values of total dialysate effluent volume in liters (V_D), dialysate urea concentration (D_{urea}), and plasma urea concentration (P_{urea}).

$$24\text{-hour } Kt/V_{urea} = (V_D)(D_{urea})/(P_{urea})(V_{urea})$$

The volume of distribution for urea (V_{urea}) is represented by the total body water and can be estimated (in liters) by the anthropometric Watson or Hume formulae. The weekly adequacy of PD can then be calculated by multiplying the 24-hour value by 7 days.

Residual renal function must be considered as it may significantly contribute to the overall solute clearance achieved by a patient. Therefore, the residual contribution needs to be added to the above calculations in patients making >100 mL of urine per day. The same equations listed above can be utilized with the 24-hour urine volume replacing the total dialysate effluent volume and the urine urea concentration replacing that of the dialysate. These urine values should be measured at a minimum of every 2 months. Steps to preserve native kidney function, such as the avoidance of nephrotoxins, should be followed in the PD population. The KDOQI guidelines recommend preference be given to ACE inhibitors and angiotensin receptor blockers (ARBs) in hypertensive patients and to be considered even in normotensive individuals in order to decrease the rate of loss of renal function. The Adequacy of Peritoneal Dialysis in Mexico (ADEMEX) study showed a statistically significant association between loss of residual renal function and death.

Ultrafiltration targets are less clearly defined. Clinical assessment of volume status often determines the need to alter the PD prescription. A minimum of 750 mL of net fluid removal per day has been associated with better outcomes in anuric patients. To enhance ultrafiltration, a higher dextrose concentration (4.25% solution) can be used, as can shorter dwell times. Also, a glucose-polymer (icodextrin) can be added to a daytime dwell to further increase fluid removal. Dietary restriction of sodium and water should be practiced in states of volume overload. Diuretics can also be employed to take advantage of residual renal function. *Ultrafiltration failure* is a term used to describe a condition of fluid overload in association with net ultrafiltration of <400 mL after a 4-hour dwell with 2 L of 4.25% dextrose solution. This can result from the rapid diffusion of the dextrose (high transporters), decreased peritoneal membrane water permeability (peritonitis, fibrosis, adhesions), or by rapid lymphatic drainage. When the management strategies described above fail to control the fluid overload, a temporary or even permanent transition to hemodialysis may be required.

COMPLICATIONS

Complications that occur in PD can be divided into three major categories: infectious, mechanical, and metabolic. Some of the common signs and symptoms found in PD patients are described in Table 26-4.

Infectious Complications

Peritonitis

Peritonitis remains a common and potentially serious complication in the PD population. Although many cases can be readily treated in the outpatient setting, recurrent episodes can threaten the long-term integrity of the peritoneal membrane. Causes most commonly involve an inadvertent break in sterile technique or migration of pathogens from the catheter site. Transvisceral passage of bacteria from diverticulitis can also result in peritonitis.

Patients typically present with cloudy peritoneal fluid, abdominal pain, and fever. The dialysate effluent, preferably from a dwell of at least 4 hours, should be evaluated by gram stain, culture, and white blood cell count with differential. A white blood cell count >100 cells/mm^3, of which at least 50% are polymorphonuclear neutrophils, is supportive of the diagnosis of microbial peritonitis. Culture of the dialysate effluent should always be sent before initiation of antibiotics, but culture results should not delay initiation of therapy.

The International Society of Peritoneal Dialysis has recommended **empiric therapy** using a combination of a first-generation cephalosporin (cefazolin or cephalothin) with ceftazidime. Routine use of vancomycin is discouraged to avoid selecting for resistance. Also, routine aminoglycoside therapy is not recommended in order to protect residual renal function. In most cases, intraperitoneal dosing of antibiotics is the preferred route of treatment. When patients are bacteremic or overtly septic, intravenous antibiotics should be administered. Suggested intraperitoneal doses for selected antibiotics are listed in Table 26-5. Those listed refer to the intermittent dosing schedules where the antibiotics are added only to the longest dwell (nighttime fill for CAPD, daytime dwell for CCPD).

Treatment strategies after the results of the gram stain and culture are available are outlined in Table 26-6. Gram-positive infections can frequently be treated with a single antibiotic agent and this can be tailored once sensitivities are available. Infections with *Pseudomonas* are particularly difficult to eradicate and a second antibiotic to which it is sensitive is recommended. In many of these cases (two-thirds in one report), catheter removal becomes necessary.

In general, the fluid should be recultured and the exit site reexamined for possible involvement if there is no clinical improvement after 4 days of therapy. The presence of an intra-abdominal abscess should be considered, particularly if the infection is polymicrobial or caused by anaerobic bacteria. Imaging or surgical exploration may be required in these cases. In general, many clinicians believe that catheter removal is indicated immediately after identification of fungal peritonitis.

Exit-Site and Tunnel Infections

Catheter infections at the exit site or within the tunnel itself are suspected when erythema and exudates are present externally. Crust formation at the exit site, however, does not

TABLE 26-4 COMMON SIGNS AND SYMPTOMS IN PD PATIENTS

Sign/Symptom	Character	Causes	Management Issues
Abdominal pain	Inflow pain	Excessively large volume of dwell Low pH of infused solution	Reduce volume of dwell Add bicarbonate to solution (10 mEq/L)
	Diffuse/rebound	Peritonitis	Check fluid cell count and differential, culture, Gram stain, empiric antibiotics
		Bowel obstruction	Abdominal or vascular imaging
		GI tract pathology (appendicitis, mesenteric ischemia)	
	Focal/localized	Abdominal hernia	Surgical correction
		Constipation	Trial of stool softener or enema
Change in dialysate	Cloudy	Peritonitis	Check fluid cell count and differential (eosinophils for allergic process), culture, gram stain, empiric antibiotics
		Allergic reaction to solution or dialysis equipment	
		Chylous leak/superior vena cava syndrome	Check triglyceride level
		Pancreatitis	Check amylase level
		GI tract pathology (appendicitis, mesenteric ischemia)	Abdominal or vascular imaging
		Fibrin strands	Add heparin (200–500 units/L) into dialysis solution for fibrin strands
	Bloody	Malignancy	Check dialysate fluid cytology
		Sclerosing encapsulating peritonitis	Abdominal imaging, with possible need for biopsy
		Gynecologic source (retrograde menstruation, cyst rupture)	
		Tuberculous peritonitis	*Mycobacterium tuberculosis* polymerase chain reaction (PCR)
Fever	Temperature >38°C	Peritonitis	Check fluid cell count and differential (eosinophils for allergic process), culture, Gram stain, empiric antibiotics
		Allergic reaction to solution or dialysis equipment	
		GI tract pathology (appendicitis, mesenteric ischemia)	Abdominal or vascular imaging
		Exit-site or tunnel infection	General fever workup as in nondialysis patients
		Nonabdominal infectious source	

TABLE 26-5 INTRAPERITONEAL DOSES OF SELECTED ANTIBIOTICS

Antibiotic	Intraperitoneal Dose
Cefazolin, cephalothin	15–20 mg/kg/bag every day
Ceftazidime	15–20 mg/kg/bag every day
Gentamicin, tobramycin	0.6 mg/kg/bag every day
Amikacin	2 mg/kg/bag every day
Vancomycin	15–30 mg/kg every 5–7 days
Ampicillin	125 mg/L/bag every day
Aztreonam	1 g/L loading, then 250 mg/L/bag every day

necessarily indicate infection, and positive cultures in the absence of other symptoms may simply indicate colonization. *Staphylococcus aureus* is the most common cause of exit-site infections. As with peritonitis, the Gram stain and culture are helpful in guiding antibiotic therapy. Gram-positive organisms can be treated with an oral cephalosporin or penicillinase-resistant antibiotic; resistant strains may require vancomycin and rifampin. Gram-negative organisms can usually be treated with oral ciprofloxacin 500 mg b.i.d. With *Pseudomonas aeruginosa*, addition of ceftazidime or an aminoglycoside may become necessary, as well as catheter removal. For infections that respond to therapy, antibiotics can be discontinued after 2 weeks. Relapsing infections or those that progress to tunnel infections may necessitate catheter removal.

Meticulous exit-site care is essential to preventing such infectious complications. Hands should be washed for 2 minutes prior to manipulating the catheter dressings or exit site. Daily application of 0.1% gentamicin cream has been shown to be effective in reducing the incidence of exit-site infections with *Staphylococcus aureus* and *Pseudomonas aeruginosa*. Catheter anchorage with tape and gauze dressings helps to prevent exit-site trauma. Vigorous scrubbing at the exit-site should be avoided.

Mechanical Complications

Outflow Failure

Outflow failure is suspected when the drain volumes are consistently and substantially less than the volumes being infused in the absence of fluid leakage. Causes include catheter kinking, constipation, adhesion formation, or fibrin plugging. Dissection of fluid along the abdominal wall can also be a cause of apparent outflow failure, manifesting as scrotal edema. Examination of the catheter, exit-site, or tunnel may reveal a mechanical obstruction to flow. Plain films of the abdomen can be helpful in evaluating the intra-abdominal course of the catheter, which should ideally be directed toward the pelvis to avoid contact with the omentum. These problems can occasionally be corrected conservatively but may require catheter replacement. Constipation should be treated with laxatives or enemas as the situation requires. Magnesium and phosphate products should be avoided in the renal failure population. Fibrin strands can sometimes be visualized in the dialysate and management includes infusion of heparin into the dialysis solution (200–500 units/L) or placement of a thrombolytic agent in the catheter lumen (tissue plasminogen activator 1 mg/mL for 1 hour). Heparin is not systemically absorbed from the peritoneal cavity, minimizing the risk of systemic anticoagulation.

Hernias

Abdominal hernias develop in 10% to 20% of patients on PD. They result from the increased intra-abdominal pressure created by the peritoneal fluid. Risk factors include large volume dwells, a sitting position during dwells, obesity, and multiparity. Any condition

TABLE 26-6 TREATMENT OF PERITONITIS

Type	Organism	Antibiotic Choices		Duration
Gram positive	Enterococcus	Ampicillin IP, consider adding aminoglycoside	Vancomycin or quinupristin/dalfopristin if resistant	14 days
	Staphylococcus aureus	First-generation cephalosporin IP with oral rifampin (600 mg/day)	Vancomycin or clindamycin if resistant	21 days
	Other gram positives	First-generation cephalosporin IP	Vancomycin or clindamycin if resistant	14 days
Gram negative	Pseudomonas/ Stenotrophomonas	Ceftazidime IP with aminoglycoside IP if urine <100 mL/day	If urine >100 mL/day, substitute aminoglycoside with oral ciprofloxacin (500 mg b.i.d.), or IV piperacillin (4 g b.i.d.), or oral TMP-SMX (double strength per day), or aztreonam IP	21 days
	Other single gram negatives	Aminoglycoside IP if urine <100 mL/day	Ceftazidime IP if urine >100 mL/day	14 days
	Multiple gram negatives or anaerobes	Cefazolin IP, ceftazidime IP, and oral metronidazole (500 mg t.i.d.)	Consider imaging and/or surgical intervention if no improvement	21 days
Fungal	Yeasts or other fungi	Oral flucytosine (load 2 g/day, maintenance 1 g/day) and oral fluconazole (200 mg/day)	If no improvement, remove catheter and continue therapy for one week after catheter removal	4–6 weeks

IP, intraperitoneal; TMP/SMX, trimethoprim-sulfamethoxazole.

that weakens the abdominal musculature, such as deconditioning, can also pose a risk for hernia formation. Diagnosis is largely clinical and treatment is typically with surgical repair. Small abdominal hernias carry the greatest risk for bowel incarceration and should be surgically corrected. In all cases, patients should be made aware of the warning signs of bowel strangulation, including the loss of reducibility and pain at the hernia site. After surgical repair of a hernia, intra-abdominal pressure must be kept as low as possible to facilitate healing. If the patient has good residual renal function it may be possible to discontinue PD altogether for 1 week, then gradually reinitiate with small volumes (1-L exchanges) for another week. Supine dialysis also helps to reduce intra-abdominal pressure. If the patient has little reserve renal function and low-volume PD is not tolerated, temporary hemodialysis may become necessary until the wound is completely healed. These principles and precautions also apply to any postoperative situation where entry into the abdominal cavity was necessary.

Fluid Leakage

Risk factors for **fluid leakage** are similar to those for hernia formation. Early leaks are those that occur in the first month after implantation and are typically found at the exit site. Late leaks can extend into the subcutaneous tissue or into the pleural space causing a hydrothorax. Clinical manifestations may be subtle and patients may present with weight gain and diminished drainage. Hydrothoraces are almost exclusively found on the right side as the left hemidiaphragm has additional coverage by the heart and pericardium. A diagnostic thoracentesis reveals markedly elevated glucose concentrations when the pleural fluid originates from the peritoneal solution. Treatment for fluid leakage entails draining the peritoneum dry for 24 to 48 hours. If the leak recurs, longer periods off PD may be required, supported with temporary hemodialysis. A hydrothorax that is symptomatic requires medical or surgical pleurodesis.

Genital edema is a specific form of fluid leakage and can occur in PD patients via a patent processus vaginalis that results in a hydrocele. Also, a defect in the abdominal wall at the catheter site may allow tracking of the dialysis solution along the anterior wall and result in scrotal edema. As with abdominal hernias, reduction in the intra-abdominal pressure with small-volume or supine PD may alleviate the symptoms. Anatomic defects, however, may need to be corrected surgically.

Sclerosing Encapsulating Peritonitis

Sclerosing encapsulating peritonitis, an uncommon clinical entity, can present with nausea, vomiting, anorexia, or decreased PD adequacy or ultrafiltration. The incidence is approximately 2.5% and it is more commonly seen in patients receiving long-term PD. It may also occur after discontinuation of PD. A bloody dialysate fluid may alert the physician to this process. The peritoneal membrane becomes thickened and rigid, with entrapment of bowel loops that can lead to symptoms of intermittent obstruction. Although the mechanism is not clearly defined, chemical irritation of the peritoneal membrane is suspected as an inciting event. Recurrent bouts of peritonitis have also been implicated. Treatment options center around bowel rest and surgical lysis of adhesions when obstruction occurs. Most patients require conversion to hemodialysis. Trials of immunosuppression using prednisolone in doses ranging from 10 to 40 mg/day have shown limited benefit.

Back Pain

In the PD population, **back pain** results from a shift in the patient's center of gravity. This can produce excess stress on the lumbar spine. Management includes bedrest in the acute situation, along with decreasing the volume of the dwells. A concomitant increase in dialysis frequency may be required to maintain adequate solute clearance. Where applicable, physical therapy with muscle-strengthening exercises may alleviate symptoms.

Metabolic Complications

Hyperglycemia

Hyperglycemia is a frequently occurring complication with PD, with as much as three-quarters of the dextrose in the dialysis solution may be absorbed during a dwell. Patients with underlying diabetes or glucose intolerance are most susceptible to such complications. This contributes to the 5% to 10% weight gain frequently observed in a patient's first year on PD.

Hyperlipidemia

An atherogenic lipid profile is also frequently encountered in PD patients. The constant diffusion of dextrose from the dialysis solution results in markedly elevated triglycerides as well as the elevation in total cholesterol and low-density lipoprotein (LDL). Smaller proteins, such as high-density lipoprotein (HDL), are preferentially lost in the dialysate, further increasing the cardiovascular risk. As with other causes of hyperlipidemia, treatment focuses on dietary modifications and exercise. HMG-coenzyme A reductase inhibitors are recommended as first-line medical therapy. Specific LDL cholesterol targets in PD patients have not been defined, and in the absence of established coronary disease or coronary disease equivalents, the accepted target is <100 mg/dL.

Protein Loss and Malnutrition

Protein loss of approximately 0.5 g/L of drainage occurs in PD, and the rate of loss may be even greater in patients with high transport membranes. This adversely affects the nutritional status of the patient. The major protein lost is albumin and thus it is not unusual for PD patients to have low albumin levels. Factors that increase the membrane's permeability, such as peritonitis, can significantly increase the total amount of protein lost, as can underlying proteinuria in the nonanuric patient. The KDOQI guidelines recommend a dietary protein intake of 1.2 to 1.3 g/kg/day for chronic PD patients.

Hypokalemia

Hypokalemia has been observed in up to one-third of PD patients. Potassium balance is determined by internal redistribution and external gains and losses. Because potassium is generally absent from standard PD solutions, there is net removal with near equilibration of blood and dialysate levels. Furthermore, the level of endogenous insulin is increased, stimulated by the continuous uptake of carbohydrates from the dialysis solution. This results in an intracellular shift of potassium and hypokalemia. Poor nutritional states in hospitalized patients are also associated with hypokalemia in the PD population. When mild, management can be conservative with loosening of dietary restrictions and oral potassium supplementation. More severe hypokalemia may require addition of potassium to the PD solution.

INDICATIONS FOR SWITCHING TO HEMODIALYSIS

Despite the safety and efficacy of PD, patients are sometimes required to switch to hemodialysis. Reasons to do so include the following:

- Consistent failure to achieve adequacy targets (Kt/V_{urea} <1.7)
- Inadequate solute transport or fluid removal
- Severe hypertriglyceridemia that is difficult to manage
- Frequent peritonitis or other infectious complications
- Irreparable mechanical problems, including sclerosing encapsulating peritonitis
- Severe protein malnutrition resistant to aggressive management

As with other forms of renal replacement, the leading causes of death for patients on PD are cardiovascular disease and infections. A statistically significant association between loss of residual renal function and mortality has been demonstrated, stressing the importance of preserving native kidney function wherever possible.

KEY POINTS TO REMEMBER

- PD is underutilized in the United States.
- High transport peritoneal membranes have poorer ultrafiltration, while low transport peritoneal membranes have slower solute transfer.
- PD orders should generally include the exchange volume, exchange frequency, dwell time, and dextrose concentration.
- Residual renal function is very important in PD patients and must be preserved whenever possible; the renal clearance of urea is added to the peritoneal clearance when calculating adequacy of treatment.
- Peritonitis must be treated early and aggressively; empiric antibiotics should be infused intraperitoneally and tailored once culture results are available.

REFERENCES AND SUGGESTED READINGS

Brown EA, Davies SJ, Rutherford P, et al. Survival of functionally anuric patients on automated peritoneal dialysis: the European APD outcome study. *J Am Soc Nephrol.* 2003;14:2948.

Churchill DN, Thorpe KE, Nolph KD, et al. Increased peritoneal membrane transport is associated with decreased patient and technique survival for continuous peritoneal dialysis patients: the Canada-USA (CANUSA) peritoneal dialysis study group. *J Am Soc Nephrol.* 1998;9:1285.

Daugirdas JT, Blake PG, Ing TS. *Handbook of Dialysis.* 3rd ed. Philadelphia: Lippincott Williams & Wilkins; 2001.

Flanigan M, Gokal R. Catheters and exit-site practices toward optimum peritoneal access: a review of current developments. *Perit Dial Int.* 2005;25:132.

Kawanishi H, Kawaguchi Y, Fukui H, et al. Encapsulating peritoneal sclerosis in Japan: a prospective, controlled, multicenter study. *Am J Kidney Dis.* 2004;44:729.

Le Poole CY, Welten AGA, Weijmer MC, et al. Initiating CAPD with a regimen low in glucose and glucose degradation products, with icodextrin and amino acids (NEPP) is safe and efficacious. *Perit Dial Int.* 2005;25:S64.

National Cholesterol Education Program (NCEP). *Third Report of the National Cholesterol Education Program (NCEP) Expert Panel on Detection, Evaluation, and Treatment of High Blood Cholesterol in Adults (Adult Treatment Panel III).* Bethesda, MD: National Heart, Lung, and Blood Institute; 2002: NIH-02-5215.

National Kidney Foundation. *KDOQI Clinical Practice Guidelines for Peritoneal Dialysis Adequacy.* 2006. www.kidney.org/professionals/kdoqi/guideline_upHD_PD_VA/pd_guide2.htm

Paniagua R, Amato D, Vonesh E, et al. Effects of increased peritoneal clearances on mortality rates in peritoneal dialysis: ADEMEX, a prospective, randomized, controlled trial. *J Am Soc Nephrol.* 2002;13:1307.

Piraino B, Bailie GR, Bernardini J, et al. ISPD guidelines/recommendations. *Perit Dial Int.* 2005;25:107.

Principles of Drug Dosing in Renal Impairment

Christine Spaeth-Kelso

Deciding the appropriate dosing strategy for medications in patients with renal impairment requires an understanding of the basic principles of pharmacokinetics and disposition, including absorption, protein binding, metabolism, and elimination.

ABSORPTION

Drug absorption may be affected in renal impairment due to disease manifestations and drug interaction. Gastric motility disturbances due to uremia or underlying conditions (e.g., diabetic gastroparesis) may result in nausea and vomiting and may adversely affect absorption. Uremia may also cause decreased absorption of medications best absorbed in acidic environments (especially iron supplements). Antacids and phosphate binders commonly used in renal failure may decrease absorption of other medications (e.g., digoxin, levothyroxine, warfarin, quinolone antibiotics, tetracycline) by binding to them via chelation.

CHANGES IN PROTEIN BINDING

Advanced renal failure, poor nutrition, catabolic states, and loss of albumin in nephrotic syndrome can all lead to hypoalbuminemia. Administration of unchanged dosages of some medications in the setting of decreased albumin levels leads to **higher "free" drug levels** due to decreased protein binding. Thus, certain acidic drugs that bind avidly to albumin (e.g., NSAIDs, penicillin, phenytoin, salicylates, and sulfonamides) have increased bioavailability due to increased free levels. Likewise, basic drugs bound to alpha$_1$-acid glycoprotein and albumin (lidocaine, phenothiazines, propranolol, quinidine, and tricyclic antidepressants) may display increased free fraction of drug.

Free levels of some drugs can be increased because of competition for protein binding sites with retained wastes in uremia. Examples include digoxin, warfarin, phenytoin, valproic acid, dihydropyridine calcium channel blockers (such as nifedipine), and NSAIDs. A classic example is with phenytoin: Traditionally, total phenytoin levels are followed in blood. In uremia, many toxins accumulate and can displace the phenytoin from albumin. Thus, although the total drug level could still be therapeutic, the free (unbound) or effective drug level may exceed the therapeutic range. Increasing the dose based on the total drug level will further increase the free drug level, putting the patient at risk for serious toxicity. Therefore, the unbound or free plasma concentration should always be measured in addition to total concentrations.

METABOLISM

Drugs with active metabolites excreted by the kidney may accumulate in renal disease (see Appendix C, Common Medications with Active Metabolites). Dosage adjustments may be necessary for these medications in order to prevent toxicity from the metabolites.

ELIMINATION

The extent to which renal disease affects the elimination of drugs depends on the percentage of drug normally excreted unchanged in the urine and the degree of renal impairment. Dosing adjustment may be necessary for several medications (see Appendixes A and B).

THERAPEUTIC DRUG MONITORING

Monitoring drug concentrations is a vital tool in preventing drug-induced nephrotoxicity with many medications, including aminoglycosides and vancomycin.

Aminoglycosides

Currently, there are two available dosing strategies for aminoglycosides: traditional and extended-interval dosing.

Traditional Dosing

- **Step I: Calculate dosing weight.** To calculate dosing weight (DW), the patient's actual body weight (ABW) must be compared with the patient's ideal body weight (IBW). Corrections need to be made if the patient is obese. The following can be used to calculate these weights:

$$\text{IBW male} = 50 \text{ kg} + 2.3 \text{ [height (in.)} - 60]$$
$$\text{IBW female} = 45.5 \text{ kg} + 2.3 \text{ [height (in.)} - 60]$$
$$\text{Obese DW} = \text{IBW} + 0.4 \text{ (ABW} - \text{IBW)}$$

The DW can now be calculated as follows:

$$\text{If ABW} > 1.2 \text{ (IBW), then DW} = \text{obese DW}$$
$$\text{If IBW} < \text{ABW} < 1.2 \text{ (IBW), then DW} = \text{IBW}$$
$$\text{If IBW} > \text{ABW, then DW} = \text{ABW}$$

- **Step 2: Calculate loading dose.** Calculation of the loading dose is based on DW. The dose may be lowered in patients with volume depletion. Gentamicin dosing can vary based on the site of infection (Table 27-1).
- **Step 3: Estimate creatinine clearance.** Creatinine clearance can be estimated using the Cockroft-Gault equation:

$$\text{Est. creatinine clearance} = \frac{(140 - \text{age}) \times \text{weight} \times 0.85 \text{ (if female)}}{72 \times \text{plasma creatinine}}$$

TABLE 27-1	TRADITIONAL DOSING: TARGET AMINOGLYCOSIDE CONCENTRATIONS			
Aminoglycoside	Site of Infection	Loading Dose (mg/kg dosing weight)	Peak (µg/mL)	Trough (µg/mL)
Gentamicin/ tobramycin	General	—	4–8	<2
	Gynecologic, eye, soft tissue	1–1.5	5–7	<2
	Lung	2	8–10	<2
	Cystic fibrosis lung	2–2.5	10–12	<2
	Urinary tract	1–1.5	3–5	<2
	CNS	2.5	8–10	<2
	Blood	2	6–8	<2
	Sepsis	2.5	6–8	<2
	Endocarditis/ synergy	1–1.5	3–5	<2
Amikacin	General	—	25–35	4–10

- **Step 4: Calculate maintenance dose.** The maintenance dose is a percentage of the loading dose (Table 27-2).
- **Step 5: Therapeutic drug monitoring.** For therapeutic drug monitoring, obtain peak and trough concentrations with the third maintenance dose. The preferred peak and trough can be selected clinically, with consideration given to the site and severity of infection, causative microorganism, minimum inhibitory concentration, immunocompetency of the patient, and intent of therapy (Table 27-1). Recheck the dosing level whenever there is a change in dosing regimen or change in renal function; recheck every 1 to 2 weeks if duration of therapy is >2 weeks.

Extended-Interval Aminoglycosides

Extended-interval dosing is equally effective and may be less toxic compared with traditional every 8-hour dosing. Extended-interval aminoglycosides take advantage of

TABLE 27-2	CALCULATION OF THE MAINTENANCE DOSE			
Creatinine Clearance (mL/minute)	Half-Life (hour)	q8h (%)	q12h (%)	q24h (%)
>90	3.1	84	100	—
80–89	3.4	80	91	—
70–79	3.9	76	88	—
60–69	4.5	—	84	—
50–59	5.3	—	79	—
40–49	6.5	—	—	92
30–39	8.4	—	—	86
25–29	9.9	—	—	81
20–24	11.9	—	—	75
<20	>12	Give loading dose, follow levels, and redose when level drops to <2 µg/mL.		

concentration-dependent killing through high peak levels and the postantibiotic effect. Calculate the patient's dosing weight (DW) as outlined above. The initial IV dosing regimen is as follows:

- Gentamicin, 5 mg/kg DW (round to nearest 50 mg)
- Tobramycin, 5 mg/kg DW (round to nearest 50 mg)
- Amikacin, 15 mg/kg DW (round to nearest 100 mg)

For therapeutic drug monitoring, obtain a single, random drug level approximately 8 to 12 hours after the initial dose. Determine the appropriate maintenance dose according to Figure 27-1. Repeat drug level as necessary. For patients with impaired renal function, estimated dosing intervals are provided in Table 27-3.

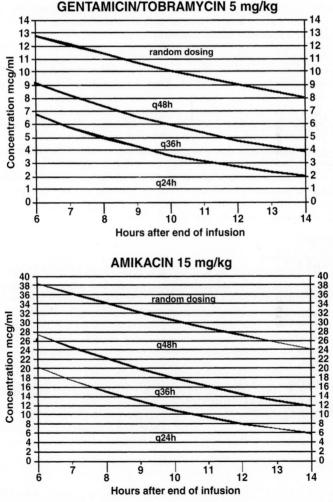

FIGURE 27-1. Nomograms depicting maintenance dose schedules for gentamicin/tobramycin and amikacin.

TABLE 27-3	ONCE-DAILY DOSING: AMINOGLYCOSIDE INTERVALS IN PATIENTS WITH IMPAIRED RENAL FUNCTION
Creatinine Clearance (mL/minute)	Usual Dosing Interval
>60	q24h
40–59	q36h
20–39	q48h
<20	Not recommended (see the section "Traditional Dosing")

Extended-interval aminoglycosides are not recommended in patients who are pregnant, patients on dialysis, or those with anasarca, creatinine clearance <20 mL/minute, endocarditis, or >20% body surface area burns.

Dialysis Patients

Patients on dialysis should be dosed using more traditional methods for aminoglycosides as opposed to extended-interval methods. Doses for gentamicin/tobramycin are 1.5 to 2 mg/kg (or 1 mg/kg if using for synergy for a gram-positive bacteremia or a UTI) and the amikacin dose is 7.5 mg/kg. Monitoring peak and trough levels in dialysis patients is recommended to prevent potential toxicity and to determine when patients need to be redosed. Desired peak levels are usually 3 to 9 μg/mL for gentamicin/tobramycin and 20 to 30 μcg/mL for amikacin, depending on the site and severity of the infection. Trough levels should be drawn immediately prior to the next dialysis session, and patients are given another dose when the trough level falls to <2 μg/mL for gentamicin/tobramycin and <10 μg/mL for amikacin. Usually, dosing frequency is every 48 hours for peritoneal dialysis, every 24 to 48 hours for patients on continuous renal replacement therapy (CRRT), and patients receiving hemodialysis are typically dosed postdialysis.

Vancomycin

Usual Dosing Regimen

Typically, the dosing regimen for vancomycin is 10 to 15 mg/kg every 12 hours and is based on body weight and renal function. Obese patients have a greater volume of distribution, and the drug may have a longer half-life. Therefore, for patients with morbid obesity, the dosing recommendation for vancomycin is 10 to 15 mg/kg of total body weight every 24 hours. Therapeutic drug monitoring should also be done in these patients. For patients with impaired renal function, estimate dosing intervals according to Table 27-4. Patients on dialysis need more-specialized dosing regimens as described below.

TABLE 27-4	VANCOMYCIN DOSING IN PATIENTS WITH IMPAIRED RENAL FUNCTION		
Body Weight (kg)	Dose (mg)	Creatinine Clearance (mL/minute)	Suggested Interval (hour)
<45	500	>60	12
45–60	750	35–60	24
60–90	1000	15–34	48
>90	1250–1500	<15	Random dosing

Therapeutic Drug Monitoring

Frequent monitoring of vancomycin levels is indicated if concomitant nephrotoxic or oto-toxic agents are being used or if there is changing renal function, suboptimal response to therapy, hemodynamic instability, or extremes of body weight. **Trough levels** (every 4–7 days) are recommended in patients receiving longer courses of therapy (>5 days) to ensure that concentrations are adequate but not excessive. Vancomycin levels are not rec-ommended for patients receiving a short course of therapy (<5 days). Levels should be obtained at steady state or immediately before administration of the third maintenance dose. Desired trough levels are three times the minimum inhibitory concentration, with 5 to 15 mg/L for bloodstream infections. Higher trough levels of 15 to 25 mg/L are recom-mended for bone, lung or CNS infections. **Peak levels** should not be routinely obtained. Occasional peak levels may be of benefit in patients with severe infections (e.g., meningi-tis, endocarditis, and osteomyelitis) or in cases where toxicity is suspected. Peaks should be obtained 1 hour after a 1-hour infusion.

Hemodialysis Patients

Dosing frequency in patients on hemodialysis depends on a few factors, the most impor-tant of which are the clearance of the dialyzer being used and residual renal function. With the newer high-clearance dialyzers, a significant amount of the drug may be cleared after a dialysis session, leading to suboptimal drug levels until the next scheduled dose. Traditional concepts of "dose and forget" regimens for vancomycin are not be applicable with the newer dialyzers, and patients may need to be dosed as frequently as every third to fifth day. Thus, at least initially, attention must be directed toward ensuring that trough levels define a dosage interval if prolonged therapy is planned. The usual practice is to redose at a level of <15 mg/L (random or predialysis). One typical regimen for vancomycin in hemodial-ysis patients using high-flux membrane dialyzers is to give a 1-g loading dose at initiation of therapy followed by supplementary doses of 500–1000 mg after each subsequent dialy-sis. One should check a predialysis vancomycin level before the third or fourth dialysis treatment on this regimen or sooner in ill patients.

KEY POINTS TO REMEMBER

- It is important to assess the patient's creatinine clearance to estimate correct dosages. Plasma creatinine levels can be misleading, especially in the elderly.
- Creatinine levels must be stable to use estimates of clearance.
- Once best-estimate dosages are instituted, levels should be followed closely, especially in patients whose renal function may be fluctuating.
- Vancomycin is extensively used in patients with ESRD on hemodialysis. It is important to note clearance of the dialyzer membrane being used. More drug is cleared with cer-tain dialyzers, requiring more-frequent dosing than the traditional once-a-week dose for the ESRD patient.

REFERENCES AND SUGGESTED READINGS

Aronoff GR, Berns JS, Brier ME, et al. *Drug Prescribing in Renal Failure: Dosing Guidelines for Adults.* 4th ed. Philadelphia: American College of Physicians; 1999.
Barclay ML, Begg EJ, Hickling KG. What is the evidence for once-daily aminoglycoside therapy? *Clin Pharmacokinet.* 1994;27:32.
Cantu TG, Yamanaka-Yuen NA, Lietman PS. Serum vancomycin concentrations: reap-praisal of their clinical value. *Clin Infect Dis.* 1994;18:533.

Cockroft DW, Gault MH. Prediction of creatinine clearance from serum creatinine. *Nephron.* 1976;16:31.

Dipiro JT, ed. *Pharmacotherapy: A Pathophysiologic Approach.* 4th ed. Stamford, CT: Appleton & Lange; 1999.

Ferriols-Lisart R, Alos-Alminana M. Effectiveness and safety of once-daily aminoglycosides: a meta-analysis. *Am J Health Syst Pharm.* 1996;53:1141.

Freeman CD, Strayer AH. Mega-analysis of meta-analysis: an examination of meta-analysis with an emphasis on once-daily aminoglycoside comparative trials. *Pharmacotherapy.* 1996;16:1093.

Hatala R, Dinh TT, Cook DJ. Single daily dosing of aminoglycosides in immunocompromised adults: a systematic review. *Clin Infect Dis.* 1997;24:810.

Leader WG, Chandler MH, Castiglia M. Pharmacokinetic optimisation of vancomycin therapy. *Clin Pharmacokinet.* 1995;28:327.

Penzak SR, Gubbins PO, Rodvold KA, et al. Therapeutic drug monitoring of vancomycin in a morbidly obese patient. *Ther Drug Monit.* 1998;20:261.

Care of the Renal Transplant Patient

28

Andrew Siedlecki and Matthew J. Koch

G iven the improvement in quality and quantity of life compared with chronic dialysis, renal transplantation is the preferred treatment for end-stage renal disease in appropriate candidates. Allograft survival time for a deceased donor kidney transplant averages more than 8 years, while that of a living donor kidney averages more than 12 years. Approximately 50% of the renal transplants done annually in the United States are from deceased donors (deceased donor allograft, or DDA), and the remainder are from living donors, either related (LRA) or unrelated (LUA). Combined kidney-pancreas (KP) transplants are also performed routinely, most often simultaneously from a deceased donor, but occasionally as a deceased donor pancreas after a living donor kidney (PAK). There are approximately 148,000 renal transplant recipients actively cared for in the U.S. health care system. This chapter provides a brief introduction for the general physician whose practice is progressively more involved in issues of pre- and posttransplant care.

PRETRANSPLANT TESTING TERMINOLOGY

Panel Reactive Antibody

Panel reactive antibody (PRA) testing is done to determine the presence of preexisting anti-HLA (human leukocyte antigen) antibodies. PRA is expressed as a percentage, reflecting the degree of sensitization to the potential donor pool. A high PRA correlates with increasing likelihood that the potential recipient will have preexisting antibodies to the donor organ. Antibody specificity is much more relevant than a PRA result.

Human Leukocyte Antigen

In kidney transplantation, six human leukocyte antigens (HLAs) (two each of the A, B, and DR classes) are most relevant, though others can play a role. A comparison of donor and recipient HLA types determines the "match," which can range from a six-antigen match to a six-antigen mismatch. HLA matching plays a role in expected graft outcome, though less so in the modern era of transplantation.

Cross Match

A cross match is a test of immunologic compatibility between the donor and recipient. Several tests are available and differ in methods and sensitivity. One or more of these may be used to help determine if a recipient has evidence for clinically significant antibodies to a potential donor.

Donor Specific Antibodies

Donor specific antibodies, or DSAs, are HLA antibodies detected in the potential recipient against HLAs present in the potential donor. These may preclude transplantation, but the significance must be interpreted in view of cross-match results. They can also develop after transplant and may contribute to acute or chronic rejection.

POSTTRANSPLANT KIDNEY DYSFUNCTION TERMINOLOGY

In the immediate posttransplant period, *delayed graft function* and *slow graft function* are the main concerns. Other causes of allograft dysfunction may occur early or late after transplantation and should be evaluated based on the time since transplantation, the presentation, and the rate of rise in the serum creatinine (Table 28-1).

Delayed Graft Function

Delayed graft function (DGF) refers to an allograft that does not immediately function following transplantation and for which dialysis is required within the first week after transplantation. It occurs more commonly in the setting of a DDA with prolonged cold ischemia time.

Slow Graft Function

There are various unofficial definitions, but slow graft function (SGF) typically refers to an allograft that functions after transplantation, but presents with a slow decrease in serum creatinine or diminished urine output prior to improved function without requirement for dialysis.

PRETRANSPLANT EVALUATION

Transplant candidates are thoroughly evaluated to determine their surgical, medical, social, and psychological fitness for transplantation. A patient with renal disease can be evaluated for transplantation at any time (ideally when the GFR is ≈ 25 mL/minute for most patients,

---

TABLE 28-1	CAUSES OF ALLOGRAFT DYSFUNCTION

Acute
- Acute interstitial nephritis (AIN)
- Acute tubular necrosis (ATN)
- Obstruction
  - Lymphocele
  - BPH
  - Bladder dysfunction
  - Ureteral stenosis
  - Nephrolithiasis
- Transplant pyelonephritis
- Acute rejection
- Vascular thrombosis
- Recurrent kidney disease
- BK nephropathy
- ITP/TTP

Chronic
- Chronic rejection
- Obstruction
- Calcineurin nephrotoxicity
- BK nephropathy
- Renal/iliac artery stenosis
- Recurrent/de novo kidney disease

dependent on the rate of progression) and can officially be "listed" when the GFR is <20 mL/minute. Allograft survival is inversely correlated with the duration of time on dialysis prior to transplant, thus early referral is encouraged. Preemptive transplantation (prior to the requirement for dialysis) is encouraged in most cases. Medical testing involves updating routine screening tests and immunizations, as well as risk-factor specific testing with particular emphasis on the cardiovascular system. In general, a potential recipient should have at least a 5-year life expectancy in order to be considered a transplant candidate. After being deemed a suitable candidate for transplantation, the patient may undergo living donor transplantation, if possible, or be placed on the deceased donor wait list. Deceased donor wait list management involves updating screening tests and repeating evaluations as indicated to help determine that transplant candidacy remains appropriate. Blood transfusions should be avoided unless absolutely necessary as sensitization to HLAs can occur. If required, leukocyte-depleted blood should be given to decrease the risk of sensitization. Currently, wait list points are accrued by time on the list as well as a component of HLA matching. The wait time for a deceased donor kidney may be several years, depending on the recipient blood group and degree of sensitization.

POSTTRANSPLANT PERIOD

Immediate Posttransplant Period (0–3 Months)

Most transplant recipients are in a state of significant immunosuppression immediately following transplantation. A potent induction agent, often a polyclonal or monoclonal lymphocyte-depleting agent, may have been utilized and the overall degree of immunosuppression is generally greater than in the chronic maintenance period. Protocols are center and patient specific, but regardless of the agent(s) used, compliance with immunosuppression and follow-up with the transplant center is extremely important during this time. Routine labs are obtained to monitor for rejection, recurrent disease, infection, and immunosuppressive drug levels. Patients with DGF may be discharged from the hospital still requiring maintenance dialysis. A period of several weeks may be required before the allograft regains adequate function and dialysis may be discontinued.

Intermediate and Long-Term Issues in Renal Transplant (>3 Months)

- Maintenance immunosuppression is adjusted based on drug levels, side effects, and the perceived risk of rejection versus infection. Antibiotic, antifungal, and antiviral (especially CMV) prophylaxis is generally given for a set period of time in the early posttransplant period.
- Continued monitoring and compliance with medications is essential for the life of the allograft.

Posttransplant Kidney Dysfunction

An acute increase of ≥20% from the baseline serum creatinine or a slowly increasing creatinine deserves further evaluation. Diagnostic tools focus on patient history, renal ultrasound, and laboratory testing, while the final assessment often requires renal biopsy. Although acute rejection (within the first year posttransplant) is uncommon—with an incidence of <10% to 15% at most transplant centers—prompt diagnosis and intervention is necessary. Rejection may be cellular and/or antibody mediated and is defined by the Banff criteria. Volume status, any history of recent illness, and medication use (particularly diuretics) should be evaluated as a possible prerenal etiology. An ultrasound should be obtained if indicated to evaluate for hydronephrosis, lymphocele, or vascular etiology. A marked increase in blood pressure, often associated with new-onset edema suggests renal or iliac artery stenosis and should be initially investigated with arterial Doppler. Urinalysis and proteinuria quantification should be assessed to evaluate for infection or recurrent disease. Immunosuppression should be reviewed, in particular calcineurin inhibitor (CNI) levels, as well as recent use of other agents with a potential for drug interaction, and overall compliance. In addition, other transplant-specific viral studies (e.g., BK virus) may be helpful. Biopsy should be expedited if there is no obvious etiology for worsening renal function. Unexplained fever or other signs or symptoms suggesting occult infection or malignancy should be thoroughly evaluated. Close communication with the transplant center is imperative to assist with timely evaluation and appropriate biopsy and immunosuppressive adjustments as indicated.

Important Drug Interactions and Immunosuppression Administration Issues

Drug interactions with CNI and sirolimus may significantly increase or decrease levels of these agents, and close review is necessary with the addition or discontinuation of any agent. Failure to do so can result in toxicity or rejection (Fig. 28-1). Immunosuppression

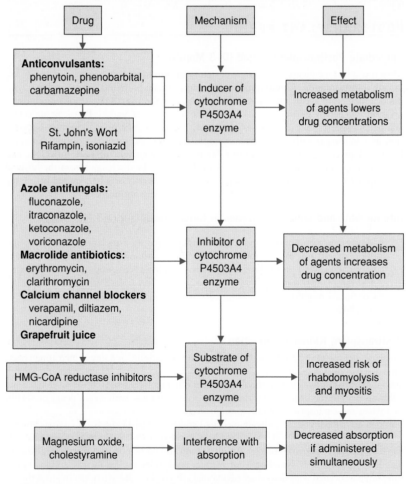

FIGURE 28-1. Cyclosporine, tacrolimus, and sirolimus drug interactions.

may need to be adjusted in the setting of significant infection, but should not be withheld completely. Routine administration of "stress-dose steroids" to patients on maintenance prednisone is rarely necessary and usually only increases the risk of infection, glucose intolerance, and poor wound healing.

For transplant recipients undergoing surgical procedures or other events that limit oral intake or gastrointestinal motility, the administration of intravenous calcineurin inhibitors is almost never necessary. Intravenous administration increases the risk of acute calcineurin toxicity and allograft dysfunction. Tacrolimus is readily absorbed and can be given following brief clamping of a nasogastric tube. Sublingual administration can also be utilized if necessary. For patients on cyclosporine, brief conversion to tacrolimus in this setting is preferable to intravenous administration. The conversion ratio of cyclosporine to tacrolimus is approximately 50:1. An equivalent steroid dose can be given intravenously, and if necessary, intravenous forms of mycophenolate or azathioprine are available, although the latter two agents can often be held briefly while continuing other maintenance immunosuppression.

Routine Health Maintenance Screening and Immunizations

Transplant recipients should continue to receive recommended vaccinations. However, **live vaccines should not be given.** Given the significant increased risk of skin cancer, routine *dermatologic screening* is recommended. Regular use of sunscreen and the avoidance of overexposure to the sun reduce cancer risk. *Cardiovascular disease* remains a leading cause of mortality following renal transplantation. Standard blood pressure and dyslipidemia guidelines should be followed. Aspirin use in appropriate patients should continue, in addition to routine cardiovascular screening (stress test) in those at high risk for cardiovascular disease. *Reduced bone mass* is a common complication related to steroid therapy. The utility of bone densitometry screening and the use of bisphosphonates to prevent fractures in this patient population remain controversial, given the potential for adynamic bone disease. Vitamin D and calcium supplementation should generally be provided, although no available treatment has demonstrated long-term efficacy in preservation of bone mass or in decreasing the risk of fractures in renal transplant recipients.

Other Long-Term Issues

Consultation with the transplant center is recommended for all immunosuppressive issues or any other concerns, especially those involving serious infection or malignancy. Other issues include the weaning of immunosuppression following a failed allograft as well as the potential need for a transplant nephrectomy for manifest or occult signs and symptoms that may relate to the transplanted kidney. Timely referral for retransplant evaluation is appropriate in those patients with an estimated GFR <30mL/minute, depending on the rate of decline in kidney function.

Maintenance Immunosuppression

Maintenance immunosuppression is often center specific and protocol driven. The combination of drugs used and initial doses or levels may be based on the use of initial induction therapy, and previous experience. The most commonly used immunosuppressive combination in the United States for renal transplantation is tacrolimus, mycophenolate, and prednisone. Variations include prednisone-free regimens that use only a CNI with an antimetabolite, or conversion from a CNI to sirolimus, usually as part of triple-maintenance immunosuppression. Most centers avoid the routine combination of a CNI with sirolimus given the increased potential for nephrotoxicity. There are no definitive studies showing the superiority of tacrolimus versus cyclosporine, sirolimus conversion from a CNI, mycophenolate versus azathioprine (or for the inclusion of an antimetabolite in a protocol that includes a CNI and prednisone), or prednisone-free versus prednisone-containing regimens in improving long-term patient or graft survival. The choice of immunosuppression is initially protocol based with subsequent tailoring to the individual patient based on risk of rejection versus opportunistic infection. Judgment is required, as no single test is available to accurately define the overall degree of immunosuppression in an individual patient.

Immunosuppressive Agents

Corticosteroids

Prednisone. Prednisone has multiple immunosuppressive and anti-inflammatory actions. Maintenance prednisone doses are usually 2.5 to 7.5 mg/day to minimize the well-known side effects of chronic use. It is unclear whether prednisone inclusion is good, bad, or indifferent for long-term patient and graft survival in the era of modern immunosuppression. The most common side effects on maintenance dosages can include cataracts, weight gain, glucose intolerance, dyslipidemia, hypertension, osteoporosis, steroid myopathy, and mood distubances.

Calcineurin Inhibitors (CNIs). Cyclosporine was the first CNI available for clinical use. No other class of drugs has had such a significant positive impact in transplantation. Calcineurin *nephrotoxicity* remains a major issue in renal and nonrenal transplantation. Therapeutic and nephrotoxic levels overlap, resulting in prolonged graft survival in most, but earlier graft impairment or loss in others. As of yet, there is no data to suggest that long-term outcomes can be improved by avoiding or minimizing CNI use, and these agents remain the backbone of most maintenance immunosuppression protocols. Drug interactions with CNI may be significant, and close attention is necessary when adding or deleting medications (Fig. 28-1).

Cyclosporine. Cyclosporine is a cyclic peptide that inhibits T-lymphocyte proliferation primarily by inhibiting the action of calcineurin phosphatase, which finally blocks the production of IL-2. Common side effects include hypertension, dyslipidemia, gingival hyperplasia, hirsutism, hyperuricemia, hyperkalemia, and hypomagnesemia. Compared with tacrolimus, neurotoxicity and glucose intolerance are less common. The original cyclosporine formulation (Sandimmune) is dependent on bile for absorption and it is not interchangeable with the new microemulsion (ME) formulation (Neoral). Available generic products are designed to be equivalent to the ME formulation. Patients should not randomly switch between the original cyclosporine and the ME formulations, or between different ME products without closely following levels, as variability in absorption may be present.

Tacrolimus. Tacrolimus acts on the calcineurin complex through a separate mechanism also resulting in suppression of IL-2 synthesis. Compared with cyclosporine, tacrolimus is more likely to cause neurotoxicity (including tremors, headache, and insomnia), glucose intolerance, alopecia, and gastrointestinal distress. Effects on blood pressure and dyslipidemia are less pronounced than with cyclosporine, while hyperkalemia is probably equivalent.

Antimetabolites

Antimetabolites include azathioprine and mycophenolate. They prevent DNA synthesis and, therefore, proliferation of B- and T- cells. **Azathioprine** is a thiopurine analog that is converted to 6-mercaptopurine and nonselectively inhibits DNA and RNA synthesis, thereby inhibiting differentiation and proliferation of T- and B-cell lymphocytes. Azathioprine has largely been supplanted by mycophenolate, although clinical data supporting this change are questionable. Currently, it is most often used as a substitute when mycophenolate is not tolerated, but an antimetabolite is still desired. Side effects of azathioprine are mostly dose related and include leukopenia and thrombocytopenia. Hepatotoxicity is rare. **Combined use of allopurinol (xanthine oxidase inhibitor) and azathioprine causes increased 6-mercaptopurine activity and potentially severe bone marrow suppression.** This combination should generally be avoided, but an azathioprine dose reduction of up to 75% with close hematologic monitoring should ensue if the two agents are used together.

Mycophenolate has largely supplanted azathioprine as the antimetabolite of choice. Short-term, prospective studies infer equivalence, while long-term retrospective data, albeit from different eras, favor mycophenolate. Mycophenolate is several times more expensive than

TABLE 28-2 IMMUNOSUPPRESSIVE DRUG INTERACTIONS

Interactions Between Immunosuppressants

Acting Drug	Increased Drug Levels	Decreased Drug Levels
Cyclosporine	Sirolimus	Mycophenolate
Sirolimus	Cyclosporine	Tacrolimus
Tacrolimus	Mycophenolate	

azathioprine. Mycophenolate is available as either a mofetil or sodium formulation. The latter is enteric coated, designed to decrease the incidence and severity of GI symptoms associated with this agent; however, the majority of GI symptoms are lower rather than upper. Mycophenolate is converted to mycophenolic acid (MPA), which causes noncompetitive reversible inhibition of inosine monophosphate dehydrogenase. This inhibition results in interference of the *de novo* pathway of purine synthesis and DNA replication of T and B cells. Primary side effects include diarrhea, nausea, gastroesophageal reflux, and myelosuppression.

Mammalian Target of Rapamycin Inhibitors

Sirolimus binds to an immunophilin and this complex attaches to and modulates the activity of the mammalian target of rapamycin (mTOR). This results in cell cycle arrest in the G1-S phase, inhibiting T and B cell proliferation. Everolimus is a second drug in this class, but it is not yet approved for use in the United States. Side effects of sirolimus include hypertriglyceridemia, hypercholesterolemia, diarrhea, leucopenia, thrombocytopenia, anemia, edema, skin rash, mouth ulcers, proteinuria, delayed wound healing, glucose intolerance, rarely pericardial or pleural effusion, and interstitial pneumonitis. Sirolimus and the CNIs are metabolized primarily by the cytochrome P450 3A4 system, thus potential drug interactions are the same (Fig. 28-1).

Sirolimus has been used in an attempt to minimize or eliminate CNI use. Significant side effects often limit tolerability and the possibility of an alternate form of nephrotoxicity, as manifested by proteinuria, is an additional concern. The use of sirolimus in conjunction with either cyclosporine or tacrolimus may increase the risk of nephrotoxicity independent of drug concentration.

Interactions Between Immunosuppressive Agents

The commonly used immunosuppressive agents may also interact with each other. Thus, drug levels and dose adjustments may be necessary when changing components of the immunosuppressive regimen (Table 28-2). Drug levels are routinely monitored for cyclosporine, tacrolimus, and sirolimus. MPA levels must be interpreted with caution.

KEY POINTS TO REMEMBER

- The availability of several individual immunosuppressive agents and potential therapeutic combinations offers the opportunity to individualize treatment based on immunologic or side-effect profile.
- Potential drug interactions should be carefully reviewed when starting or stopping any medication in a patient on immunosuppression.
- Any decrease in renal function should be thoroughly and promptly evaluated.
- Close communication with the transplant center should continue to assist with appropriate care of the transplant recipient.

REFERENCES AND SUGGESTED READINGS

Kasiske B, Cosio FG, Beto J, et al. Clinical practice guidelines for managing dyslipidemias in kidney transplant patients: a report from the Managing Dyslipidemias in Chronic Kidney Disease Work Group of the National Kidney Foundation Kidney Disease Outcomes Quality Initiative. *Am J Transplant.* 2005;4[Suppl 7]:13–53.

Kasiske BL, Cangro CB, Hariharan S, et al. The evaluation of renal transplantation candidates: clinical practice guidelines. *Am J Transplant.* 2001;1[Suppl 2]:3–95.

Meier-Kriesche HU, Li S, Gruessner RW, et al. Immunosuppression: evolution in practice and trends, 1994–2004. *Am J Transplant.* 2006;6(5 Pt 2):1111–1131.

Ojo AO, Hanson JA, Meier-Kriesche H, et al. Survival in recipients of marginal cadaveric donor kidneys compared with other recipients and wait-listed transplant candidates. *J Am Soc Nephrol.* 2001;12(3):589–597.

Solez K, Colvin RB, Racusen LC, et al. Banff '05 meeting report: differential diagnosis of chronic allograft injury and elimination of chronic allograft nephropathy ("CAN"). *Am J Transplant.* 2007;7(3):518–526.

Red Flag Drugs That May Cause Renal Impairment

A

Antimicrobials	Chemotherapy	Immunosuppressive drugs
Acyclovir	Carboplatin	Cyclosporine
Aminoglycosides	Cisplatin	Tacrolimus
Amphotericin	Methotrexate (high dose)	Neurologic drugs
Cephalosporins	Mitomycin	Lithium
Cidofovir	Nitrosoureas	Phenobarbital
Ciprofloxacin	Diuretics	Phenytoin
Foscarnet	Loop diuretics	Rheumatologic drugs
Methicillin	Mannitol (high dose)	Penicillamine
Pentamidine (IV)	Thiazide	Gold
Sulfonamides	Cardiovascular drugs	Drugs of abuse
TMP	ACE inhibitors	Amphetamine
Vancomycin	Dopamine (high dose)	Cocaine
Analgesics	Hydralazine	Heroin
Acetaminophen	Norepinephrine	Phencyclidine
NSAIDs		

Mechanisms of Nephrotoxicity and Alternatives to Some Common Drugs

B

Drug	Mechanism	Alternatives/comments
ACE inhibitors	Hemodynamic	Beta blockers, calcium channel blockers
Acetaminophen	ATN	Avoid doses >4 g/day
Acyclovir	ATN	Hydration, dose adjustment
Aminoglycosides	ATN	Monitor serum concentration, nontoxic substitutes
Amphotericin	ATN	Saline loading, lipid products, continuous infusion
Carboplatin	ATN	Hydration
Cephalosporins	Interstitial nephritis	Alternative antibiotics
Cimetidine	Interstitial nephritis	Proton pump inhibitor
Ciprofloxacin	Interstitial nephritis	Alternative antibiotics
Cisplatin	Tubular necrosis	Hydration, carboplatin
Cyclosporine	Hemodynamic, chronic interstitial nephritis	Monitor levels, sirolimus
Foscarnet	ATN	Dose adjust, ganciclovir
Ketorolac	Hemodynamic	Acetaminophen, opiate analgesic
Gold	Glomerulopathy	Methotrexate, hydroxychloroquine
High-dose mannitol	Hemodynamic	Avoid doses >200 g/day
Hydralazine	Glomerulopathy	ACE inhibitors
Lithium	Glomerulopathy, interstitial nephritis	Monitor levels, valproic acid
Loop diuretics	Interstitial nephritis	Non–sulfa-containing diuretics

Drug	Mechanism	Alternatives/comments
Methicillin	Interstitial nephritis	Vancomycin
Methotrexate	Tubular obstruction	Adjust dosage, urinary alkalinization, allopurinol
NSAIDs	Hemodynamic, interstitial nephritis	Acetaminophen, tramadol, opiate analgesics
Penicillamine	Glomerulopathy	Methotrexate, hydroxychloroquine
Pentamidine	Tubular necrosis	TMP-SMX, dapsone
Phenytoin	Interstitial nephritis, glomerulopathy	Alternative anticonvulsant
Phenobarbital	Interstitial nephritis	Alternative anticonvulsant
Sulfonamides	Tubular obstruction, interstitial nephritis	Non–sulfa-containing antibiotic
Tacrolimus	Hemodynamic, interstitial nephritis	Monitor levels, sirolimus
Thiazides	Interstitial nephritis	Alternative diuretics

ATN, acute tubular necrosis.

Common Medications with Active Metabolites

Drug	Metabolite	Cumulative Toxicity
Acetaminophen	N-acetyl-p-benzoquinoneimine	Hepatotoxicity, acute tubular necrosis
Allopurinol	Oxypurinol	Bone marrow suppression
Chlorpropamide	2-Hydroxychloropropramide	Hypoglycemia
Meperidine	Normeperidine	Seizures
Primidone	Phenobarbital	Oversedation, coma
Procainamide	N-acetyl-procainamide	Arrhythmia, hypotension, respiratory failure
Nitroprusside	Thiocyanate	Lactic acidosis, hallucinations, coma, tinnitus
Morphine	6-Morphine glucuronide	Oversedation, coma

Dosing Adjustments for Antimicrobials

Name	Usual Dose	Creatinine Clearance (mL/min)			Dialysis
		>50	10–50	<10	
Antibiotics					
Amoxicillin	250–500 mg q8h	No change	q8–12h	q24h	HD: dose after HD CAPD: 250 mg q12h
Ampicillin	250 mg–2 g q6h	No change	q8–12h	q24h	HD: dose after HD CAPD: 250 mg q12h
Ampicillin/ sulbactam	1.5–3 g q6h	No change	q8–12h	q24h	HD: dose after HD CAPD: q24h
Aztreonam	2 g q8h	No change	50–75%	25%	HD: extra 0.5 g after HD CAPD: 25%
Cefazolin	1–2 g q8h	No change	q12h	q24h	HD: 1 g after HD CAPD: 0.5 g q12h
Cefepime	1–2 g IV q8h	No change	q12–24h	q24h	HD: 1–1.5 g after HD CAPD: 1–2 g q48h
Cefotaxime	1–2 g q8h	q8–12h	q12–24h	q24h	HD: 1 g after HD CAPD: 0.5–1 g qd
Cefotetan	1–2 g q12h	No change	50%	25%	HD: 1 g after HD CAPD: 1 g qd
Ceftazidime	1–2 g q8h	q8–12h	q24–48h	q48h	HD: 1 g after HD CAPD: 0.5 g qd
Cefuroxime	0.75–1.50 g q8h	q8h	q8–12h	q24h	HD: dose after HD CAPD: q24h
Ciprofloxacin PO	250–750 mg q12h	No change	(<30) q24h	q24h	HD, CAPD: 250–500 mg after dialysis
Ciprofloxacin IV	200–400 mg q12h	No change	(<30) q24h	q24h	HD, CAPD: 200–400 mg after dialysis

Dosing Adjustments for Antimicrobials

Name	Usual Dose	Creatinine Clearance (mL/min)			Dialysis
		>50	10–50	<10	
Levofloxacin PO, IV	250–500 mg qd	No change	250 mg q24–48h	250 mg q48h	HD, CAPD: 250 mg q48h
Gatifloxacin PO, IV	400 mg q24h	No change	200 mg q24h	200 mg q24h	HD, CAPD: 200 mg after dialysis
Gemifloxacin	320 mg q24h	No change	160 mg q24h	160 m g q24h	HD: dose after dialysis; CAPD: 160mg q24h
Clarithromycin	500 mg q12h	No change	75%	50%	HD: dose after dialysis; CAPD: no change
Erythromycin	250–500 mg q6h	No change	No change	50%	No change
TMP-SMX	5 mg/kg TMP component q6–8h	No change	(<30) 50% q12h	Not recommended	HD: 50%
TMP-SMX PO	1 tab b.i.d.	No change	(<30) 50%	Not recommended	HD: 50%
Telithromycin	800 mg q24h	No change	(<30): 600 mg q24h	600 mg q24h	HD: Give after HD
Daptomycin	4–6 mg/kg q24h	No change	(<30): 4–6 mg/kg q48h	4–6 mg/kg q48h	HD: 4–6 mg/kg q48h, give after HD CAPD: 4–6 mg/kg q48h
Imipenem	500 mg IV q6h	No change	250 mg q6–12h	125–250 mg q12h	HD: dose after HD CAPD: 125–250 mg q12h
Meropenem	1 g IV q8h	No change	1 g q12h	0.5 g q12h	HD: dose after HD CAPD: 0.5 g q12h
Ertapenem	1 g q24h	No change	(<30) 500 mg q24h	500 mg q24h	HD: 500 mg q24h
PCN G	0.5–4 mU q4h	No change	75%	25–50%	HD: dose after HD CAPD: 25–50%

Piperacillin	3–4 g q4–6h	No change	q6–8h	q8h	HD: dose after HD CAPD: q8h
Piperacillin/ tazobactam	3.375 g q6h	No change	2.25 g q6h	2.25 g q8h	HD: 2.25 g q8h + 0.75 g after HD; CAPD: 2.25 g q8h
Ticarcillin/ clavulanate	3.1 g q4h	No change	2 g q4–8h	2 g q12h	HD: extra 3.1 g after HD CAPD: 2 g q12h
Tetracycline	250–500 mg q6h	q8–12h	q12–24h	q24h	Avoid
Antifungals					
Amphotericin	0.4–1 mg/kg/day	No change	No change	q24–48h	HD: no change CAPD: q24–48h
Fluconazole	200–400 mg qd	No change	50%	50%	HD: extra 200 mg after HD CAPD: 50%
Itraconazole	100–200 mg q12h	No change	No change	50%	HD, CAPD: 100 mg q12–24h
Voriconazole IV	6 mg/kg q12h × 2 then 4 mg/kg IV q12h	No change	Not recommended (toxic vehicle may accumulate, use PO route)	Not recommended (toxic vehicle may accumulate, use PO route)	Not recommended (toxic vehicle may accumulate, use PO route)
Voriconazole PO	200 mg PO b.i.d. (if >40 kg); 100 mg PO b.i.d. (if <40 kg)	No change	No change	No change	No change

(continued)

Name	Usual Dose	Creatinine Clearance (mL/min)			Dialysis
		>50	10–50	<10	
Antivirals					
Acyclovir PO	200–800 mg q4–6h	No change	(<25) q8h	q12h	HD: after HD
Acyclovir IV	5–12.4 mg/kg q8h	No change	q12–24h	2.5 mg/kg q24h	HD: after HD CAPD: 2.5 mg/kg q24h
Amantadine PO	100 mg b.i.d.	q24–48h	q48–72h	q7d	No change
Cidofovir induction	5 mg/kg q1wk	No change	0.5–2 mg/kg q1wk	0.5 mg/kg q1wk	Limited data
Cidofovir maintenance	5 mg/kg q2wk	No change	0.5–2 mg/kg q2wk	0.5 mg/kg q2wk	Limited data
Entecavir	0.5–1 mg q24h	No change	(CrCl 30–49): 50% of usual dose (CrCl 10–29): 30% of usual dose	10% of regular dose	HD: Give 10% of regular dose after HD
Famciclovir	500 mg q8h	No change	q12–24h	250 mg q24h	HD: after HD CAPD: no data
Ganciclovir IV	5 mg/kg q24h	2.5–5 mg/kg q24h	0.6–1.25 mg/kg q24h	0.625 mg/kg 3×/wk	HD: 0.6 mg/kg after HD CAPD: 0.625 mg/kg 3×/wk
Ganciclovir PO	1 g t.i.d.	0.5–1 g t.i.d.	0.5–1 g qd	0.5 g 3×/wk	HD: 0.5 g after HD
Valacyclovir	1 g q8h	No change	q12–24h	0.5 g q24h	HD: after HD CAPD: 0.5 g q24h
Valganciclovir	900 mg q12–24h	No change	450 mg q24–48h	Not recommended	—

CAPD, continuous ambulatory peritoneal dialysis; HD, hemodialysis

Dosing Adjustments for Antiretrovirals

E

Name	Usual Oral Dose	Creatinine Clearance (mL/min)			Dialysis
		>50	10–50	<10	
Didanosine (ddI, Videx)	>60 kg, 400 mg qd <60 kg, 250 mg qd	No change	50% of usual dose	25% of usual dose	HD, CAPD: 25%
Lamivudine (3TC, Epivir)	150 mg b.i.d.	No change	150 qd	50 mg qd	HD: 25–50 mg qd CAPD: no data
Stavudine (d4T, Zerit)	>60 kg, 40 mg b.i.d. <60 kg, 30 mg b.i.d.	No change	50% q12–24h	50% q24h	HD, CAPD: 25%
Zidovudine (AZT, Retrovir)	300 mg b.i.d.	No change	No change	300 mg qd	HD: 300 mg qd CAPD: 300 mg qd
Zalcitabine (ddC, Hivid)	0.75 mg t.i.d.	No change	0.75 mg b.i.d.	0.75 mg qd	HD: 0.75 mg qd CAPD: no change
Tenofovir (Viread)	300 mg q24h	No change	Not recommended <60 mL/min	Not recommended	Not recommended

CAPD, continuous ambulatory peritoneal dialysis; HD, hemodialysis

Note:

Combination products: use separate products and adjust each as necessary. Combivir (AZT + 3TC), Trizivir (Abacavir + AZT + 3TC).

No recommendation or no dosing adjustment necessary:

Nucleoside reverse transcriptase inhibitors (NRTI): abacavir (Ziagen), emtricitabine (Emtriva)

Non-nucleoside reverse transcriptase inhibitors (NNRTI): nevirapine (Viramune), delavirdine (Rescriptor), efavirenz (Sustiva)

Protease inhibitors: atazanavir (Reyataz), amprenavir (Agenerase), indinavir (Crixivan), saquinavir (Invirase, Fortovase), ritonavir (Norvir), nelfinavir (Viracept), lopinavir + ritonavir (Kaletra), tipranavir (Aptivus), darunavir (Prezista)

Fusion inhibitor: enfuvirtide (Fuzeon)

Index

Page numbers followed by *f* refer to figures; page numbers followed by *t* refer to tables.

Acid(s), 78–81
  bases and, balance with, 79–81
    regulation of, 79–81
  bicarbonate reabsorption for, 80
Acid base disorders, 78–92. *See also* Anion gap
    metabolic acidosis; Metabolic acidosis;
    Metabolic alkalosis; Nongap metabolic
    acidosis
  causes of, 90–91
    from medicine changes, 90–91
  compensatory responses for, 80*t*, 81
  evaluation of, 81–82
  map for, 82*f*
  metabolic acidosis, 83–87
    anion gap, 83–85
    anion gap acidosis, 83–85
    differential diagnosis of, 83*t*
    nongap, 83, 85–87
    nongap acidosis, 85–87
    treatment of, 87
  metabolic alkalosis, 87–89
    diagnosis of, 88–89
    initiation of, 87–88
    maintenance of, 87–88
    treatment for, 89
    types of, 88–89, 88*t*
  primary, 81–82
  respiratory acidosis, 89–90
    acute, 90
    chronic, 90
  respiratory alkalosis, 90
    acute, 90
    chronic, 90
  simple, 81*t*
  stepwise approach to, 78
Acidemia, 78–79
Acquired cystic kidney disease, 218–219
  diagnosis of, 219
    ADPKD *v.*, 219
  incidence rates for, 218–219
  management of, 219
  screening for, 219
  symptoms of, 219
Acromegly, 73
Acute Dialysis Quality Initiative (ADQI), 94
  dialysis dosing guidelines under, 157
Acute interstitial nephritis (AIN),
    135–141
  acute pyelonephritis and, 141
  causes of, 135, 136*t*, 138*t*, 140*t*

definition of, 135
diagnosis of, 135, 137
  through biopsies, 135, 137
epidemiology of, 135
management of, 137, 141
  with corticosteroids, 137
pathogenesis of, 135
symptoms of, 135, 137
Acute kidney injury (AKI), 94–100, 107–119.
    See also Acute interstitial nephritis;
    Atheroembolic renal disease; Contrast-
    induced nephropathy; Crystalline
    nephropathies; Renal replacement
    therapies
  ADQI and, 94
  atheroembolic renal disease, 121–124
  cardiorenal syndrome, 112–113
  CIN, 144–148
    atheroembolic renal disease *v.*, 145
    epidemiology of, 145–147
    pathogenesis of, 144
    prevention of, 147–148
    risk factors for, 144–145, 145*t*
  classification for, 95*t*
  diagnosis of, 95, 97–100
    blood counts in, 99
    chemistry panels in, 99
    contemporary biomarkers in, 99–100
    renal ultrasound, 99
    serological profiles in, 99, 100*t*
    of tissues, 99
    urinalysis in, 97–98, 98*t*
  epidemiology for, 94–95
  hepatorenal syndrome, 111–112
    causes of, 111
    definition of, 111
    diagnosis of, 111–112
    pathogenesis of, 111
    symptoms of, 111–112
    treatment for, 112
    types of, 111
  incidence rates for, 94
  intrinsic, 121–141
    causes of, 122*t*
    glomerulus, 122*t*
    interstitial causes of, 122*t*, 134–141
    microvascular causes of, 121–125, 122*t*, 126*t*
    scleroderma renal crisis, 124
    tubular causes of, 122*t*, 125, 128–129,
      132–134

Acute kidney injury (AKI) (*continued*)
  patient evaluation with, 95–96
    infection history in, 96
    medication use in, 96
    urine patterns in, 96
    volume status in, 96
  physical examinations for, 97
    of abdomen, 97
    of cardiac system, 97
  postrenal, 113–119
    acidosis and, 116
    causes of, 114*t*, 115, 115*t*
    classification of, 113
    clinical manifestations of, 115–116
    definition of, 113
    diagnosis of, 116–118
    epidemiology of, 113
    hypertension and, 116
    management of, 118
    nephrolithiasis and, 116
    obstructive nephropathy and, 113
    obstructive uropathy and, 113
    pathophysiology of, 115
    polycythemia and, 116
    polyuria and, 118
    prognosis for, 119
    UTIs and, 116
  prerenal, 107–111
    ADH and, 107
    adrenergic system and, 107
    azotemia in, 108*f*
    causes of, 109–110, 109*t*
    definition of, 107
    diagnosis of, 110
    FENa in, 110
    FEUrea in, 110
    pathogenesis for, 107–109
    renin-angiotensin-aldosterone system and,
      108
    symptoms of, 110
    treatment for, 111
  renal replacement therapy for, 151–157
    ADQI guidelines for, 157
    CRRT, 151–156
    IHD, 151
    indications for, 152*t*
    modalities of, 151–157, 153*t*
    nomenclature for, 154*t*
    PD, 151
    SLED, 151, 156–157
  risk factors for, 97
  staging systems for, 95*t*
Acute Kidney Injury Network (AKIN), 94
Acute pancreatitis. *See* Pancreatitis, acute
Acute renal failure. *See* Renal failure, acute
Acute tubular necrosis (ATN), 100–104
  causes of, 101*t*
  management of, 102–104

  with acid-base/electrolyte disturbances,
    103–104
  through circulatory volume restoration,
    102
  with DA, 103
  through diuretics, 102–103
  with experimental agents, 103
  with fenoldopam, 103
  through medication adjustment, 104
  through nephrotoxin withdrawal, 102
  through nutritional support, 104
  nephrotoxic injury and, 101–102
  pathogenesis of, 100–101
  phases of, 104
  rhabdomyolysis and, 101–102
Acyclovir crystals, 6
ADH. *See* Antidiuretic hormone
ADHR rickets. *See* Autosomal-dominant
  hypophosphatemic rickets
ADPKD. *See* Autosomal dominant polycystic
  kidney disease
ADQI. *See* Acute Dialysis Quality
  Initiative
Adrenergic system, 107
AIN. *See* Acute interstitial nephritis
AKIN. *See* Acute Kidney Injury
  Network
AKI. *See* Acute kidney injury
Albumin, 22–23
  proteinuria testing for, 22–23
  in urine dipstick testing, 22
Albuminuria, 195*t*
  microalbuminuria, 194
Aldosterone, 53*t*
  hypokalemia from, 57*t*
  in renin-angiotensin-aldosterone system,
    108
Alkalemia, 79
Amikacin, 289*t*
Ammonium biurate crystals, 6
Amphotericin, 57
Amyloidosis, 190
  primary, 190
  secondary, 190
Anemia, 253–254
  CKD and, 253–254
    ESAs and, 253–254
    iron deficiencies in, 254
  pathophysiology of, 253
Aneurysms, 214–215, 214*t*
Anion gap metabolic acidosis, 83–85
  DKA, 84
  lactic acidosis, 83–84
  nongap *v.*, 83
  renal failure and, 85
  salicylate overdose and, 85
  starvation ketoacidosis, 84
Antegrade pyelography, 118

Anticoagulation, 152–153
  during hemodialysis, 269
Antidiuretic hormone (ADH), 35
  prerenal AKI and, 107
Anti-GBM disease. *See* Antiglomerular
      basement membrane disease
Antiglomerular basement membrane
      (anti-GBM) disease, 187–188
  epidemiology of, 187–188
  renal pathology of, 188
  symptoms of, 187
  treatment for, 188
Antiphospholipid syndrome (APS), 121, 124
  catastrophic, 124
APS. *See* Antiphospholipid syndrome
Arginine vasopressin (AVP), 35. *See also*
      Antidiuretic hormone
Arteriovenous fistulas, 19
ASRVD. *See* Atherosclerotic renal vascular
      disease
Asymptomatic hematuria, 163
Asymptomatic proteinuria, 163
Atheroembolic renal disease, 121–124
  CIN *v.*, 145
  definition of, 121
  diagnosis of, 122–123
    with biopsies, 123
  incidence rates for, 122
  management of, 123–124
  pathogenesis of, 121–122
  symptoms of, 122–123, 123*t*
Atherosclerotic renal vascular disease (ASRVD),
      202
ATN. *See* Acute tubular necrosis
Autosomal-dominant hypophosphatemic
      (ADHR) rickets, 76
Autosomal dominant polycystic kidney disease
      (ADPKD), 212–217
  characteristics of, 216*t*
  definition of, 212
  diagnosis of, 213, 215–216
    acquired cystic kidney disease *v.*, 219
    through medical history, 213
    through physical examinations, 213
    through screening, 215
    through ultrasound, 215, 215*t*
  etiology of, 212–213
  manifestations of, 214–215
    cerebral aneurysms as, 214–215, 214*t*
    extrarenal, 214–215
    renal, 214
  mechanisms of, 213
  pathogenesis of, 212–213
  physiology, 213
  prognosis after, 217
  risk factors for, 217*t*
  symptoms of, 213
  treatment for, 216–217

AVP. *See* Arginine vasopressin
Azotemia, 108*f*

Barium toxicity, 56
Bases, 78–81
  acids and, balance with, 79–81
  regulation of, 79–81
Beer potomania, 39
Beta$_2$-andregenic agents, 53–54
Bilirubin crystals, 6
Biophosphonates, 66
  hyperphosphatemia from, 73
Biopsies
  for AIN, 135, 137
  for atheroembolic renal disease,
      123
  renal, 15–19
  for SLE, 183–184
Blood pH, 78–79, 79*t*
  acidemia and, 78–79
  alkalemia, 79
Blood urea nitrogen (BUN), 9
BUN. *See* Blood urea nitrogen

Calcific uremic arteriolopathy as, 270
Calcineurin inhibitors (CNIs), 298
Calcitonin, 66
Calcitriol, 63
  phosphorus regulation by, 71
Calcium, 62–63
  calcitriol and, 63
  fluxes in levels of, 64*t*
  homeostasis for, 62
  in neuromuscular function, 62
  PTH and, 62–63
  regulation of, 62–63
Calcium crystals, 6
  oxalate, 6
  with phosphates, 6
Calcium metabolism disorders, 63–70. *See also*
      Hypercalcemia; Hypocalcemia
  hypercalcemia, 63–67
    acute, 65–66
    causes of, 63–65, 64*t*
    chronic, 66–67
    familial hypocalciuric, 64
    lab studies for, 65
    malignant, 67
    symptoms of, 65
    treatment for, 65–67
  hypocalcemia, 67–70
    acute symptomatic, 69–70
    causes of, 67–69, 68*t*
    chronic, 70
    familial, 67
    lab studies for, 69
    management of, 69–70
    symptoms of, 67

Cancers. *See* Tumors
CAPD. *See* Continuous ambulatory peritoneal dialysis
Captopril plasma renin activity, 207
Cardiorenal syndrome (CRS), 112–113
    features of, 112
    pathogenesis of, 113
    treatment for, 113
Casts
    epithelial cell, 5
    fatty, 5
    granular, 5
    hyaline, 5
    red cell, 5
    waxy, 5
    white cell, 5
Cation-exchange resins, 54
CCPD. *See* Continuous cycling peritoneal dialysis
Cholesterol crystals, 6
Chronic glomerulonephritis, 164
Chronic kidney disease (CKD), 250–258
    anemia and, 253–254
    dialysis access in, 256
    GFR and, 11, 11t
    hypertension and, 251–253
    immunizations with, 256
        for influenza, 256
        for pneumococcus, 256
    incidence rates for, 250
    lab workup for, 252t
    lipid management in, 255–256
    MDRD and, 250
    NKF guidelines for, 250
    nutritional issues in, 257–258
        goals and, 257t
    during pregnancy, 229–230
    prognosis after, 258
    RAAS and, 253
    renal osteodystrophy and, 254–255
        acidosis in, 255
        secondary hyperparathyroidism and, 254–255
        vitamin deficiency in, 255
    renal replacement therapies for, 258
    staging of, 11t, 250
    transplant suitability with, 257
Churg-Strauss syndrome (CSS), 187
CIN. *See* Contrast-induced nephropathy
Cirrhosis, 40
Cisplatin, 57
CKD. *See* Chronic kidney disease
CNIs. *See* Calcineurin inhibitors
Cockcroft-Gault formula, 10
Computed tomography (CT)
    for AKI, 118
    for hematuria, 32
    for RAS, 206

    for renal colic, 242
    for RVTHN, 206
C1Q nephropathy, 174
Continuous ambulatory peritoneal dialysis (CAPD), 277
Continuous cycling peritoneal dialysis (CCPD), 277
Continuous renal replacement therapy (CRRT), 151–156
    anticoagulation in, 152–153
        issues with, as complication, 156
    complications from, 154–156
        arrhythmias as, 155
        central venous catheter issues as, 155–156
        electrolyte disturbances as, 156
        hypotension as, 155
        hypothermia as, 156
    drug dosing in, 154, 155t
    fluids in, 152
    principles of, 151–152
    regimen for, 154
Contrast-induced nephropathy (CIN), 144–148
    atheroembolic renal disease *v.,* 145
    epidemiology of, 145–147
        concomitant medications and, 146
        contrast media for, 147
        statins and, 146
    pathogenesis of, 144
    prevention of, 147–148
        through alternative therapies, 148
        through intravenous volume expansion, 147
        through NAC, 147–148
    risk factors for, 144–145, 145t
        diabetes mellitus, 144–145
        pre-existing renal impairment as, 144
        score predictions among, 146t
Corticosteroids, 137, 168
    CNIs, 298
    cyclosporine, 298
    for posttransplant patient care, 298
    prednisone, 298
    tacrolimus, 298
Creatinine production, 8–9, 8–12
    clearance time periods for, 12
    GFR for, 8, 9f, 10–12
    as marker, 8–9
    markers for, 8–9, 12
    with plasma, 9, 9f
    during pregnancy, 223, 224t
    rates of, 8
Creatinine production in, plasma levels in, 9, 9f
Cross matches, 293
CRRT. *See* Continuous renal replacement therapy

CRS. *See* Cardiorenal syndrome
Crystalline nephropathies, 125, 128–129, 132–133
  causes of, 130*t*
  definition of, 125
  ethylene glycol intoxication, 128–129
    diagnosis of, 128–129
    management of, 132–133
    ultrasound for, 129
  management of, 129, 132–133
  myeloma cast nephropathy, 133–134
    definition of, 133
    diagnosis of, 133–134
    epidemiology of, 133
    management of, 134
    pathogenesis of, 133
    symptoms of, 133–134
  pathogenesis of, 125, 128
  TLS, 69, 125, 128
    management of, 132
    pathophysiology of, 128
    risk factors for, 128
  TLS as, 125, 128
CSS. *See* Churg-Strauss syndrome
CT. *See* Computed tomography
Cyclosporine, 298
Cystic diseases of the kidney. *See* Acquired cystic kidney disease; Autosomal dominant polycystic kidney disease; Cysts, renal; Glomerulocystic disease; Medullary cystic kidney disease; Medullary sponge kidney
Cystine crystals, 6
  in nephrolithiasis, 236
Cystinuria, 247–248, 247*f*
Cysts, renal, 217–218
  classification system, 218*t*
  evaluation of, 217–218
    through ultrasound, 217–218
  management of, 218
  symptoms of, 217
Cytoscopy, 32

DA. *See* Dopamine
Delayed graft function (DGF), 294
DGF. *See* Delayed graft function
Diabetes
  insipidus, 44
  mellitus, 144–145
Diabetic ketoacidosis (DKA), 84
Diabetic nephropathy, 193–199
  causes of, 193–194
    histopathology of, 193–194
    pathophysiology of, 193
  complications of, 198–199
    acute renal failure as, 198–199
    hyperkalemia as, 199
    hypoglycemia as, 198

  definition of, 193
  diagnosis of, 196–197
  evaluation of, 195–196
    through lab analysis, 196
    medical history in, 195–196
    through physical examination, 196
  incidence rates for, 193
  during pregnancy, 231
  risk factors for, 195
  screening for, 194
    microalbuminuria in, 194
  symptoms of, 194
  treatment for, 197–198
    albuminuria as marker in, 198
    glycemic control in, 197
    hypertension and, 197
Dialysis. *See also* Continuous renal replacement therapy (CRRT); Hemodialysis; Peritoneal dialysis
  for CKD, 256
  for hypercalcemia, 66
  IHD, 151
  PD, 151, 273–284
    adequacy parameters for, 278–279
    complications from, 279, 281, 283–284
    dosing in, 281*t*
    hemodialysis switching from, 284
    mechanisms of, 274–277, 275*f*
    modalities of, 277–278
    patient selection for, 273
    patient symptoms of, 280*t*
    physiology of, 274
    prescriptions for, 278
  pregnancy and, 231
    management principles during, 232*t*
  SLED, 151, 156–157
Disorders. *See* Calcium metabolism disorders; Phosphorus metabolism disorders; Potassium balance disorders; Water balance disorders
Diuretics, 40, 65
  ATN management through, 102–103
  thiazide, 40, 65
    for nephrolithiasis, 245
DKA. *See* Diabetic ketoacidosis
Donor specific antibodies, 293–294
Dopamine (DA), 103
Drug dosing, 286–291
  absorption in, 286
  in CRRT, 154, 155*t*
  elimination after, 287
  maintenance schedule calculations for, 288*t*, 289*f*
  metabolism as factor for, 287
  protein binding changes and, 286
  therapeutic monitoring for, 287–291
    for aminoglycosides, 287–290, 288*t*, 290*t*
    for vancomycin, 290–291, 290*t*

Electron microscopy, for glomerular disease, 162
Epithelial cells, 4–5
  casts in, 5
  oval fat bodies in, 5
  renal tubular, 4–5
  squamous, 4
  transitional, 4
Erythropoiesis-stimulating agents (ESAs), 253–254
ESAs. *See* Erythropoiesis-stimulating agents
Ethylene glycol intoxication, 128–129, 132
  diagnosis of, 128–129
  management of, 132
  ultrasound for, 129

Familial hypocalcemia, 67
Familial hypocalciuric hypercalcemia, 64
Fatty casts, 5
Fatty liver, acute, 228
FENa. *See* Fractional excretion of sodium
Fenoldopam, 103
FEUrea. *See* Fractional excretion of urea
FGF-23. *See* Fibroblast growth factor 23
Fibroblast growth factor 23 (FGF-23), 72
Fibromuscular dysplasia (FMD), 202–203, 209
  treatment of, 209
FMD. *See* Fibromuscular dysplasia
Focal segment glomerulosclerosis (FSGS), 171–174
  C1Q nephropathy and, 174
  histological variants of, 172*t*
  primary, 172–173
    outcomes of, 172
    symptoms of, 172
    treatment of, 173
  secondary, 173–174
    genetic causes of, 173–174
    HIV infection and, 173
    pharmacological associations with, 173
    sickle cell disease and, 174
    treatment of, 174
Fractional excretion of sodium (FENa), 110
Fractional excretion of urea (FEUrea), 110
FSGS. *See* Focal segment glomerulosclerosis

Gallium nitrate, 66
Gentamicin, 289*t*
GFR. *See* Glomerular filtration rate
Glomerular disease(s), 159–169
  classification of, through imaging studies, 159–160, 162
    with electron microscopy, 162
    with immunofluorescence, 162
    with light microscopy, 159–160, 161*f*, 162
  complications of, 167–169
    from corticosteroid therapy, 168

    infection as, 167
    from medications, 168–169
  definition of, 159
  lab evaluation for, 164–165
    algorithm for, 167*f*
    specialized, 165–166
    with ultrasound, 165
    with urinalysis, 165
  physical exams for, 162–163
  primary, 159, 160*t*, 171–180
    definition of, 171
    FSGS, 171–174
    IgA nephropathy, 179–180
    membranous nephropathy, 176–178
    minimal change disease, 174–175
    MPGN, 178–179
  proteinuria, 23
  secondary, 159
  spectrum of, 164*f*
  symptoms of, 162–164
    for asymptomatic hematuria, 163
    for asymptomatic proteinuria, 163
    for chronic glomerulonephritis, 164
    for nephritic syndrome, 164
    for nephrotic syndrome, 163–164
    for RPGN, 164
  treatment principles for, 166, 168
Glomerular diseases, primary, 159, 160*t*, 171–180. *See also* Focal segment glomerulosclerosis
  definition of, 171
  FSGS, 171–174
    C1Q nephropathy and, 174
    histological variants of, 172*t*
    primary, 172–173
    secondary, 173–174
  IgA nephropathy, 179–180
    diagnosis of, 180
    incidence rates for, 179
    pathology of, 180
    progression of, 180
    secondary causes of, 180
    symptoms of, 179–180
    treatment for, 180
  membranous nephropathy, 176–178
    epidemiology for, 176
    pathogenesis of, 176
    pathology for, 176–177
    secondary causes of, 176
    symptoms of, 176
    treatment outcomes for, 177–178
  minimal change disease, 174–175
    incidence rates for, 174
    pathology of, 175
    secondary causes for, 175
    symptoms of, 174
    treatment outcomes for, 175
    variants of, 175

MPGN, 178–179
    classification of, 178–179
    pathogenesis of, 178–179
    pathology of, 178–179
    symptoms of, 178
    treatment of, 179
Glomerular filtration rate (GFR), 8, 9*f,* 10–12
    CKD and, 11, 11*t*
    clearance estimates in, 10–11
    Cockcroft-Gault formula in, 10
    creatine production and, 8, 9*f,* 10–12
    definition of, 10
Glomerular proteinuria, 23
Glomerulocystic disease, 219–220
    evaluation of, 219–220
    symptoms of, 219
Glomerulonephritis, chronic, 164. *See also*
        Poststreptococcal glomerulonephritis;
        Systemic lupus erythematosis
    PSGN and, 185–186
    SLE and, 183–185
Glucocorticoids, 66
Granulomatous disease as, 65
Gross hematuria, 27

HELLP. *See* Hemolysis, elevated liver enzymes,
        low platelets syndrome
Hematuria, 15, 27–33
    asymptomatic, 163
    AUA guidelines for, 27
    causes of, 28
    clinical follow-up for, 33
    definition of, 27
    detection of, 27–28
        through dipstick testing, 27–28
        through urinalysis, 28
    evaluation of, 28, 30, 32–33
        through imaging, 32–33
        through lab evaluation, 30, 31*f,* 32
        through medical history, 28
        through physical examination, 28, 30
    gross, 27
    incidence rates for, 27
    microscopic, 27
        causes of, 29*t*
        risk factors for, 30*t*
    from MSK, 221
    screening for, 27
Hemodialysis, 54, 260–277
    access to, 261–265
    administration modalities for, 261–265
    anticoagulation during, 269
        with heparin, 269
    complications of, 263–265, 269–271
        calcific uremic arteriolopathy as, 270
        cardiovascular, 270–271
        dialyzer reactions as, 270
        from infections, 264–265

        nephrogenic systemic fibrosis as, 270
        skin diseases as, 269
        for urea clearance, 269
    electrolyte balances for, 268
    IHD, 151
    initiation of, 260–261
    mechanisms for, 264*f,* 265–266, 268–269
        maintenance guidelines in, 267*t*
        prescriptions as part of, 265–266
    mortality rates with, 260
    PD switching to, 284
Hemoglobin, 3
    in urine, 3
Hemolysis, elevated liver enzymes, low platelets
        (HELLP) syndrome, 121, 124, 227
    management of, 227
    TTP-HUS and, 189–190
        renal pathology of, 189
        treatment for, 189–190
Hemolytic-uremic syndrome (HUS), 121,
        124
    TTP-HUS and, 188–190
        epidemiology of, 188–189
        in pregnancy, 227
Henderson-Hasselbach equation, 79
Heparin, 269
Hepatorenal syndrome, 111–112
    causes of, 111
    definition of, 111
    diagnosis of, 111–112
    pathogenesis of, 111
    symptoms of, 111–112
    treatment for, 112
        with MARS, 112
        with TIPS, 112
    types of, 111
HIV. *See* Human immunodeficiency virus
HLAs. *See* Human leukocyte antigens (HLAs)
Hormones. *See* Antidiuretic hormone;
        Parathyroid hormone
HRHA. *See* Hyporeninemic hypoaldosteronism
Human immunodeficiency virus (HIV), 173
Human leukocyte antigens (HLAs), 293
Hungry bone syndrome, 68–69
    hypophosphatemia from, 75
HUS. *See* Hemolytic-uremic syndrome
Hyaline casts, 5
Hypercalcemia, 63–67
    acute, 65–66
        treatment for, 65–66
    causes of, 63–65, 64*t*
        bone resorption increase as, 63–64
        granulomatous disease as, 65
        hyperparathyroidism as, 63
        immobilization as, 64
        intestinal absorption increase as, 64–65
        Milk-Alkali syndrome as, 64
        renal excretion decrease as, 65

Hypercalcemia (*continued*)
    thiazide diuretics as, 65
    thyrotoxis as, 64
    tumors as, 63–64
    vitamin intoxication as, 65
  chronic, 66–67
  familial hypocalciuric, 64
  hypercalcuria from, 238
  lab studies for, 65
  malignant, 67
  symptoms of, 65
  treatment for, 65–67
    with biphosphonates, 66
    with calcitonin, 66
    with dialysis, 66
    with gallium nitrate, 66
    with glucocorticoids, 66
Hypercalcuria, 237–238
  diagnosis of, 237t
  from hypercalcemia, 238
  idiopathic, 238
Hyperglycemia, from PD, 284
Hyperkalemia, 48–55. *See also*
    Hypoaldosteronism
  aldosterone levels in, 53t
  causes of, 49–52, 50t
    decreased cellular uptake as, 49
    hypoaldosteronism as, 51–52
    potassium movement out of cells as,
      49–50
    pseudohyperkalemia as, 52
    renal excretion decreases as, 50–51
  chronic, 54–55
  definition of, 48–49
  from diabetic nephropathy, 199
  electrocardiographic changes in, 49
  evaluation of, 52
    through medical history, 52
    through physical exam, 52
    through urinalysis, 52
  exogenous potassium administration in,
    49
  renin levels in, 53t
  symptoms of, 49
  treatment for, 52–54, 53t
    with beta$_2$-andregenic agents, 53–54
    with calcium gluconate, 53
    with cation-exchange resins, 54
    through hemodialysis, 54
    with insulin, 53
    through renal elimination, 54
    with sodium bicarbonate, 54
Hyperlipidemia, 284
Hypernatremia, 43–46
  causes of, 44–45
    pregnancy as, 44–45
  etiology of, 43–44, 44f
    diabetes insipidus in, 44
    evaluation of, 43–44
    pathogenesis for, 43
    symptoms of, 43
    treatment for, 45–46
Hyperoxaluria, 238–239
  causes of, 238t
  dietary, 238
  enteric, 239
  primary, 239
  treatment for, 245–246
Hyperparathyroidism, 63
  secondary, 254–255
Hyperphosphatemia, 72–74
  acute, 74
  causes of, 72–74, 73t
    acromegly as, 73
    biophosphonates as, 73
    hypoparathyroidism as, 73
    phosphate intake increases as, 73
    pseudohypoparathyroidism as, 73
    transcellular shifts as, 73
    tumoral calcinosis, 73
  chronic, 74
  lab studies for, 73–74
  management of, 74
  symptoms of, 73
Hypertension, 116
  CKD and, 251–253
  diabetic nephropathy and, 197
  in hemodialysis patients, 270–271
  pathophysiology of, 251
  during pregnancy, 224–225
    chronic, 224–225
    drug options for, 225
    treatment of, 225
  RAS and, 203
  RVTHN and, 203–204
Hyperthyroidism, 56
  primary, 76
  secondary, 76
Hypertonic hyponatremia, 38–39
  mannitol solutions and, 39
Hyperuricemia, 240–241
Hyperuricosuria, 239–241
Hypoaldosteronism, 51–52
  causes of, 51t
  HRHA, 51t
Hypocalcemia, 67–70
  acute symptomatic, 69–70
  causes of, 67–69, 68t
    acute pancreatitis as, 67
    hungry bone syndrome as, 68–69
    hypomagnesemia, 67
    hypoparathyroidism as, 67
    pseudohypoparathyroidism as, 68
    rhabdomyolysis as, 69
    septic shock as, 69
    TLS as, 69

vitamin deficiencies as, 68
chronic, 70
familial, 67
lab studies for, 69
management of, 69–70
symptoms of, 67
Hypocitraturia, 239
treatment for, 245
Hypoglycemia, 198
Hypokalemia, 55–59
causes of, 55–57, 56t
amphotericin as, 57
barium toxicity as, 56
cellular intake changes as, 55–56
cisplatin as, 57
extrarenal losses as, 57
hyperthyroidism as, 56
hypomagnesemia as, 57
hypothermia as, 56
primary aldosterone as, 57t
renal excretion increases as,
56–57
thiazide agents as, 57
chronic, 59
definition of, 55
evaluation of, 57–58, 58f
mild, 55
from PD, 284
severe, 55
rhabdomyolysis from, 55
symptoms of, 55
treatment of, 58–59
with potassium replacement, 59
Hypomagnesemia, 57
hypocalcemia from, 67
Hyponatremia, 35–43. See also Hypotonic
hyponatremia
acute, 35–36
acute renal failure and, 40
causes of, 37–40
hypertonic hyponatremia as, 38–39
hypotonic hyponatremia as, 39–40
pseudohyponatremia as, 37–38
thiazide diuretics as, 40
cirrhosis and, 40
complications of, 36
neurological, 36
congestive heart failure and, 40
definition of, 35
evaluation of, 36–37, 38f
clinical, 36
lab, 36–37
nephrotic syndrome and, 40
SIADH and, 40–41
causes of, 37t
treatment for, 41–43
Hypoparathyroidism, 67
hyperphosphatemia from, 73

Hypophosphatemia, 74–77
causes of, 74–76
extracellular phosphate redistribution as,
74–75
hungry bone syndrome as, 75
hyperthyroidism as, 76
intestinal absorption decreases as, 75
refeeding syndrome as, 75
renal excretion increases as, 76
vitamin deficiencies from, 75
lab studies for, 76
management of, 76–77
moderate, 76–77
rickets from, 76
ADHR, 76
XLH, 76
severe, 77
symptoms of, 76
Hyporeninemic hypoaldosteronism (HRHA),
51
Hypotension, 155
in hemodialysis patients, 270–271
after renal biopsies, 19
Hypothermia, 56, 156
Hypotonic hyponatremia, 39–40
urine osmolality and, 39–40
volume depletion and, 40

IgA nephropathy, 179–180
diagnosis of, 180
incidence rates for, 179
pathology of, 180
progression of, 180
secondary causes of, 180
symptoms of, 179–180
treatment for, 180
IHD. See Intermittent hemodialysis
Imaging studies
for AKI, 116–118
for RAS, 205–206
for RVTHN, 205–206
Immunizations, 256
during posttransplant patient care, 297
Immunofluorescence, for glomerular disease,
162
Infections
AKI and, in patient history, 96
from glomerular diseases, 167
during hemodialysis, 264–265
from PD, 279, 281
UTIs, 116
Influenza, 256
Informed consent, 16
Insulin, 53
phosphorus regulation through, 71
Intermittent hemodialysis (IHD), 151
Intravenous urography (IVU), 117
for hematuria, 32

Ischemic nephropathy, 203
Isotope renography, 117
IVU. *See* Intravenous urography

Ketones, 4
Kidney dialysis. *See* Dialysis; Hemodialysis
Kidneys, function of, 8–12. *See also* Acute
    kidney injury; Renal biopsies;
    Urinalysis; Urine
  creatinine production in, 8–12
    clearance time periods for, 12
    GFR for, 8, 9*f*, 10–12
    markers for, 8–9, 12
    with plasma, 9, 9*f*
    rates of, 8
  GFR for, 8, 9*f,* 10–12
    CKD and, 11, 11*t*
    clearance estimates in, 10–11
    Cockcroft-Gault formula in, 10
    creatine production and, 8.10–12, 9*f*
    definition of, 10
  urea in, 9
    BUN and, 9
Kidney stones. *See* Nephrolithiasis

Lactic acidosis, 83–84
LCDD. *See* Light chain disposition disease
Leucine crystals, 6
Leukocyte esterase, 3–4
Light chain disposition disease (LCDD),
    190
Light microscopy, for glomerular diseases,
    159–160, 162

Magnetic resonance angiography (MRA)
  for RAS, 206
  for RVTHN, 206
Malnutrition
  from PD, 284
  severe, 39
MARS. *See* Molecular Adsorbent Recirculating
    System
MCKD. *See* Medullary cystic kidney disease
MDRD study. *See* Modification of Diet in
    Renal Disease study
Medullary cystic kidney disease (MCKD),
    220
  evaluation of, 220
  management of, 220
  pathophysiology of, 220
  symptoms of, 220
Medullary sponge kidney (MSK), 220–221
  complications of, 221
    hematuria as, 221
    nephrolithiasis as, 221
    UTIs as, 221
  diagnosis of, 221
  nephrolithiasis from, 221, 239–240

pathophysiology of, 221
  symptoms of, 221
  treatment for, 221
Membranoproliferative glomerulonephritis
    (MPGN), 178–179
  classification of, 178–179
  pathogenesis of, 178–179
  pathology of, 178–179
  symptoms of, 178
  treatment of, 179
    alternative therapies in, 179
Membranous nephropathy, 176–178
  epidemiology for, 176
  pathogenesis of, 176
  pathology for, 176–177
  secondary causes of, 176
  symptoms of, 176
  treatment outcomes for, 177–178
Metabolic acidosis, 83–87. *See also* Nongap
    metabolic acidosis
  anion gap, 83–85
    DKA, 84
    lactic acidosis, 83–84
    nongap *v.,* 83
    renal failure and, 85
    salicylate overdose and, 85
    starvation ketoacidosis, 84
  differential diagnosis of, 83*t,* 88–89
  nongap, 83, 85–87
    anion gap *v.,* 83
    RTA, 85–87, 86*t*
  treatment of, 87
Metabolic alkalosis, 87–89
  diagnosis of, 88–89
  initiation of, 87–88
  maintenance of, 87–88
  treatment for, 89
  types of, 88–89, 88*t*
    chloride-resistant, 88–89
    chloride-responsive, 88
    unclassified, 89
Microalbuminuria, 194
Microscopic polyangiitis (MPA),
    187
Milk-Alkali syndrome, 64
Minimal change disease, 174–175
  incidence rates for, 174
  pathology of, 175
  secondary causes for, 175
  symptoms of, 174
  treatment outcomes for, 175
  variants of, 175
Modification of Diet in Renal Disease
    (MDRD) study, 10
  CKD and, 250
  urine collection *v.,* 12*t*
Molecular Adsorbent Recirculating System
    (MARS), 112

MPA. *See* Microscopic polyangiitis
MPGN. *See* Membranoproliferative
    glomerulonephritis
MRA. *See* Magnetic resonance angiography
MSK. *See* Medullary sponge kidney
Myeloma cast nephropathy,
    133–134
  definition of, 133
  diagnosis of, 133–134
  epidemiology of, 133
  management of, 134
  pathogenesis of, 133
  symptoms of, 133–134

NAC. *See* N-acetylcysteine
N-acetylcysteine (NAC), 147–148
National Kidney Foundation (NKF), CKD
    guidelines for, 250, 251*t*
Nephritic syndrome, 164
Nephrogenic systemic fibrosis, 270
Nephrolithiasis, 116, 235–248
  definition of, 235
  epidemiology of, 235
  hypercalciuria and, 237–238
    diagnosis of, 237*t*
    from hypercalcemia, 238
    idiopathic, 238
  hyperoxaluria and, 238–239
    causes of, 238*t*
    dietary, 238
    enteric, 239
    primary, 239
    treatment for, 245–246
  hyperuricemia and, 240–241
  hyperuricosuria and, 239–241
  hypocitraturia and, 239
    treatment for, 245
  incidence rates for, 235
  lab follow-up for, 243
  from MSK, 221, 239–240
  pathogenesis of, 240–241
    for struvite stones, 241
    for uric acid stones, 240–241
  physical chemistry of, 236–237
    formation product in, 236
    solubility product in, 236
    urinary saturation in, 236–237
  during pregnancy, 229
  renal colic and, 242–243
    imaging modalities for, 242
    treatment of, 243
  stone composition in, 235–236
    from calcium salts, 235
    cystine, 236
    struvite, 235
    from uric acid, 235
  symptoms of, 241–242
  treatment for, 240*t*, 243–248

    for cystine stones, 247–248
    through diet, 245
    through oral phosphates, 245
    for struvite stones, 246–247
    through thiazide diuretics, 245
    for uric acid stones, 246
Nephrotic syndrome, 15
  definition of, 21
  hyponatremia and, 40
  proteinuria and, 21
  symptoms of, 163–164
NIPD. *See* Nocturnal intermittent peritoneal
    dialysis
Nitrites, 3–4
NKF. *See* National Kidney Foundation
Nocturnal intermittent peritoneal dialysis
    (NIPD), 277
Nongap metabolic acidosis, 83, 85–87
  RTA, 85–86
    characteristics of, 86*t*
    types of, 85–87

Obstructive nephropathy, 113
Obstructive uropathy, 113. *See also* Acute
    kidney injury
  during pregnancy, 229
Oval fat bodies, 5
Overflow proteinuria, 23

Pancreatitis, acute, 67
Panel reactive antibody (PRA), 293
Parasites, in urine, 7
Parathyroid hormone (PTH), 62–63
  phosphorus regulation by, 71
Patient care, 293–299
  posttransplant, 294–299
    allograft dysfunction in, 294*t*,
      295–296
    antimetabolites use for, 298–299
    corticosteroid use for, 298
    drug interactions during, 296–297,
      296*f*, 299
    immunizations during, 297
    maintenance immunosuppression in,
      297–298, 299*t*
    screening during, 297
    terminology for, 294
  pretransplant, 293–295
    evaluation in, 294–295
    terminology in, 293–294
  pretransplant terminology in,
    293–294
  after renal biopsies, 18
Pauci-immune glomerulonephritis, 186
PD. *See* Peritoneal dialysis
Percutaneous transluminal renal angioplasty
    (PTRA), 208–209
  risks of, 209

Peritoneal dialysis (PD), 151, 273–284
  adequacy parameters for, 278–279
  complications from, 279, 281,
      283–284
    infections as, 279, 281
    mechanical, 281, 283
    metabolic, 283–284
  dosing in, 281*t*
  hemodialysis switching from, 284
  mechanisms of, 274–277, 275*f*
    catheters, 274
    equilibration tests, 276–277
    membrane types, 276–277, 277*t*
    solutions, 275–276, 275*t*, 276*t*
    transfer sets, 274
  modalities of, 277–278
    CAPD, 277
    CCPD, 277
    NIPD, 277
  patient selection for, 273
  patient symptoms in, 280*t*
  physiology of, 274
  prescriptions for, 278
Peritonitis, 279, 281
  treatment for, 282*t*
Phosphorus, 71–72
  homeostasis for, 71, 72*f*
  hyperphosphatemia, 72–74
    management of, 74
  regulation of, 71–72
    by calcitriol, 71
    by FGF-23, 72
    through insulin, 71
    through PTH, 71
Phosphorus metabolism disorders, 71–77.
      See also Hyperphosphatemia;
      Hypophosphatemia
  hyperphosphatemia, 72–74
    acute, 74
    causes of, 72–74, 73*t*
    chronic, 74
    lab studies for, 73–74
    symptoms of, 73
  hypophosphatemia, 74–77
    causes of, 74–76
    lab studies for, 76
    management of, 76–77
    moderate, 76–77
    rickets from, 76
    severe, 77
    symptoms of, 76
Physiologic buffer systems, 79
  Henderson-Hasselbach equation in, 79
Pneumonia, 256
Polycythemia, 116
Polydipsia, primary, 39
Polyuria, 118

Poststreptococcal glomerulonephritis (PSGN),
      185–186
  incidence rates for, 185
  renal pathology for, 185–186
  symptoms of, 185
  treatment for, 186
Potassium, 48
  for hypokalemia, as treatment, 59
  movement out of cells of, 49–50
  in plasma, 48
  regulation of, 48
Potassium balance disorders, 48–59. *See also*
      Hyperkalemia; Hypokalemia
  hyperkalemia, 48–55
    aldosterone levels in, 53*t*
    causes of, 49–52, 50*t*
    chronic, 54–55
    definition of, 48–49
    electrocardiographic changes in, 49
    evaluation of, 52
    exogenous potassium administration in,
      49
    renin levels in, 53*t*
    symptoms of, 49
    treatment for, 52–54, 53*t*
  hypokalemia, 55–59
    causes of, 55–57
    chronic, 59
    definition of, 55
    evaluation of, 57–58, 58*f*
    mild, 55
    severe, 55
    symptoms of, 55
    treatment of, 58–59
PRA. *See* Panel reactive antibody
Prednisone, 298
Preeclampsia, 124, 225–226
  complications of, 226*t*
  etiology of, 225–226
  incidence rates for, 225
  risk factors for, 226*t*
  symptoms of, 226
Pregnancy. *See also* Hemolysis, elevated liver
      enzymes, low platelets syndrome;
      Preeclampsia
  acute fatty liver of, 228
  acute renal failure in, 227
    causes of, 228*t*
  CKD during, 229–230
  complications of, 232
  creatinine production during, 223, 224*t*
  diabetic nephropathy during, 231
  dialysis and, 231
    management principles during, 232*t*
  hypernatremia from, 44–45
  hypertension during, 224–225
    chronic, 224–225

drug options for, 225
treatment of, 225
immunosuppressive drug management during, 232
nephrolithiasis during, 229
obstructive uropathy during, 229
proteinuria during, 229
treatment of, 229
renal biopsies during, 16
renal changes during, 223–224
anatomic, 223
hemodynamic, 223–224
physiologic, 223–224
renal cortical necrosis during, 228
after renal transplants, 231
SLE during, 229–230
diagnosis of, 230
treatment of, 230
TTP-HUS in, 227
Prescriptions
for hemodialysis, 265–266
for PD, 278
Primary glomerular diseases. *See* Glomerular diseases, primary
Primary polydipsia. *See* Polydipsia, primary
Proteinuria, 15, 21–25. *See also* Urine dipsticks
classification of, 23–24
orthostatic, 24
persistent, 24
transient, 23–24
glomerular, 23
mechanisms of, 23–24
nephrotic syndrome and, 21
overflow, 23
during pregnancy, 229
treatment of, 229
symptoms of, 24
testing parameters for, 21–23, 25, 25*f*
with albumin evaluation, 22–23
with microalbumin-to-creatinine ratio, 23
with spot urine protein-to-creatinine ratio, 22
with 24-hour urine collection, 23
with urine dipstick, 21–22, 22*t*
tissue, 23
tubular, 23
Pseudohyperkalemia, 52
Pseudohyponatremia, 37–38
Pseudohypoparathyroidism, 68
hyperphosphatemia from, 73
PSGN. *See* Poststreptococcal glomerulonephritis
PTH. *See* Parathyroid hormone
PTRA. *See* Percutaneous transluminal renal angioplasty

RAAS. *See* Renin-angiotensin-aldosterone system
Rapidly progressive glomerulonephritis (RPGN), 164
RAS. *See* Renal artery stenosis
RBCs. *See* Red blood cells
Red blood cells (RBCs), 4
in urinalysis, 4
Red cell casts, 5
Refeeding syndrome, hypophosphatemia from, 75
Renal angiography
for RAS, 206
for RVTHN, 206
Renal artery stenosis (RAS), 202–209
causes of, 202–204
ASRVD, 202
FMD as, 202–203, 209
epidemiology of, 202–203
hypertension and, 203
imaging studies for, 205–206
CT in, 206
MRA in, 206
renal angiography in, 206
ultrasound in, 205–206
incidence rates for, 203
ischemic nephropathy and, 203
pathophysiology of, 203–204
symptoms of, 204
testing for, 204–207
diagnostic, 204–206
functional, 207
treatment for, 205*f*, 207–209
intervention indications in, 208
PTRA in, 208–209
with revascularization, 205*t*, 206*t*
stent placement in, 208–209
through surgery, 209
Renal biopsies, 15–19
allograft, 19, 19*t*
indications for, 19*t*
complications from, 18–19, 18*t*
arteriovenous fistulas as, 19
hypotension as, 19
pain as, 19
contraindications for, 17*t*
indications for, 15, 16*t*
acute renal failure as, 15
hematuria as, 15, 27–33
nephrotic syndrome as, 15
proteinuria as, 15
procedure evaluations for, 15–18
anesthesia in, 17
informed consent in, 16
patient positioning in, 17
postbiopsy care in, 18
with pregnancy, 16
preprocedures in, 15–16, 16*t*

Renal colic, 242–243
  imaging modalities for, 242
    CT in, 242
    ultrasound in, 242
  treatment of, 243
Renal cortical necrosis, 228
Renal cysts. See Cysts, renal
Renal failure, acute, 15. See also Acute kidney
        injury
  anion gap acidosis and, 85
  from diabetic nephropathy, 198–199
  hyponatremia and, 40
  in pregnancy, 227
    causes of, 228t
Renal osteodystrophy, 254–255
  acidosis in, 255
  secondary hyperparathyroidism and,
        254–255
  vitamin deficiency in, 255
Renal replacement therapies, 151–157. See also
        Continuous renal replacement therapy;
        Hemodialysis
  ADQI guidelines in, 157
  for CKD, 258
  CRRT, 151–156
    anticoagulation in, 152–153
    complications from, 154–156
    drug dosing in, 154, 155t
    fluids in, 152
    principles of, 151–152
    regimen for, 154
  IHD, 151
  indications for, 152t
  modalities of, 151–157
    comparisons among, 153t
  nomenclature for, 154t
  PD, 151
  SLED, 151, 156–157
Renal transplants
  for CKD, 257
  patient care after, 293–299
  pregnancy after, 231
Renal tubular acidosis (RTA), 85–87
  characteristics of, 86t
  types of, 85–87
Renin, 53t
Renin-angiotensin-aldosterone system (RAAS),
        108
  in CKD and, 253
Renovascular hypertension (RVHTN),
        202–209
  characteristics of, 204t
  hypertension and, 203–204
  imaging studies for, 205–206
    CT in, 206
    MRA in, 206
    renal angiography in, 206
    ultrasound, 205–206

pathophysiology of, 203–204
  symptoms of, 204
  testing for, 204–207
    diagnostic, 204–206
    functional, 207
  treatment for, 205f, 207–209
    intervention indications in, 208
    PTRA in, 208–209
    stent placement in, 208–209
Respiratory acidosis, 89–90
  acute, 90
  chronic, 90
Respiratory alkalosis, 90
  acute, 90
  chronic, 90
Rhabdomyolysis, 55
  ATN and, 101–102
  hypocalcemia from, 69
  pathogenesis of, 101
  symptoms of, 101–102
RPGN. See Rapidly progressive
        glomerulonephritis
RTA. See Renal tubular acidosis
RVTHN. See Renovascular hypertension

Scleroderma renal crisis, 124
Screening
  for acquired cystic kidney disease, 219
  for ADPKD, 215
  for diabetic nephropathy, 194
  for hematuria, 27
  for posttransplant patient care, 297
Septic shock, 69
SGF. See Slow graft function
Sickle cell disease, 174
SLE. See Systemic lupus erythematosis
SLED. See Sustained low-efficiency dialysis
Slow graft function (SGF), 294
Sodium bicarbonate, 54
Staging, of CKD, 250
Starvation ketoacidosis, 84
Statins, 146
Surgery, conventional, for RAS, 209
Sustained low-efficiency dialysis (SLED), 151,
        156–157
Syndromes. See Milk-Alkali syndrome;
        Nephrotic syndrome
Systemic lupus erythematosis (SLE),
        183–185
  biopsies for, 183–184
  classification of, 184t
  incidence rates for, 183
  maintenance therapy for, 185
  during pregnancy, 230–231
    diagnosis of, 230
    treatment for, 230
  renal pathology for, 183–184
  treatment for, 184–185

Tacrolimus, 298
Thiazide agents, 40, 65
  hypokalemia as, 57
  for nephrolithiasis, 245
Thrombotic-thrombocytopenic purpura (TTP)
    syndrome, 121, 124
  TTP-HUS and, 188–190
    epidemiology of, 188–189
    in pregnancy, 227
    renal pathology of, 189
    treatment for, 189–190
Thyrotoxis, 64
TIPS. See Transjugular intrahepatic
    portosystemic shunt
Tissue proteinuria, 23
TLS. See Tumor lysis syndrome
Tobramycin, 289t
Transjugular intrahepatic portosystemic shunt
    (TIPS), 112
Transplants. See Renal transplants
Triple phosphate crystals, 6
TTP syndrome. See Thrombotic-
    thrombocytopenic purpura syndrome
Tubular proteinuria, 23
Tumoral calcinosis, 73
Tumor lysis syndrome (TLS), 69, 125,
    128
  management of, 128
  pathophysiology of, 128
  risk factors for, 128
Tumors, as hypercalcemia cause, 63–64
Tyrosine crystals, 6

Ultrasound
  for ADPKD, 215, 215t
  for AKI, 99, 117, 117f
  for ethylene glycol intoxication,
    129
  for glomerular diseases, 165
  for hematuria, 32
  for RAS, 205–206
  for renal colic, 242
  for renal cysts, 217–218
  for RVTHN, 205–206
Urea, 9
  BUN and, 9
Ureterorenoscopy, 32–33
Urinalysis, 1–7. See also Urine dipsticks
  for AKI, 97–98, 98t
  albumin in, 22
  chemical properties in, 3–4
  definition of, 1
  for glomerular diseases, 165
  for hyperkalemia, 52
  through microscopic exam, 4–7
    of casts, 5
    of cells, 4–5
    of crystals, 6

  of organisms, 6–7
  physical properties in, 1–3
  specimen collection for, 1, 12t
    procedures for, 2t
Urinary tract infections (UTIs), 116
  from MSK, 221
Urine, 1–7. See also Casts; Hematuria;
    Proteinuria
  casts in, 5
  chemical properties in, 3–4
    glucose presence, 3
    hemoglobin presence, 3
    ketones, 4
    leukocyte esterase, 3–4
    nitrites, 3–4
    pH, 3
    protein presence, 3
  crystals in, 6
    acyclovir, 6
    ammonium biurate, 6
    bilirubin, 6
    calcium, 6
    cholesterol, 6
    cystine, 6
    leucine, 6
    triple phosphate, 6
    tyrosine, 6
  epithelial cells in, 4–5
  MDRD study and, 12t
  organisms in, 6–7
    bacteria, 6
    fungal, 6
    parasites, 7
  osmolality for, 39–40
    increased, 39–40
    low, 39
  physical properties of, 1–3
    clarity, 2
    color, 1–2
    odor, 2
    specific gravity, 2–3
  RBCs in, 4
  WBCs in, 4
Urine dipsticks, 21–22
  detection scale for, 22t
  for hematuria, 27–28
  positive/negative tests with,
    21–22
UTIs. See Urinary tract infections

Vancomycin, 290–291, 290t
Vitamins
  hypercalcemia and, 65
  hypocalcemia and, 68
  hypophosphatemia and, 75
  renal osteodystrophy and, from deficiency of,
    255
Voiding cystourethrography, 118

Water balance disorders, 35–46. *See also*
  Hypernatremia; Hyponatremia
ADH and, 35
hypernatremia, 43–46
  causes of, 44–45
  etiology of, 43–44, 44*f*
  evaluation of, 43–44
  pathogenesis for, 43
  symptoms of, 43
  treatment for, 45–46
hyponatremia, 35–43
  acute, 35–36
  acute renal failure and, 40
  causes of, 37–40
  cirrhosis and, 40
  complications of, 36
  congestive heart failure and, 40
  definition of, 35

evaluation of, 36–37, 38*f*
nephrotic syndrome and, 40
SIADH and, 40–41
treatment for, 41–43
Waxy casts, 5
WBCs. *See* White blood cells
Wegener's granulomatosis (WG),
  186–187
  epidemiology of, 186
  renal pathology of, 186
  symptoms of, 186
  treatment for, 186–187
WG. *See* Wegener's granulomatosis
White blood cells (WBCs), in urinalysis, 4
White cell casts, 5

X-linked hypophosphatemic (XLH)
  rickets, 76